HEPATOBILIARY MRI
A Text-Atlas at Mid and High Field

HEPATOBILIARY MRI
A Text-Atlas at Mid and High Field

DONALD G. MITCHELL, M.D.

Associate Professor of Radiology
Director of MRI, Department of Radiology
Thomas Jefferson University Hospital
Jefferson Medical College
Philadelphia, Pennsylvania

DAVID D. STARK, M.D.

Professor of Radiology
Director of MRI
University of Massachusetts Medical Center
Worcester, Massachusetts

With Contributions by

PETER F. HAHN, M.D., Ph.D.

Assistant Professor of Radiology
Harvard Medical School
Massachusetts General Hospital
Boston, Massachusetts

*With 1190 Illustrations
Including 21 in Color*

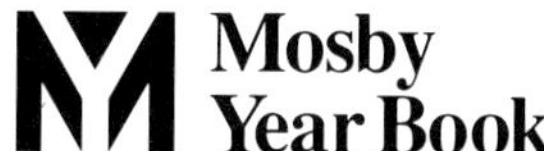

Mosby
Year Book

St. Louis Baltimore Boston Chicago London Philadelphia Sydney Toronto

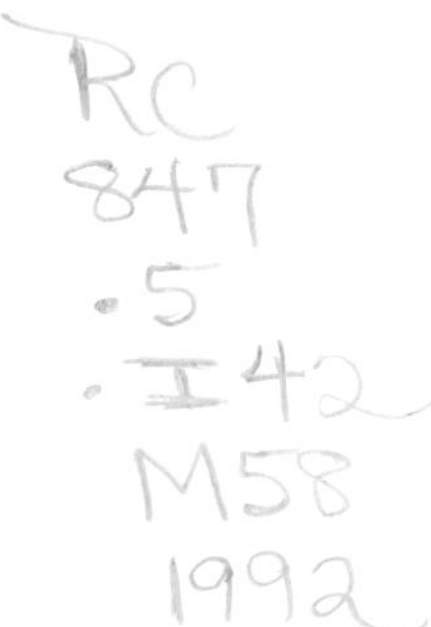

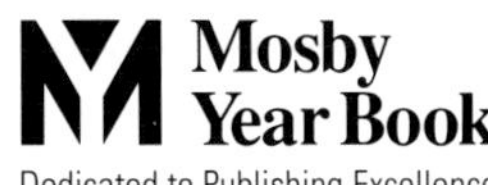
Mosby Year Book
Dedicated to Publishing Excellence

Publisher: George S. Stamathis
Editor: Anne S. Patterson
Assistant Editor: Maura K. Leib
Project Manager: Carol Sullivan Wiseman
Production Editor: Diana Lyn Laulainen
Book and Cover Design: Gail Morey Hudson

Printed in the United States of America

Mosby–Year Book, Inc.
11830 Westline Industrial Drive
St. Louis, Missouri 63146

Library of Congress Cataloging in Publication Data

Mitchell, Donald G.
    Hepatobiliary MRI : a text-atlas at mid and high field / Donald G.
  Mitchell, David D. Stark ; with contributions by Peter F. Hahn.
        p.   cm.
    Includes bibliographical references and index.
    ISBN 0-8016-6804-2 : $90.00
    1. Liver—Magnetic resonance imaging. 2. Biliary tract—Magnetic
  resonance imaging. I. Stark, David D. II. Hahn, Peter F.
  III. Title.
    [DNLM: 1. Biliary Tract Diseases—diagnosis—atlases. 2. Liver
  Diseases—diagnosis—atlases. 3. Magnetic Resonance Imaging—
  method—atlases. 4. Tomography, X-Ray Computed—methods—atlases.
  WI 17 M681h]
  RC847.5.I42M58   1992
  616.3′6207548—dc20
  DNLM/DLC   92-8554
  for Library of Congress   CIP

92 93 94 95 96 CL/MY 9 8 7 6 5 4 3 2 1

To
Deborah, Susan, Rebecca,
Elizabeth, and Elizabeth

Preface

Diagnosing liver disease is a unique challenge for imaging because the homogeneous hepatic parenchyma is actually a blend of hepatobiliary and reticuloendothelial tissue. Furthermore, both of these components are perfused by two separate but adjacent circulations, the hepatic arterial and portal venous systems. The liver is also unusual in that venous drainage does not parallel arterial anatomy. A variety of radiographic, scintigraphic, and sonographic strategies have been devised to investigate certain components of this complex organ, but no single technique has emerged as the method of choice in every respect.

Magnetic resonance imaging (MRI), the newest modality to be used for hepatic imaging, is perhaps the most versatile. In the past few years, it has shown great potential for diagnosing a wide range of diffuse and focal hepatic diseases, exploiting its ability to selectively image free water, fat, iron, and blood flow. Pharmaceutical contrast enhancement extends this potential for selective investigation of hepatobiliary, reticuloendothelial, and vascular disorders.

In this book, we review the current role of MRI relative to other modalities in hepatic diagnosis, particularly CT.

Donald G. Mitchell
David D. Stark

Acknowledgments

Hepatobiliary MRI grew out of work begun by the authors for *Magnetic Resonance Imaging,* 2nd edition, by David D. Stark and William G. Bradley, also published by Mosby–Year Book. Some of the illustrations and tables in this book have also appeared in two chapters of *Magnetic Resonance Imaging:* "Liver," by Donald G. Mitchell and David D. Stark, and "Biliary System, Pancreas, Spleen, and Alimentary Tract," by Peter F. Hahn, David D. Stark, and Karl Glastad.

Most of the pathologic correlation was provided by Drs. Juan Palazzo and Rafael Rubin. Most photographic work was by Fred Ross and Ken Goodman. Pamela Bittle assisted with manuscript preparation. Much clinical follow-up was obtained by Theresa Matteucci. Chief Technologists Lucille Aquilone and Peter Natale were also invaluable.

Simon Vinitski, Ph.D., has contributed substantively toward understanding and improving abdominal MRI at 1.5 T; he is directly responsible for the high quality of many of these images. This work also would not have been possible without a department chairman as supportive as David C. Levin, M.D.

Other individuals have contributed substantially toward generating clinical material used in this volume. Although all of these cannot be mentioned, special thanks goes to interventional radiologist Marcelle Shapiro, M.D., who organized the pancreatic imaging project that is the source of most of the 1.5 T images of pancreatic cancer shown here. Hepatic surgeon Michael Moritz, M.D. and hepatologists Santiago Munoz, M.D., Paul Martin, M.D., and Hie-Won Y. L. Hann, M.D. were and continue to be especially valuable clinical colleagues.

Donald G. Mitchell
David D. Stark

Contents

HEPATOBILIARY MRI
A Text-Atlas at Mid and High Field

PART

I

TECHNIQUE, ANATOMY, AND COMPARISON WITH X-RAY COMPUTED TOMOGRAPHY

As with any imaging modality, success depends primarily on the use of proper technique. The best possible image-interpretation skills may not be sufficient if the images are inadequate. On the other hand, a high-quality examination can be interpreted with the help of an expert consultant or after reference to an appropriate book or journal article.

We do not consider it appropriate to include a chapter on basic physics, since this subject demands more than cursory treatment. The interested reader is advised to refer to a basic MRI textbook or physics primer, if necessary, to acquire a preliminary background in MRI physics. In this section we assume some knowledge about MRI and how images are formed. We thus explore in-depth the various techniques that are useful in hepatic imaging and discuss the factors that determine image quality.

First, we consider the important determinants of tissue contrast and how this can be optimized in conventional (breathing-averaged) MRI techniques. More than any other factor, motion artifact has limited success of MRI in the abdomen, and its suppression is essential before MRI can be considered useful. More recently, breath-hold techniques have been introduced that may, in the near future, replace breathing-averaged techniques as the standard of reference for abdominal MRI.

Next, we consider the important issue of field strength. Although a wide range of field strengths can be used to obtain adequate images of the liver, field strength influences the techniques that may be optimal on a given system. We also consider the important potential of chemical shift techniques and contrast enhancement.

Although the anatomy depicted by MRI is the same as that seen by other modalities, we review this briefly. Finally, we compare MRI with x-ray computed tomography (CT) for hepatic diagnosis, discussing the inherent advantages and disadvantages of each and reviewing critically some recent comparative studies.

Breathing-Averaged Techniques

TISSUE CONTRAST

Although animal models of hepatic metastases are effective and practical for comparing pulse sequences,[68] a readily available contrast phantom that models physiologic motion is preferable. Furthermore, the use of normal volunteers facilitates comparative evaluation of the signal-to-noise ratio (SNR) and contrast-to-noise ratio (CNR) performances of different machines and field strengths. The spleen in normal human subjects has relaxation times (T1 and T2) and proton density similar to those of hepatic metastases,[38,563] and both contain little or no MR-observable lipid. Additionally, the spleen is a large homogeneous organ from which reproducible image intensity data can be measured, and it is located on the same transverse sections as the liver. Although lesions in individual patients often have signal intensity different from that of the spleen, pulse sequence performance can be assessed using the spleen-liver CNR as an approximate model for cancer-liver contrast.[237,501] For contrast enhancement, however, the spleen is not a suitable model for hepatic metastases, since the spleen has a much larger blood pool and is an active reticuloendothelial organ.

Compared with liver tissue, most tumors have increased free water and thus have prolonged T1 and T2 relaxation times. Although hydrogen density may be slightly higher, T1 and T2 relaxation times appear far more important for determining contrast.[580,582] In general, T1 contrast causes lesions to be dark, whereas T2 contrast causes lesions to be bright. Thus it is usually undesirable to have both T1 and T2 differences influence image contrast, since they may compete with each other and may cause lesions and liver to be isointense.

T1-WEIGHTED IMAGES
Spin Echo

Spin-echo technique is used at most centers to obtain T1-weighted images. To optimize T1 contrast in spin-echo images, it is essential to use TR less than the T1s of the tissues of interest. The optimum TR is typically between 250 and 500 msec, depending on field strength. The shortest possible TE should be used to minimize contributions to image contrast from T2 differences (Fig. 1-1).[203,358,501] Additional benefits of reducing TE include an increased number of sections available for a given TR, and reduced motion artifact. Motion artifact is reduced because there is less time for phase changes to accumulate from motion.

TE can be reduced by increasing the rate of sampling for analog-to-digital conversion (the sampling bandwidth)[358] or by asymmetric sampling of the echo. Both methods reduce SNR, but since averaging, thick sections (e.g., 7 to 10 mm), and large field of view (e.g., greater than 32 cm^2) are usually used to image the liver, SNR is rarely a problem on T1-weighted images.

Early reports on hepatic MRI were compromised by machine restrictions that limited the minimum TR to

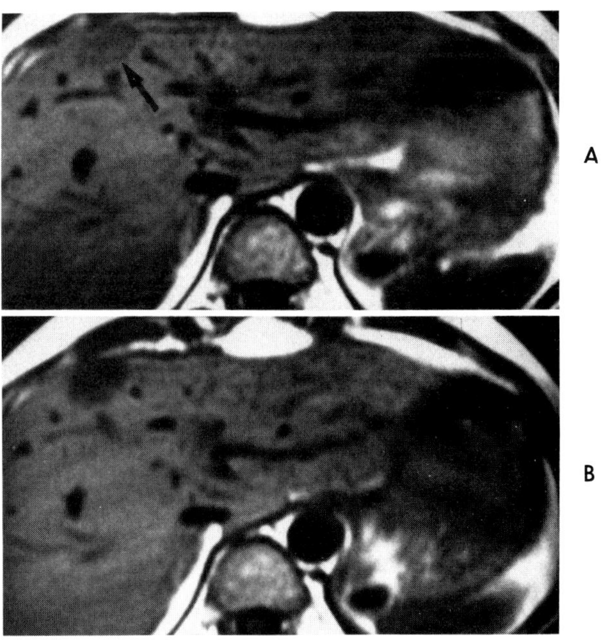

Fig. 1-1 Improved conspicuity of a metastasis on T1-weighted images (TR = 400 msec) at 1.5 T by reducing TE. Lesion *(arrow)* in medial segment of left lobe is subtle with TE = 20 msec *(top)* but obvious with TE = 12 msec *(bottom)*. (From Mitchell, D.G., Vinitski, S., Saponaro, S., et al.: Radiology 178:67-71, 1991.)

Table 1-1 Quantitative Analysis of Pulse Sequence Performance

				Performance rank	
Pulse sequence	n	Liver SNR	Cancer-liver magnitude CNR	CNR	Confidence factor
SE 1500/30	7	19.9	1.9 ± 0.9	19	
SE 1500/30 PC	7		3.0 ± 2.4	15	
SE 1500/60	7	13.3	3.5 ± 3.0	14	
SE 1500/90	6	9.5	5.5 ± 4.2	10	
SE 2000/30	27	17.2	2.4 ± 2.1	18	10
SE 2000/30 PC	25		4.2 ± 3.1	13	8
SE 2000/60	33	11.8	4.7 ± 3.6	11	9
SE 2000/60 PC	6		6.9 ± 2.7	7	
SE 2000/90	27	8.7	7.5 ± 5.3	5	7
SE 2000/120	5	6.0	7.7 ± 3.4	4	
SE 2000/180	4	3.7	4.2 ± 2.0	12	
IR 1500/450/30	33	16.5	6.2 ± 3.6	9	5
IR 1500/450/30 PC	1		1.6	20	
IR 1500/450/18	35	17.8	7.9 ± 4.2	3	3
IR 1500/280/18	30	11.3	7.2 ± 3.7	6	2
SE 500/30	37	25.5	6.4 ± 4.1	8	6
SE 500/30 PC	6		2.9 ± 2.1	17	
SE 260/30	32	24.8	8.1 ± 4.6	2	4
SE 260/30 PC	5		3.2 ± 0.9	15	
SE 260/18	39	27.4	10.3 ± 5.2	1	1

Data are normalized to reflect a standard 9-minute scan time for all pulse sequences. n, Number of patients studied; imaging performed at 0.6 T.
SNR, Signal-to-noise ratio.
CNR, Contrast-to-noise ratio is also known as signal difference-to-noise ratio SD/N. $CNR = SD/N = S_{tumor} - S_{liver\ noise}$
PC, Phase-contrast "opposed-phase" image, obtained using the chemical shift imaging method of Dixon.
Confidence factor, the ratio of the mean CNR to its standard deviation, is calculated only when number of patients (n) is ≥ 25.
(From Stark, D.D., et al: Radiology 159: 365-370, 1989.)

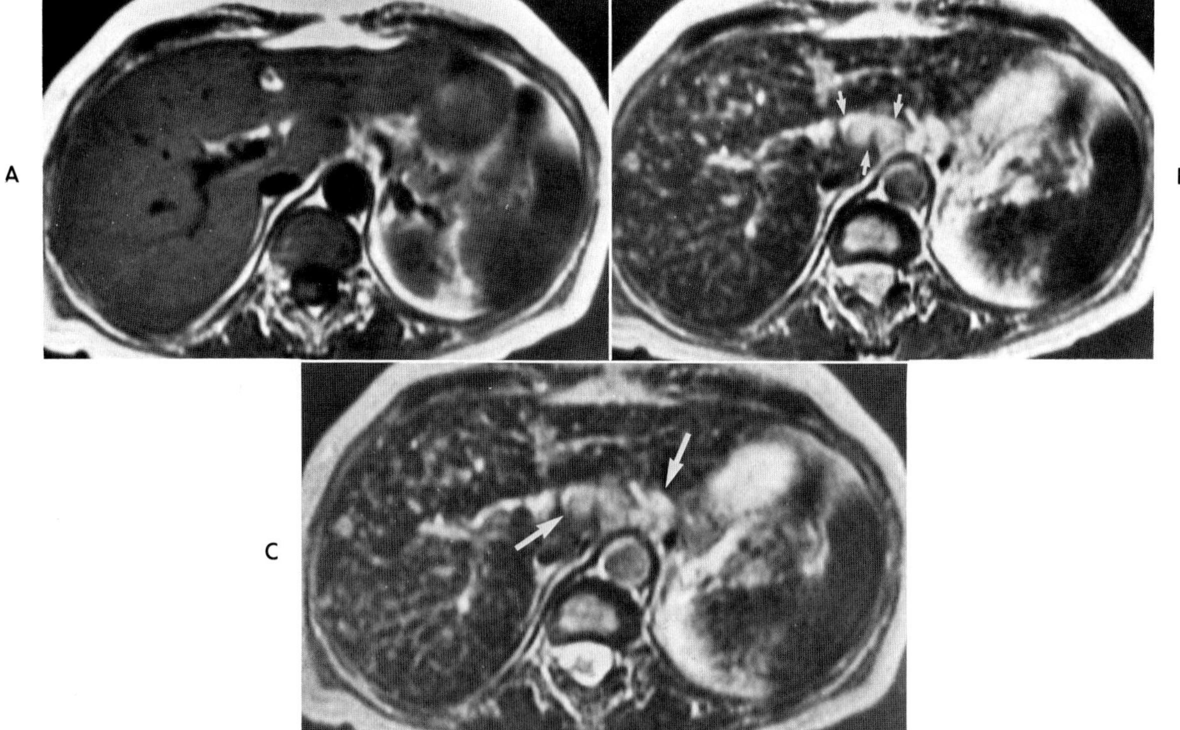

Fig. 1-2 Intrahepatic and extrahepatic metastases in a woman with metastatic breast carcinoma depicted at 1.5 T. **A,** Axial SE 500/20 image. **B** and **C,** On the T2-weighted images (SE 2500/50 and SE 2500/100, respectively), numerous tiny lesions are seen throughout the liver, some as small as 1 to 2 mm. Large lymphatic metastases in the gastrohepatic ligament *(arrows)* are nearly isointense with fat on this image and were isointense with liver on **A.** Confident diagnosis can be reached by comparison of the two images. Because of transfusional iron overload, the liver has decreased signal, causing contrast between liver and lesion to be more optimal with the TE of 50 msec than the TE of 100 msec.

500 msec and the minimum TE to 30 msec.[94,166,364] SE 500/30 images contain significant contributions from T1 and T2 differences, resulting in poor image contrast (Table 1-1). Pulse sequences such as these should not be referred to as *T1 weighted.*

T1-weighted images are important for lesion detection, especially at low field and mid field. Additionally, T1-weighted images are more effective than T2-weighted images for distinguishing perihepatic lymph nodes from fat (Fig. 1-2).

Inversion Recovery

As opposed to spin-echo imaging, in which T1 contrast depends on different rates of relaxation during a short TR, T1 contrast in inversion recovery images depends primarily on the inversion time (TI).[56] The initial 180-degree inversion pulse inverts the longitudinal magnetization. During the TI, which is the interval between this 180-degree pulse and the subsequent 90-degree excitation pulse, longitudinal magnetization recovers, depending on the T1 relaxation time. Initially, recovery is from negative magnetization towards zero, followed by recovery towards the original positive equilibrium value. If an appropriate TI is chosen so that recovery of longitudinal magnetization has reach zero for a given tissue (i.e., the "null point"), this tissue will have virtually no signal in the resulting image (Fig. 1-3).

A unique form of signal ambiguity can occur with inversion recovery technique. Two tissues may have different T1s but may be isointense on an inversion recovery image, depending on the TI. The tissue with short T1 (e.g., liver) may have recovered beyond the null point, whereas the tissue with long T1 (e.g., lesion) may not have reached the null point. Since most inver-

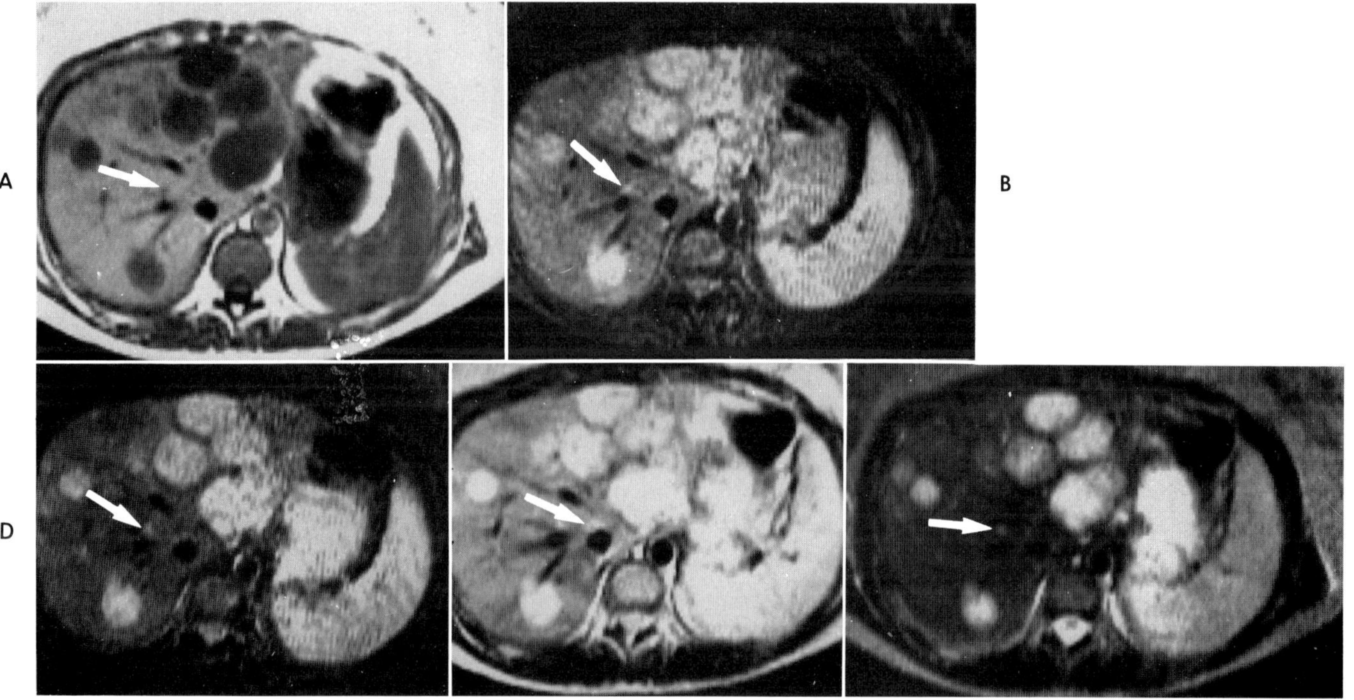

Fig. 1-3   Comparison of spin-echo and inversion recovery images at 0.6 T. **A,** MR image at SE 275/14 shows multiple metastases as hypointense high-contrast lesions (CNR = −21.2). Note the similar signal intensity of metastases and spleen. Not all metastases show the same level of soft-tissue contrast. Small metastases *(short arrow)* are indistinguishable from hepatic vessel *(long arrow)*. Note excellent anatomic detail (liver SNR = 65.2). **B,** MR images at IR 1500/30/80 and **C,** IR 1500/60/80 show absence of fat signal. Both images show metastases as high-intensity lesions (IR 1500/30/80, CNR = +12.0; IR 1500/60/80, CNR = +13.6). Small metastases are easily distinguishable from vessels. Anatomic detail in both IR images is inferior to that in SE 275/14 images (IR 1500/30/80, liver SNR = 21.7; IR 1500/60/80, liver SNR = 18.6). **D,** MR images at SE 2350/60 and **E,** SE 2350/180 also display metastases as high–signal-intensity lesions (SE 2350/60, CNR = +9.3; SE 2350/180 CNR = +15.0). Anatomic detail is only slightly inferior (SE 2350/60, liver SNR = 20.5; SE 2350/180, liver SNR = 5.3) compared with that in IR images. (From Dousset, M., Weissleder, R., Hendrick R.E., et al.: Radiology 171:327-33, 1989.)

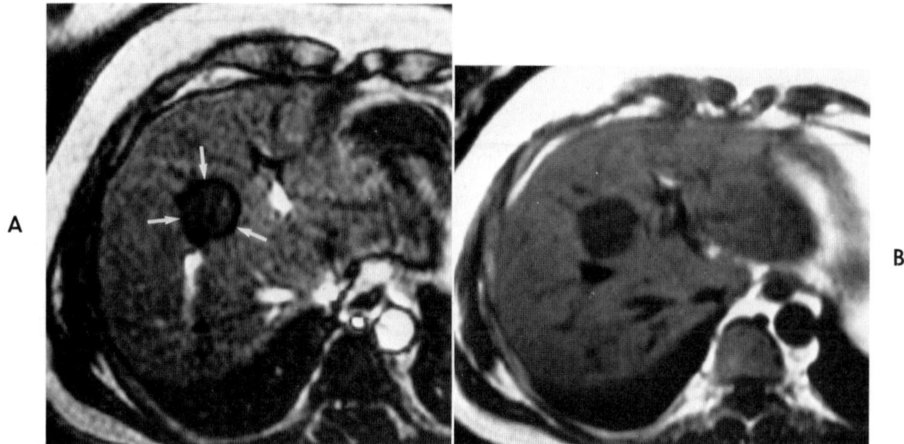

Fig. 1-4 Bounce-point artifact from inversion recovery technique at 1.5 T in a patient with cavernous hemangioma. **A,** Snapshot inversion recovery image (TI = 500 msec, centric view order) (see Chapter 3, Ultrashort TR Images). The black rim *(arrows)* surrounding the lesion is a bounce-point artifact. This occurs because liver and lesion have T1 relaxation times that are on opposite sides of the null point of the inversion recovery curve. **B,** Corresponding SE 400/12 image. There is no peripheral rim.

sion recovery images are reconstructed based on phase-insensitive magnitude intensity values, negative and positive intensities cannot be distinguished.

A signal void occurs at the boundary between two isointense tissues that are on different sides of the null point (Fig. 1-4). This artifact is sometimes referred to as the *bounce-point artifact,* and one must be aware that it does not represent a real structure. Bounce-point artifacts occur commonly at the periphery of liver lesions that have especially long T1, such as cysts, hemangiomas, and some metastases. Although they can artifactually mimic a tumor capsule and therefore lead to an erroneous impression of hepatocellular carcinoma, they allow detection of lesions that would otherwise be isointense. Therefore once one is familiar with this artifact, it should be considered a fortunate occurrence because it prevents hepatic lesions from being missed on inversion recovery images with intermediate TI.

Standard T1-weighted inversion recovery sequences use a TI similar to the T1 of the longer of the two tissues being compared (e.g., liver lesion). As with T1-weighted spin-echo images, the shortest possible TE should be used, whereas TR is usually long to maximize SNR and number of sections. Inversion recovery sequences such as these allow stronger T1 weighting than with spin-echo sequences.[431] It is possible to choose a TI so that normal liver is suppressed, maximizing contrast relative to pathology.[278,400,404]

Short TI (tau) inversion recovery (STIR) images differ from most other images in that tissues with long T1 are bright, rather than dark. As with other sequences, however, tissues with long T2 are bright. Thus long T1

and long T2, characteristic of most liver lesions, both contribute to signal intensity. T1 and T2 contrast are therefore additive rather than competitive.[56] Because significant but opposing T1 and T2 contrast is present between liver and most lesions, STIR is especially promising for the liver (see Figs. 1-4 and 1-5).[55,106,206] Additionally, perihepatic lymph nodes are conspicuously bright on STIR images, although their intensity is similar to liver on conventional T1-weighted images and similar to fat on T2-weighted images.[484] An additional benefit of STIR is suppression of signal from fat, which decreases motion artifacts.[55,56,106] As with SE sequences, T2 weighting can be increased by using longer TE,[106] but images such as these are rarely acquired because SNR and the number of sections are even less than with short TE STIR.

Other considerations have limited the use of inversion recovery for the liver. Inversion recovery images take longer to acquire than T1-weighted spin-echo images and therefore have lower SNR per unit of time (see Table 1-1). Additionally, fewer sections per acquisition can usually be acquired for a given TR. Although the flip angle of the inversion and excitation pulses can be varied to increase the number of sections or decrease the TR,[566] this has not been applied in clinical imaging.

T2-WEIGHTED IMAGES

With long TR and long TE, most focal lesions are more intense than liver parenchyma because of the increased free water within them. Lesions are typically visible on long TR/TE spin-echo images, but reproducible high quality images are harder to obtain than with

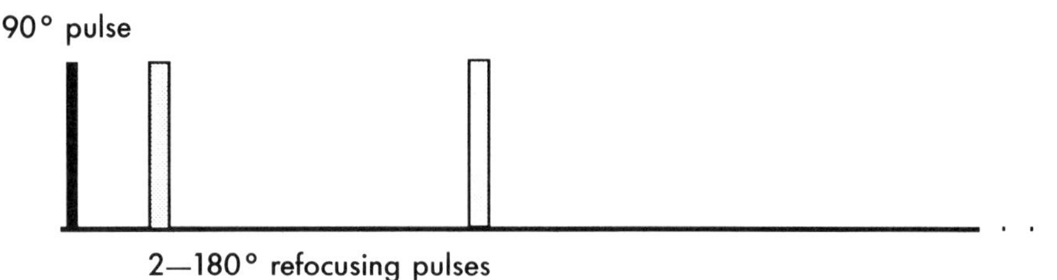

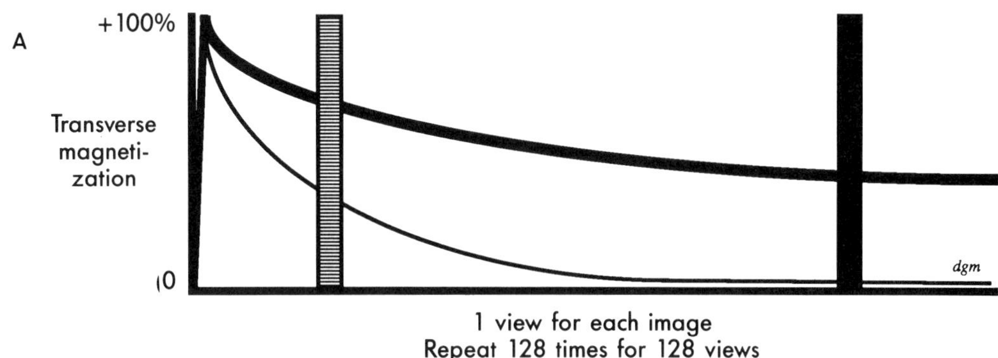

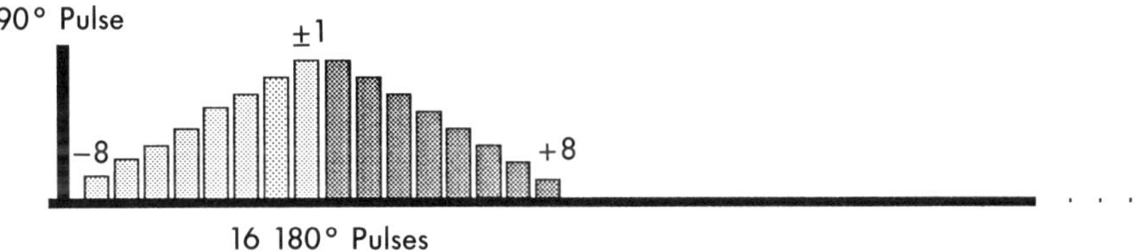

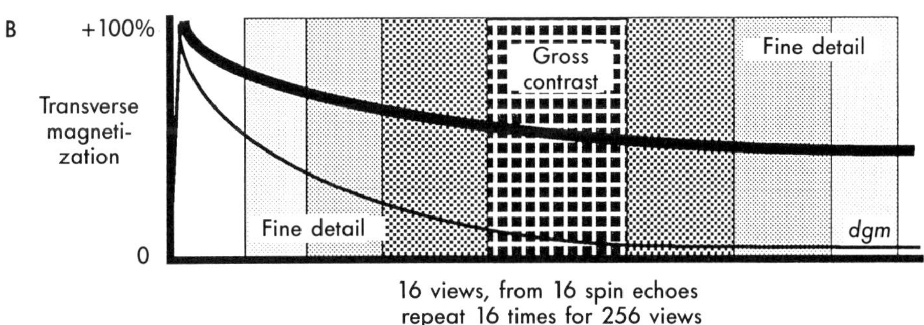

Fig. 1-5   Diagrammatic comparison between conventional and conjugate (fast) spin-echo techniques. **A,** With conventional double–spin-echo technique, two echoes are formed from two 180-degree refocusing pulses and are used for one phase-encode value in each of two images. Transverse magnetization is decreased on the second echo, accentuating contrast between tissues with long T2 *(thick curve)* and short T2 *(thin curve)*. **B,** With fast spin-echo technique, 16 180-degree pulses are used to form 16 echoes, which supply 16 phase-encode values for the image. To construct an image with a matrix of 256 × 256, this need to be repeated only 16 times. The high-order views, which use the strongest phase-encoding gradients, contribute to fine detail, whereas gross tissue contrast depends primarily on the central views, which use the weakest phase-encoding gradients.

short TR/TE techniques (see Figs. 1-4 and 1-5). Because of the long TR, averaging is not a practical technique for eliminating motion artifacts. To compound this problem, long TE reduces SNR and renders the image more vulnerable to phase errors from motion. T2-weighted spin-echo images are quite important, however, for detecting and confirming liver lesions, especially at high field, and for characterizing hepatic pathology at all field strengths.

SNR can be increased in long TE images by reducing the rate of sampling for analog-to-digital conversion (sampling bandwidth).[179,202,357,567] This may be useful at middle or low field strength if SNR limits the adequacy of long TR/TE images. SNR is rarely a problem for imaging the liver at high field strength, however, even with long TE. This is because large fields of view, 7 to 10-mm thick sections, and at least two averages, as are typically obtained for imaging the liver, all contribute to high SNR. The disadvantages of reduced sampling bandwidth (increased artifact from chemical shift and motion and decreased number of sections) thus outweigh its advantages for imaging the liver at high field strength.[357]

Examination time of T2-weighted spin-echo images can be reduced by decreasing the TR, maintaining contrast by optimizing the excitation flip angle.[182,355,414,426,547] For double (or even number) echo techniques, this involves reducing the angle, whereas for single (or odd number) echo techniques, flip angle is increased.

Conjugate Spin-Echo Train Techniques

Faster and better T2-weighted images can be obtained if multiple spin echoes are acquired after each excitation pulse. Rather than using these echoes to form separate images with different degrees of T2 weighting, as in conventional multiecho imaging, each echo can be used as a different phase-encoding view in the same image (Figs. 1-5 to 1-7).

The original version of this technique, referred to as *RARE (Rapid Acquisition with Relaxation Enhancement)*, was a heavily T2-weighted snapshot technique with low resolution and low SNR.[205] However, segmented or multishot versions of RARE appear more useful for clinical imaging. In a recent implementation of this technique, referred to by one equipment vendor as *fast spin echo*, 16 views are acquired after each excitation, allowing acquisition of T2-weighted images in one sixteenth of the time for a given TR.[210,331] In practice the time savings is usually less than this because less slices per repetition time may be obtained when the echo train is long.

Tissue contrast in conjugate spin-echo train techniques depends on the order of phase encoding. The "central" phase encode views, where the phase encoding gradient strength is close to 0, determine tissue con-

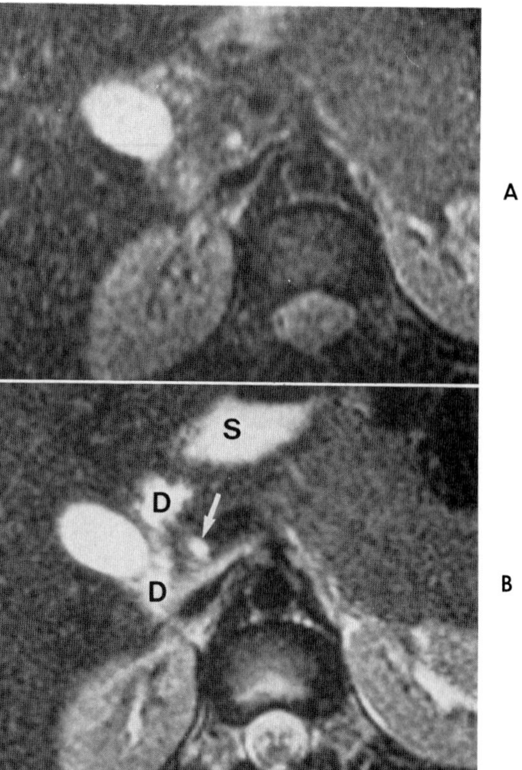

Fig. 1-6 Comparison between conventional and conjugate (fast) spin-echo T2-weighted images at 1.5 T. **A,** Axial conventional SE 2500/100 image with two signal averages, 256 × 128 matrix, has limited SNR and resolution but is otherwise adequate. Imaging time was 11 minutes. **B,** Image at an identical location using conjugate technique, with an echo train of 16 echoes after each excitation. TR/TE = 4000/102 msec, four signal averages, 256 × 256 matrix, imaging time for 13 sections = 4 minutes. SNR and resolution are improved. Note the improved clarity of fluid in stomach *(S)* and duodenum *(D)* because of the longer TR. This improves depiction of the pancreas. Note the higher signal of the common bile duct *(arrow)* and cerebrospinal fluid because of the longer TR.

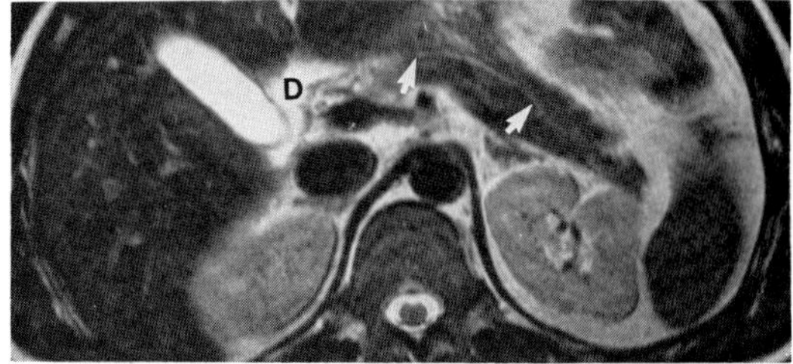

Fig. 1-7 Improved SNR, contrast, and resolution using conjugate (fast) spin-echo technique at 1.5 T. TR/TE = 5500/102 msec, using an echo train of 16 echoes per excitation, four signal averages, 512 × 256 matrix. Note the clarity of the duodenum *(D)* and the pancreatic duct *(arrows)*. Other abdominal structures are also clear. Fat has higher intensity than on conventional SE images with comparable TR and TE.

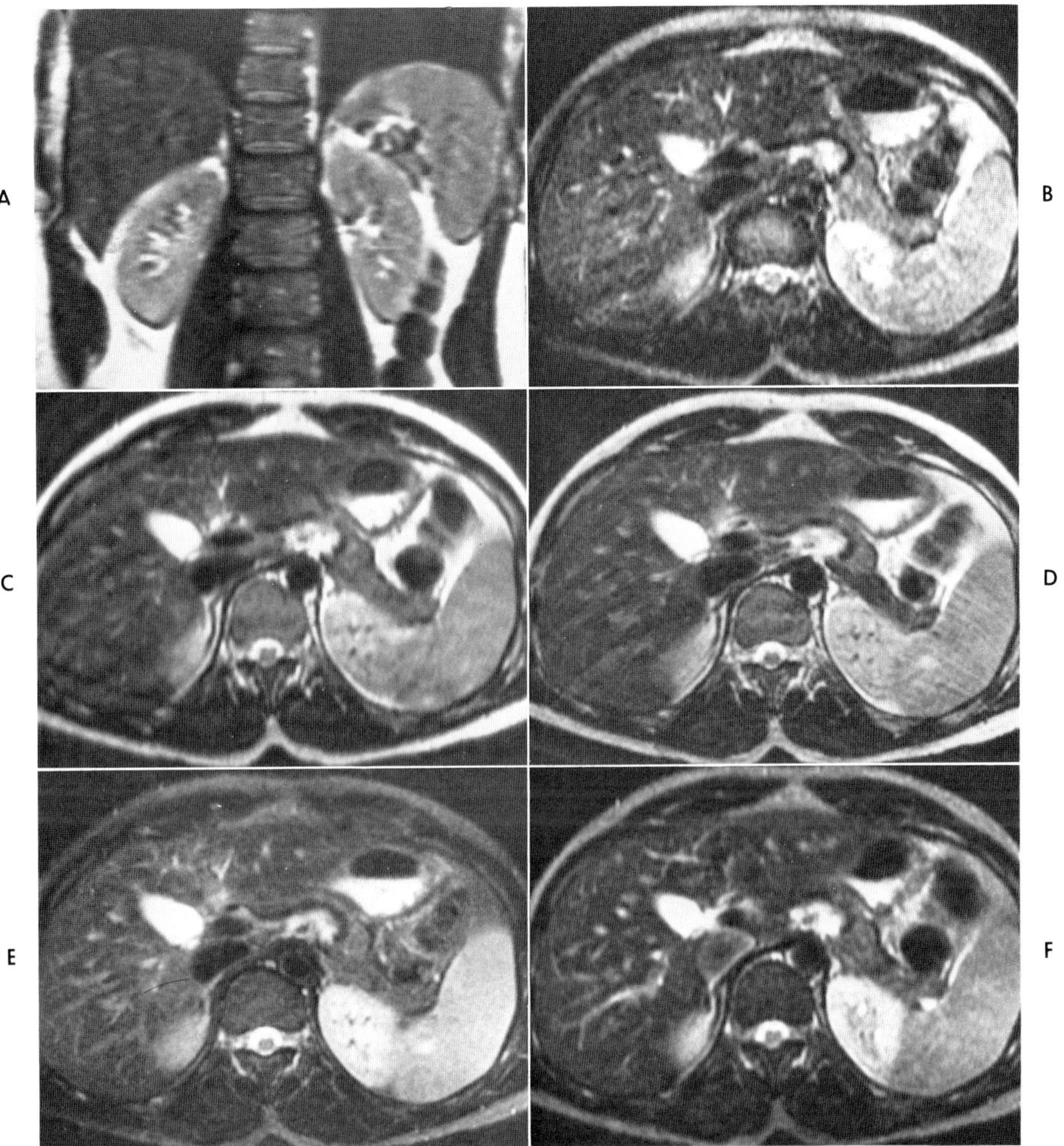

Fig. 1-8   Conjugate (fast) spin-echo technique, using a train of 16 echoes and various resolution parameters. **A,** Coronal T2-weighted localizer image (TR/TE = 1500/102 msec) acquired using a 256 × 128 matrix and one signal average. Eight images were acquired during a 33-second suspended respiration. **B,** Axial fast SE 1500/102 image (256 × 128, NSA = 1), four images acquired during a 19-second suspended respiration. **C,** TR/TE = 4000/102 msec, matrix = 256 × 128, four signal averages. Twelve images were acquired in 2 minutes. SNR is better, but motion artifact is severe. **D,** Fast SE 4000/102 image with 256 × 256 matrix and four signal averages, acquiring 12 images in 4 minutes. Motion artifact and resolution are improved. **E,** As in **D,** with fat suppression. Although fat suppression is only partially effective, motion artifact is reduced. **F,** Conventional SE 3000/100 image using 256 × 128 matrix and two signal averages, with respiratory-ordered phase encoding and gradient moment nulling to reduce motion artifact (see Chapter 2). In 14 minutes, 22 locations were acquired.

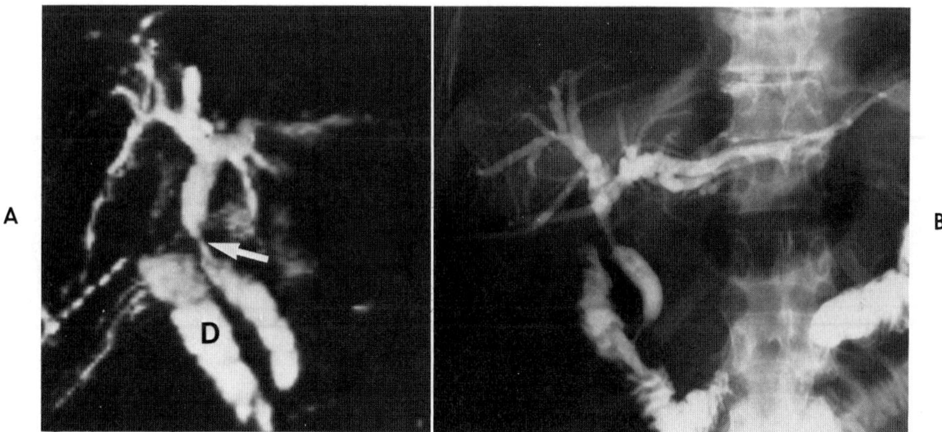

Fig. 1-9 MR cholangiographic image at 1.5 T of a woman with a common hepatic duct stricture *(arrow)*. D = duodenum. Bile ducts are depicted because of the long T2 of bile; no contrast agent was given **A,** Right anterior oblique projection image of the biliary system, reconstructed from contiguous 3-mm thick coronal conjugate (fast) spin-echo images using integration reconstruction algorithm (TRAP). TR/TE = 4000/160 msec, matrix = 256 × 256, field of view = 28 cm. **B,** Corresponding image from radiographic cholangiography. (Courtesy Eric Outwater, M.D.)

trast, whereas the "high order" phase encoding views (high positive and high negative phase encoding gradient strength) contribute to spatial resolution (see Fig. 1-7). The central phase encoding views can thus be acquired from echoes with the desired TE, referred to as the *effective TE*. The resulting tissue contrast is similar to that of a conventional SE image at that TE but echoes at different TE contribute to the image.

Interestingly, fat has higher signal than it would have with conventional SE technique at comparable TR and TE. The basis for this has not been determined but may be due to contribution to the image from short TE echoes or to elimination of mechanisms of lipid signal loss related to long interecho intervals with conventional technique. The images are also less sensitive to diffusion and susceptibility effects, so iron overload may be less apparent.

Conjugate spin-echo train images can be used to acquire up to six T2-weighted images of diagnostic quality within a breath-hold. These images have acceptable resolution (e.g., 256 × 128) but low SNR, and there is often some artifact in the phase-encode axis even without motion (Fig. 1-8). Newly introduced phased-array coils shaped to the body may improve SNR and therefore the quality of breath-hold conjugate spin-echo train images.

Alternatively, the time advantage can be "traded in" to obtain higher quality breathing-averaged T2-weighted images within a slightly decreased acquisition time. Since the number of slices per TR is limited by long echo trains, TR is often increased beyond what is practical for routine SE imaging. It is thus possible to completely eliminate contamination from T1 contrast, enhancing the difference between soft tissue and fluid, such as cerebrospinal fluid, bile, and intestinal lumen (Figs. 1-6 to 1-9). Averaging also becomes a practical approach to reducing motion artifact. For instance, one successful application of the spin-echo train technique for abdominal imaging involves TR = 4000 to 5000 msec, effective TE = 102 msec, acquisition matrix = 512 × 256 and four signal averages, for a total acquisition time of approximately 6 minutes.

High-resolution images with long TR may be especially valuable for imaging the pancreas and biliary system. Even small biliary ducts are depicted clearly because of less T1 contamination and higher resolution. The borders of the pancreas are also more distinct because of the higher intensity of fat on these images.

Motion Artifact

Once a certain threshold of contrast has been achieved, suppression of motion-induced artifacts is likely to be the major determinant of the optimum pulse sequence on a given system.[204,352] Although these artifacts are most severe at high field, they can degrade images at virtually any field strength (Fig. 2-1). There are numerous strategies for reducing artifact from motion (Table 2-1), many of which can be used together.

AVERAGING

Averaging is a powerful method for suppressing motion artifacts on short TR sequences.[496] An added benefit of averaging is increased SNR, which is especially important at low and mid field. Its major disadvantage is increased examination time. Averaging is not practical for conventional long TR techniques but can be used when examination time is decreased by conjugate spin-echo train techniques (e.g., RARE, fast spin echo) (see Chapter 1, T2-Weighted Images).

The motion-artifact reducing benefits of averaging are related to the total number of phase-encode views acquired, not merely to the number of times a complete set of views is repeated. For instance, resolution along the phase-encode axis can be doubled (e.g., from 128 to 256) and the number of excitations decreased (e.g., from 4 to 2) without increasing motion artifact. Although SNR is less with the latter technique, this is more than offset by the added resolution. Additionally, truncation (i.e., Gibbs) artifact, a ring-down artifact at high contrast borders, is reduced when resolution is increased.

RESPIRATORY AND CARDIAC MONITORING

Respiratory gating is rarely used because it requires long TR, preventing T1 weighting.[120] Changing the order in which phase-encoding views are acquired to match the respiratory cycle is a more practical method of compensating for respiratory motion.[16] Respiratory-ordered phase encoding (ROPE, Exorcist) is most effective with short TR/TE sequences. With long TR sequences, variations in the respiratory cycle have a greater effect, decreasing the effectiveness of reordered

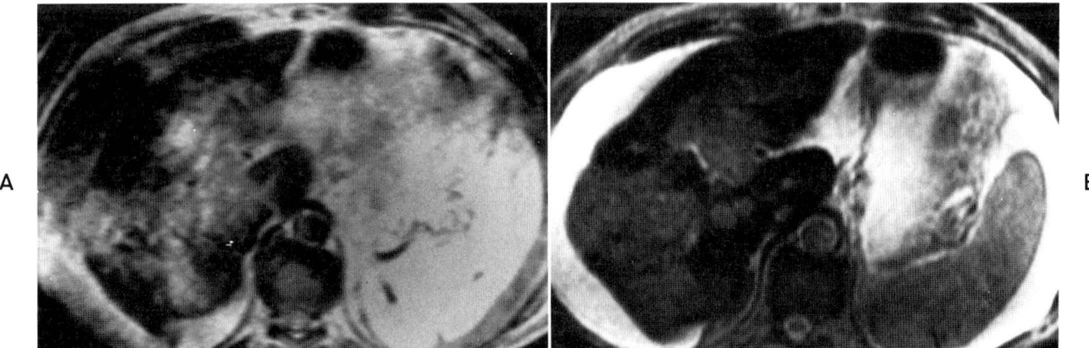

Fig. 2-1 Multifocal hepatocellular carcinoma with portal vein invasion, examined at 0.5 and 1.5 T. Proper technique is more important than field strength. **A,** T2-weighted image (SE 2000/60) at 0.5 T. Note the severity of motion-induced artifact **B,** Corresponding image at 1.5 T (SE 2500/100). Motion artifact is suppressed by reordered phase encoding, gradient moment nulling, and spatial presaturation. The portal vein is filled and expanded with tumor, and several smaller nodules are noted. There is abundant ascites. Motion artifact is a problem at mid and high field, and appropriate measures to reduce it should be used.

Table 2-1   Motion-Artifact–Suppression Techniques

Technique	Mechanisms	Comments
Averaging	Decreases conspicuity of random motion and increases SNR	Time consuming
Respiratory gating	Acquires all signals from the same point in the respiratory cycle	Requires long TR
Respiratory-ordered phase encoding	Changes order of phase encoding views to reduce ghost artifacts	Reduces view-to-view artifacts; no disadvantages
Cardiac gating	Acquires all signals from the same point in the cardiac cycle	Variable heart rate causes artifacts from variable TR
Gradient moment nulling	Reduces artifact from within-view motion	Powerful technique for long TE images
Spatial presaturation	Reduces vascular signal and ghosts	Slightly less images per TR, otherwise no disadvantages
Fat suppression	Reduces artifact from moving fat, improves dynamic range	Causes artifacts from magnetic field heterogeneity
Suspended respiration	Eliminates respiratory artifact and blurring	Requires special software; CNR may be limited

phase encoding. Additionally, within-view phase changes are greater with long TE, and these are not compensated for by reordered phase encoding.

A novel technique of respiratory monitoring uses MR data itself to detect bulk motion. For instance, the first echo of a double-echo sequence can serve as a "navigator echo," allowing reconstruction of the image relative to the abdominal viscera rather than to the imager couch.[118,130,261] This technique can correct for motion-induced artifact from within-view and view-to-view changes, as well as motion-induced blurring.

Cardiac gating is widely available but has limited applications for imaging the abdomen. Vascular pulsation artifact is controlled quite well by a combination of gradient moment nulling and presaturation (see next section), so cardiac gating is not necessary. Additionally, cardiac gating restricts the TR to a multiple of the R-to-R interval, rendering it difficult to implement for short TR techniques. Finally, slight irregularities in cardiac rate present in normal individuals lead to variable TR throughout image acquisition. This produces image blurring and artifacts from view-to-view intensity changes. Although cardiac gating is essential for imaging the heart and is quite helpful elsewhere in the chest, it is not helpful for most abdominal imaging.

GRADIENT MOMENT NULLING

Gradient moment nulling (flow compensation, motion artifact suppression technique [MAST]) corrects for phase changes within each view that are caused by motion while gradients are applied. These phase changes are eliminated by altering the gradient waveform.[180,405]

This altered gradient waveform takes more time, lengthening the minimum TE. Gradient moment nulling is therefore not appropriate for T1-weighted images but is more effective than reordered phase encoding for reducing motion artifact on T2-weighted images (Fig. 2-2).[353] The two techniques should be used together for T2-weighted images, however, because they are synergistic. Gradient moment nulling reduces artifact from within-view phase changes, whereas reordered phase encoding reduces artifact from between-view intensity changes.

Gradient moment nulling can also be accomplished by exploiting the phenomenon of *even echo rephasing,* whereby phase errors accumulated for the first echo are corrected for the second echo.[119,354] Even when gradient moment nulling is used, motion artifact can be decreased further if the first echo is half as long as the second echo (e.g., TE = 50 and 100 msec).[353]

The major disadvantage of gradient moment nulling is the increased intravascular signal that results in an undesirable feature for most applications of T2-weighted SE images. Signal within intrahepatic vessels renders small liver lesions less obvious. Additionally, ghosting from pulsatile flow may actually be increased by gradient moment nulling, even if correction for higher orders of motion, such as acceleration and pulsatility, is done. This is because the increased intravascular signal within vessels resulting from gradient moment nulling may vary from view to view, depending on velocity. Fortunately, this ghosting can be virtually eliminated by presaturating blood flowing into the stack of imaging sections (Fig. 2-3).[353]

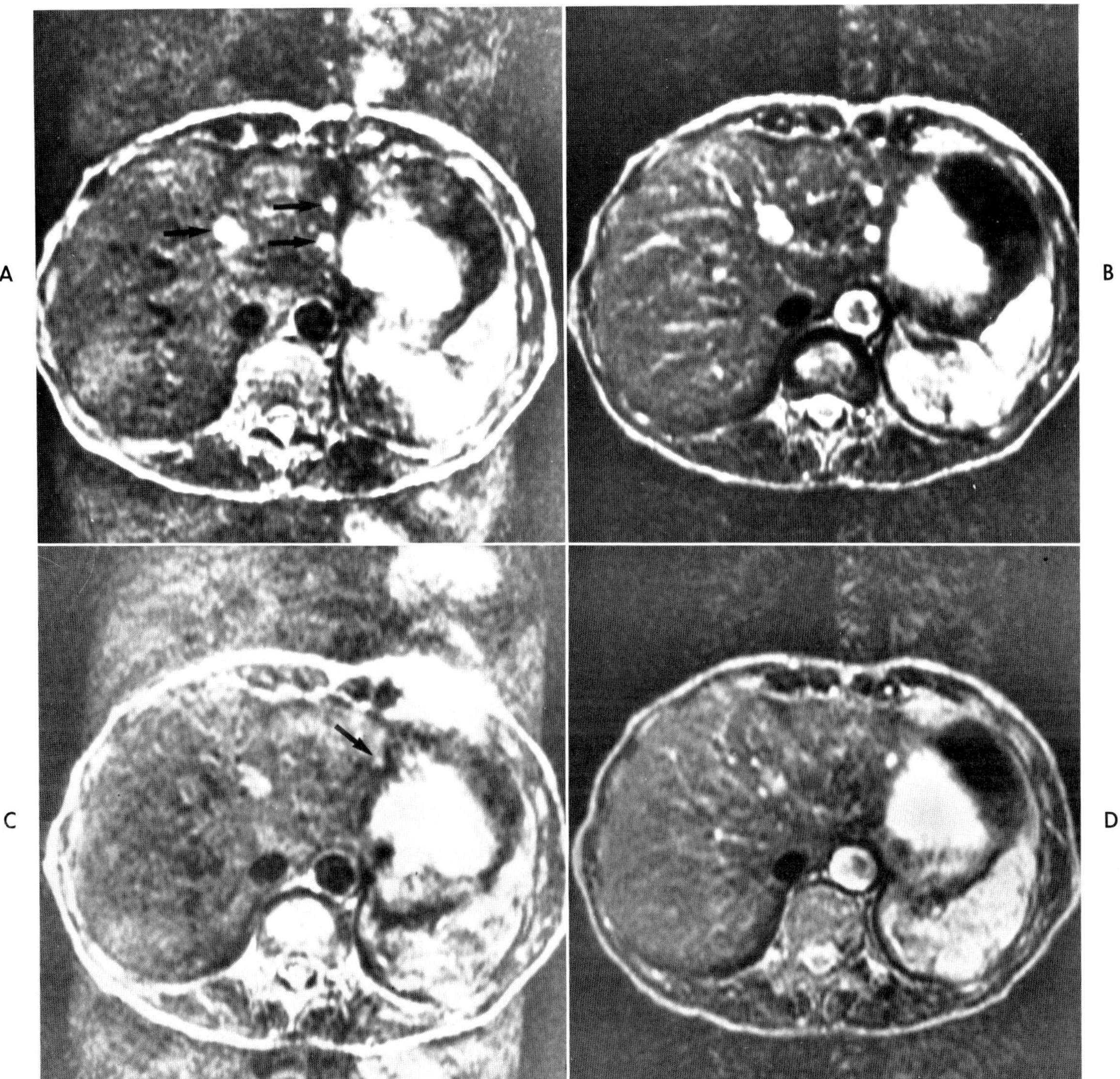

Fig. 2-2   Superiority of gradient moment nulling over reordered phase encoding for motion artifact suppression on T2-weighted images at 1.5 T. **A,** Axial MR image (SE 2500/80) with reordered phase encoding depicting three liver lesions *(arrows),* in spite of severe motion artifact. **B,** With gradient moment nulling but without reordered phase encoding (all other parameters identical), artifact is substantially reduced. Note that ghost artifact from pulsatile flow in the aorta is still severe. **C,** Twelve-mm cephalad to **A,** a fourth liver lesion *(arrow)* is identified only in retrospect. **D,** With gradient moment nulling, this 3-mm lesion is obvious. (From Mitchell, D.G., Vinitski, S., Burk, D.L., et al.: Radiology 169:155-160, 1988.)

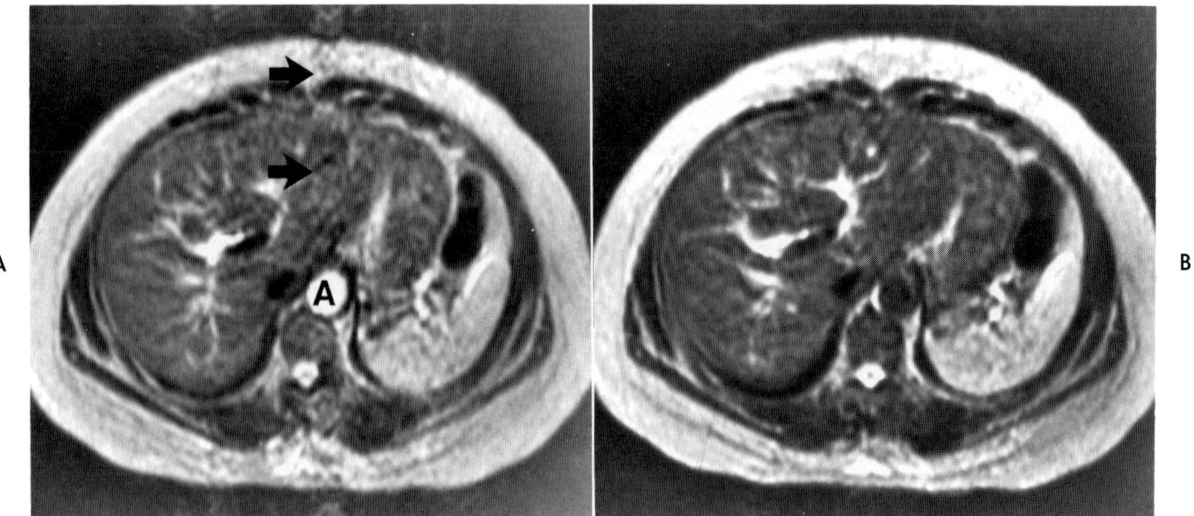

Fig. 2-3   Combined artifact-reducing effects of gradient moment nulling and spatial presaturation at 1.5 T. **A,** With gradient moment nulling (SE 2500/80) ghost artifact is minimal, except from pulsatile flow in the aorta. Note the high signal of intrahepatic vessels. **B,** With spatial presaturation (all other parameters identical), signal in and artifact from the aorta are decreased, but intrahepatic vascular signal is unaffected. (From Mitchell, D.G., Vinitski, S., Burk, D.L., et al.: Radiology 169:155-160, 1988.)

SPATIAL PRESATURATION

Spatial presaturation is a highly effective technique for decreasing intravascular signal and ghosting from major vessels that are perpendicular to the plane of imaging, such as the aorta and inferior vena cava.[111,129] Combining spatial presaturation with gradient moment nulling virtually eliminates vascular ghosts (see Fig. 2-3). Signal within intrahepatic vessels, the splenic vein, and other vessels oriented within the imaging plane, may be unaffected by standard spatial presaturation.[353] For this reason, T2-weighted images with gradient moment nulling are unreliable for evaluating vessels. Correlation with other sequences, such as T1-weighted images with spatial presaturation and gradient-echo images with gradient moment nulling, is therefore essential. An alternative is to selectively presaturate blood in the portal vein with an appropriately located oblique presaturation pulse.[115,397] This approach is not suitable for screening examinations, since oblique presaturation pulses are likely to obscure some pertinent anatomy.

SUPPRESSING SIGNAL FROM FAT

Suppressing signal from fat eliminates ghost artifacts that arise from motion of fat. Fat can be suppressed in inversion recovery sequences by choosing an appropriately short TI (usually between 100 and 150 msec, depending on field strength) (see Figs. 1-4 and 1-5)[56] or in spin-echo sequences by chemical shift fat-suppression techniques (see Chapter 5, Chemical Shift Imaging).* This does not eliminate motion artifact completely, however, since most abdominal motion is from cephalocaudad visceral excursions.[479,515] For instance, the liver moves up to 2 cm with each breath.

---

*141, 254, 357, 443, 517, 518

Breath-Hold Techniques

In the abdomen, rapid imaging can be defined as any single-slice or multislice technique that can be acquired during suspended respiration, eliminating respiratory artifact.[54,70,112,579] One disadvantage of breath-holding for single-slice techniques is that slice misregistration artifact may cause small lesions to elude detection. Ultrafast techniques, however, allow an entire liver to be imaged within a single suspended respiration, eliminating slice misregistration artifacts. If images are acquired within 1 second or less, even ghosting from pulsatile flow may be eliminated.

Acquisition time may be reduced by decreased averaging, increasing the number of sections acquired per repetition time, decreasing repetition time, and/or acquiring more than one phase encoding view per excitation.

DECREASED AVERAGING

Most rapid techniques use two or less averages. If TR is short enough (e.g., $\leq$ 250 msec), and half-Fourier data sampling is used for one excitation, it is possible to obtain a set of T1-weighted spin-echo images during a single breath-hold (rapid acquisition spin echo [RASE]). These images have reduced SNR, but respiratory artifact can be eliminated.[307,342] Although these images are superior to SE images obtained without effective suppression of motion artifacts,[342] their clinical utility relative to optimized conventional images has not been established. The major potential of rapid spin-echo images may be for effective use of dynamic contrast enhancement.[343] Gradient-echo techniques (see next section) may yield images with higher SNR in less time, but chemical shift and vascular artifact may be problematic.

INCREASED SECTIONS PER REPETITION TIME

If the 180-degree refocusing pulse is eliminated and echoes are formed by gradient reversal, more images with higher SNR can be obtained for a given TR (Figs. 3-1 and 3-2). If TE is minimized, SNR and number of images for a given TR increase even further.[113] If TE is short enough, within-view phase errors can be virtually eliminated. However, view-to-view changes because of pulsatile flow usually produce ghost artifacts with mul-

tislice techniques (Fig. 3-3). This artifact is not exacerbated by administration of paramagnetic contrast agents and is not reduced by gradient moment nulling. Additionally, one must be aware that fat-water cancellation may occur on gradient-echo images, depending on TE (see Chapter 5, Chemical Shift Imaging).[581]

SHORT TR "ANGIOGRAPHIC" IMAGES

Single-slice gradient-echo images with short TR and reduced flip angle are usually suboptimal for depicting abdominal pathology, but such images can be quite useful for vascular imaging.[158] These images are most successful when gradient moment nulling is used to compensate for constant velocity motion, and TE is minimized. Ghost artifact from pulsatile flow in the aorta may be reduced by using a low flip angle.[530] Usually, between two and five such images may be acquired per suspended respiration. Although axial images are optimal in most cases, coronal and sagittal images may also be useful.

It is important to remember that the major mechanism causing high signal of flowing blood is inflow of unsaturated spins. For this reason, these sequences are often referred to as *time-of-flight* techniques. Their sensitivity to flow is greatest when the direction of flow is perpendicular to the plane of the image. For this reason, the splenic vein, right portal vein, and main hepatic veins may not be uniformly hyperintense.

Although vascular anatomy can be delineated clearly by tomographic flow-sensitive images, the data from these images can be combined to produce projection MR angiographic images, frequently using a maximum-intensity projection algorithm (Fig. 3-4). The in-plane resolution and image quality are best if the acquisition and projection planes are the same, but projection onto other planes allows a rotating movie-type format. Saturation pulses can eliminate unwanted vessels from the projection or to allow measurement of velocity (Fig. 3-5).[115]

One must be aware that some information is lost when data from multiple images are condensed into one, and artifacts are introduced by the maximum intensity projection algorithm. Additionally, ascites may have high signal that is depicted on MR angiograms as

Text continued on p. 20.

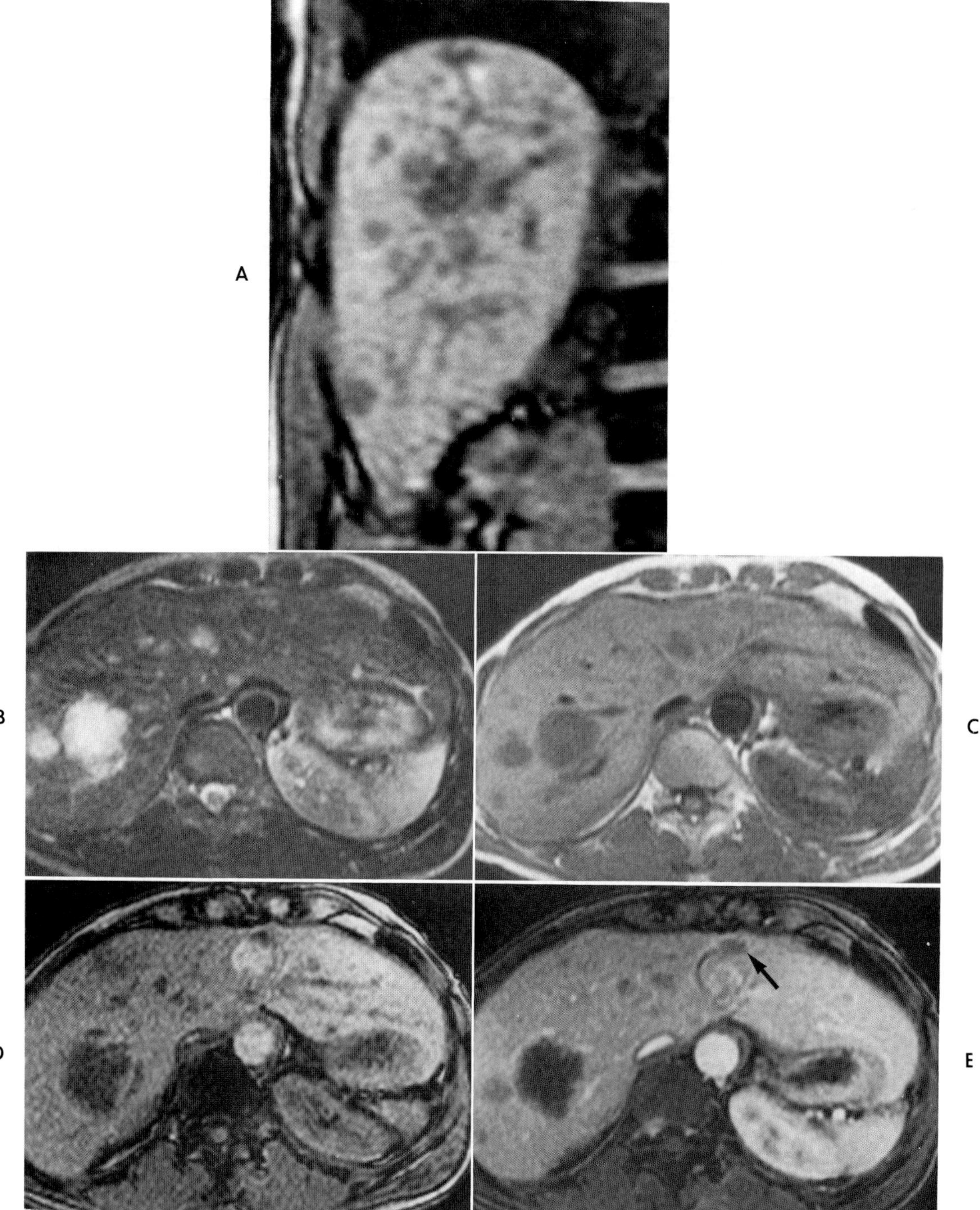

Fig. 3-1   Multislice spoiled gradient-echo technique at 1.5 T, allowing acquisition of 12 axial images during a single 14-second suspended respiration. **A,** Coronal localizer image depicts numerous metastases. **B,** Even more lesions are depicted on this SE 3000/100 image. **C,** Axial SE 400/12 image depicts several lesions. **D,** Corresponding spoiled gradient-echo image with TR/TE = 102/2.3 msec, flip angle = 90-degree. Although there is no respiratory artifact, some lesions are obscured by low SNR, and it is difficult to distinguish low-intensity vessels from lesions. Flow artifact degrades depiction of the left lobe. **E,** Same technique as in **D,** less than 1 minute after administration of a bolus of gadopentatate dimeglumine, 0.1 mmol/kg. More lesions are seen, and vessels have high signal. Artifact from the aorta is not worse, and a lesion *(arrow)* in this region is depicted more clearly than on other images.

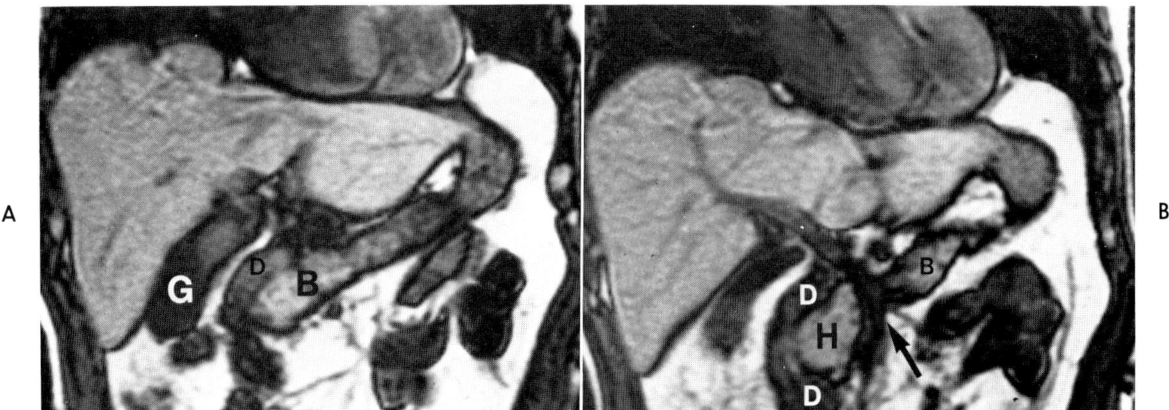

Fig. 3-2   Coronal images of the pancreas and the duodenum *(D)* (TR/TE/flip angle = 102/
2.3/90-degrees). Twelve images were acquired during a single 14-second suspended respiration. **A,** The pancreatic body *(B)* is sharply delineated due to lack of motion-induced artifact. *G* = gallbladder. Artifactual edge enhancement is due to phase cancellation at bound-
aries between water and fat due to the TE of 2.3 msec (see Chapter 5, Chemical Shift Imaging). **B,** Posterior to **A,** the superior mesenteric vein *(arrow)* divides the pancreatic body *(B)*
from the head *(H)*.

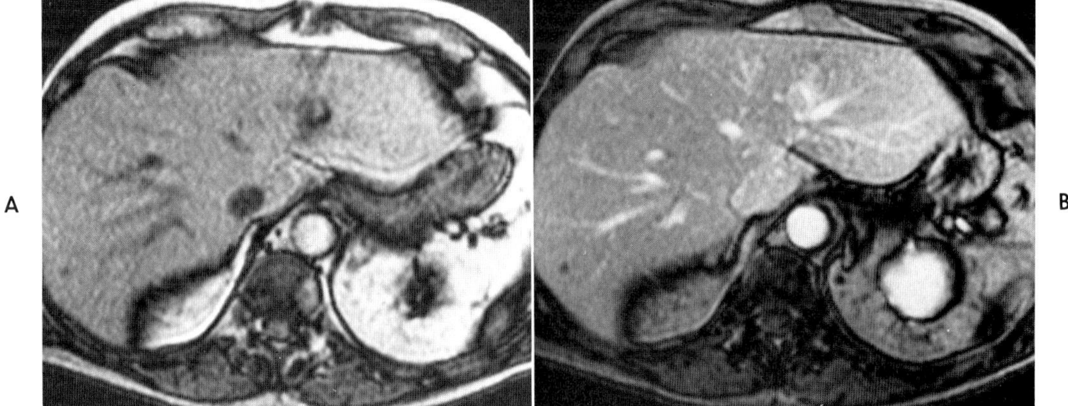

Fig. 3-3   Artifact from the aorta on multislice short TE gradient-echo images does not increase after contrast administration. (1.5T). **A,** Axial image (TR/TE/flip angle = 102/2.3/90
degrees). Pulsation artifact from the aorta obscures part of the left lobe. **B,** After administration of gadopentatate dimeglumine, 0.1 μmol/kg, the artifact is less conspicuous. This is because view-to-view intensity changes are not increased by enhancement and because within-view phase changes are minimal with TE = 2.3 msec. Note small cyst in posterior right
lobe.

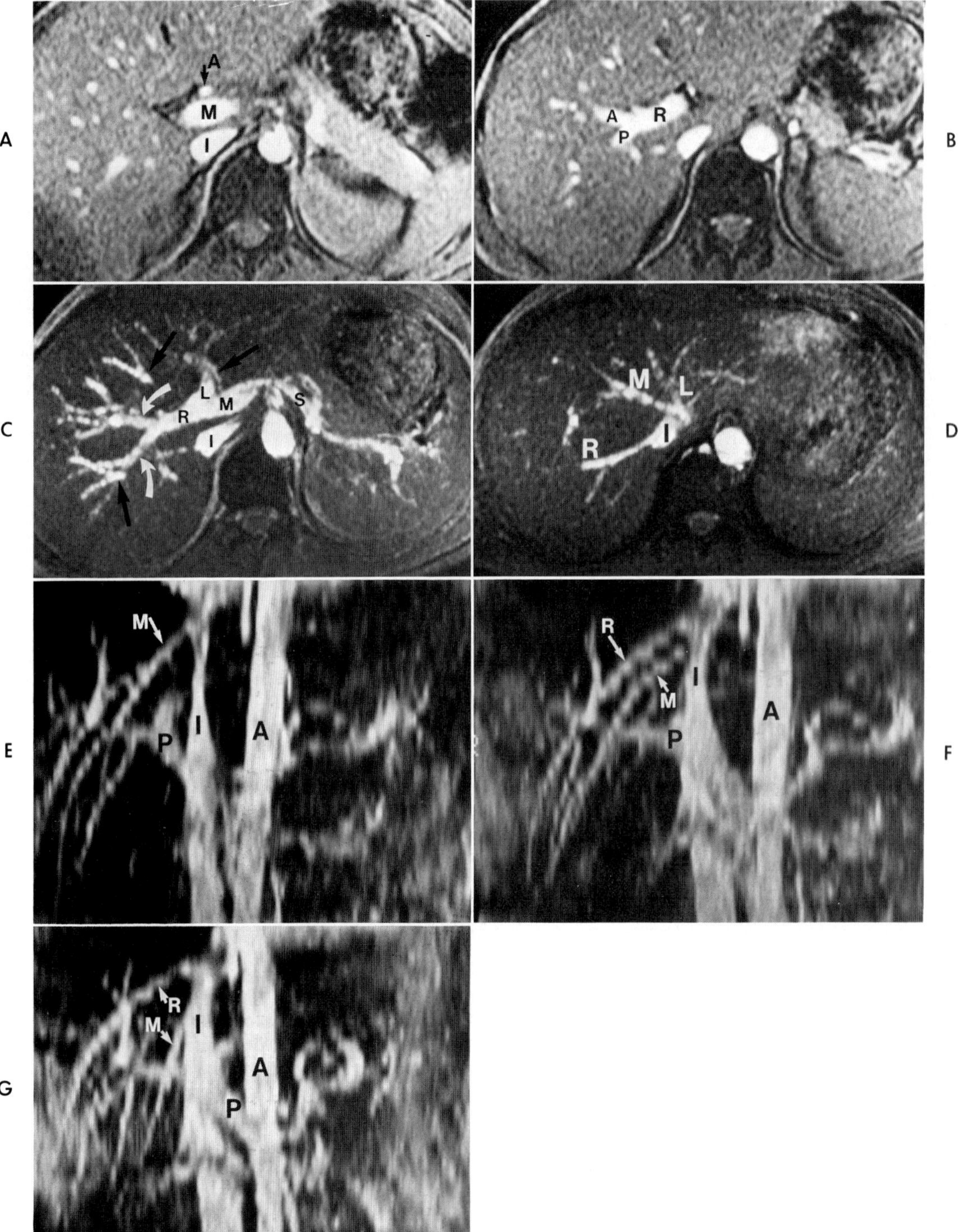

Fig. 3-4 Two-dimensional time-of-flight (2D-TOF) MR angiography at 1.5 T. **A** to **B,** Two representative sections from a set of contiguous spoiled gradient-echo images, 7-mm thick. TR/TE/flip angle = 27/6.3/20 degrees. With one signal averaged, four sections were acquired during each 13-second suspended respiration. **A,** view at the level of the main portal vein *(M),* which is situated between the main hepatic artery *(A)* and the inferior vena cava *(I).* **B,** Right portal vein *(R),* bifurcating into anterior *(A)* and posterior *(P)* segmental branches. The left portal vein extends superiorly, and is not visualized on this section. **C,** Composite image consisting of eight contiguous sections, including the splenic vein *(S)* and the main *(M),* right *(R),* and left *(L)* portal veins. *Curved white arrows* = segmental portal vein branches, *black arrows* = hepatic veins. *I* = inferior vena cava. **D,** Composite image at the level of the hepatic venous confluence showing the right *(R),* middle *(M),* and left *(L)* hepatic veins. *I* = inferior vena cava. **E** to **G,** Three of a total of 19 maximum intensity projections (MIPs) of the two-dimensional data set, projected at 10-degree increments around a 180-degree axis. *A* = aorta, *I* = inferior vena cava, *P* = main portal vein, *M* = middle hepatic vein, *R* = right hepatic vein. **E,** Right posterior oblique projection. **F,** Anteroposterior (coronal) projection. **G,** Left posterior oblique projection.

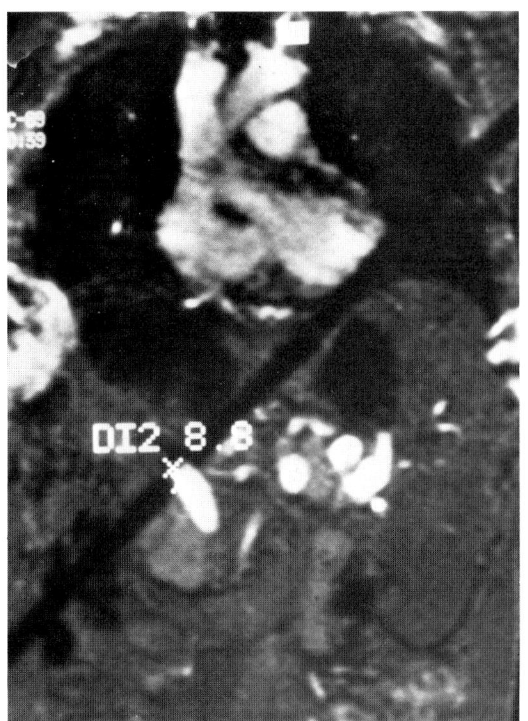

Fig. 3-5 Coronal MR angiogram at 1.5 T, demonstrating use of an oblique saturation pulse to estimate portal vein velocity by measuring the distance unsaturated blood travels into the saturation band. Notice that the saturation band has eliminated signal from intrahepatic portal veins. (Courtesy Robert Edelman)

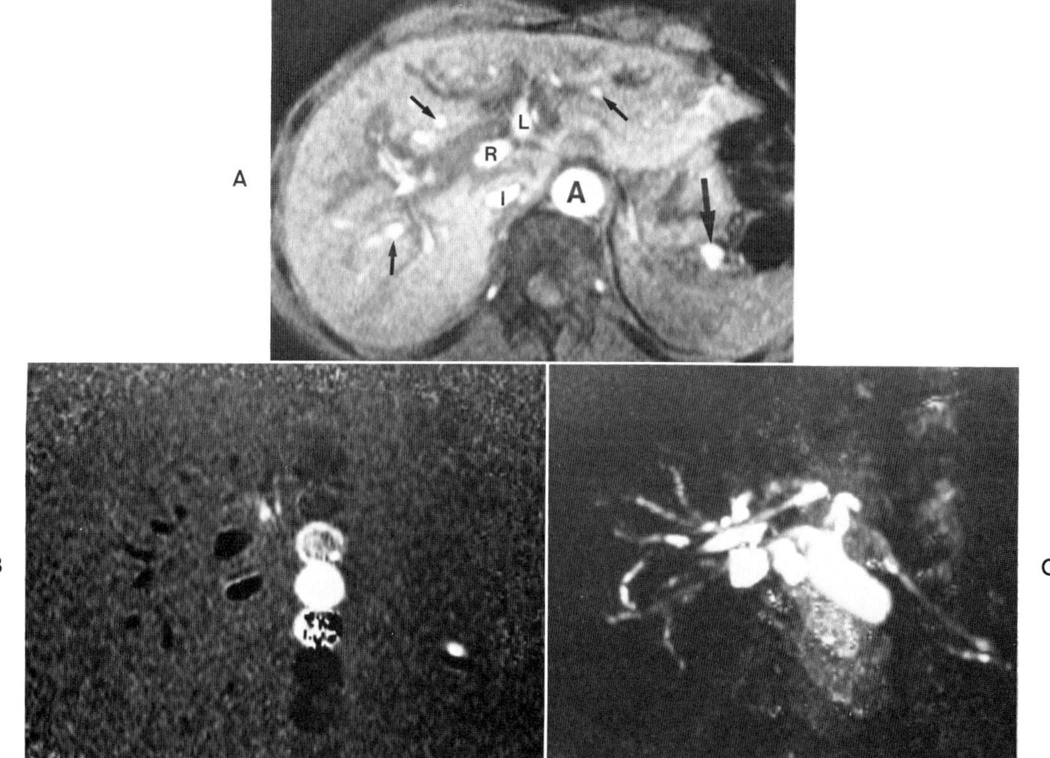

Fig. 3-6 Two-dimensional phase-contrast (2D-PC) MR angiography at 1.5 T in a patient with sclerosing cholangitis at the level of the proximal right *(R)* and left *(L)* portal veins. TR/TE flip angle = 20/8.6/20 degrees. *A* = aorta, *I* = inferior vena cava, *small arrows* = hepatic vein branches, *large arrow* = splenic artery and vein. **A,** Magnitude image. Vessels have high signal because of inflow enhancement (time-of-flight effect). **B,** Phase-contrast image corresponding to **A.** Phase shifts are encoded in the slice-select axis. Subtraction of flow-compensated and flow-encoded images results in subtraction of static tissue and depiction of only phase shifts along the slice-select axis. Flow towards the head is black, flow towards the feet is white, and background and static tissue are grey. The phase shifts in the aorta vary from view to view, resulting in severe ghosting. **C,** Composite axial phase-contrast MR angiogram using magnitude reconstruction results in nearly total suppression of static tissue.

if it were blood flow.[570] Therefore findings depicted on a projection MR angiogram must be verified by examining the pertinent tomographic sections.

Phase-contrast techniques represent phase changes from motion. Phase changes may be positive or negative relative to stationary tissue, which has no phase change. Intensity is proportional to the velocity of flow along the flow encoding axis. In two-dimensional phase-contrast techniques, flow in one direction is dark, flow in another direction is bright, and background is depicted as grey (Fig. 3-6).[433] Although time-of-flight techniques are most sensitive to flow perpendicular to the plane of the image, phase-contrast techniques can depict flow along any of the three axes of the image. Phase-contrast data can be encoded in color and superimposed on a grey scale magnitude image to depict unambiguously the direction and velocity of flow relative to stationary anatomy (Fig. 3-7) (see also Color Plate I). Phase-contrast techniques also allow measurement of flow velocity and volume.[108]

Time-of-flight and phase-contrast flow images may also be acquired using three-dimensional techniques, but these are difficult to implement with breath-holding and are therefore more vulnerable to motion-induced artifact. Additionally, most three-dimensional time-of-flight techniques are less sensitive to slow flow, where only a small fraction of blood in the imaging slab can be replaced by unsaturated spins.

ULTRASHORT TR IMAGES

When TR and TE are minimized, images can be acquired in less than a second. Ultrashort TR techniques have been implemented for real-time MR fluoroscopy, where the image is continually updated as new phase-encoding views are acquired.[127,216]

Heavily T1-weighted single-slice images can be obtained rapidly by snapshot inversion recovery techniques, such as turboFLASH. In this magnetization-prepared technique an ultrashort TR/TE gradient-echo sequence is preceded by a single 180-degree inversion pulse (Figs. 1-5, and 3-8 to 3-12).[69,92,181,368] Because TR is so short, the central phase-encoding views are acquired before periodic changes in signal intensity within a voxel can occur. Motion may thus cause some blurring, but ghost artifacts do not occur, even with highly pulsatile aortic flow (see Fig. 3-9).

Text continued on p. 25.

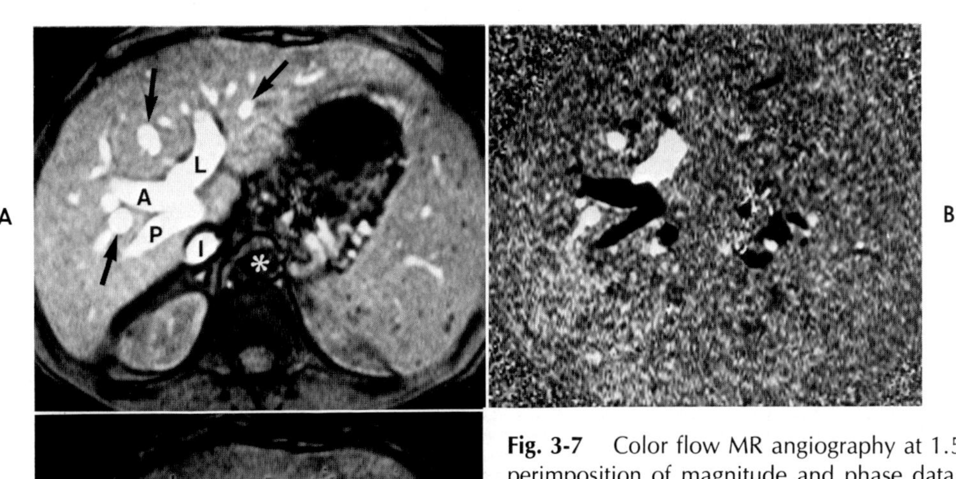

Fig. 3-7   Color flow MR angiography at 1.5 T, produced by unambiguous superimposition of magnitude and phase data from 2D-PC images, showing the anterior *(A)* and posterior *(P)* branches of the right portal vein and the left portal vein *(L)*. *I* = inferior vena cava. A saturation pulse was applied superiorly to eliminate signal from the aorta *(asterisk)*. *Arrows* = hepatic vein branches. **A,** Magnitude image. **B,** Corresponding phase image. Flow towards the right is black, flow towards the left is white, and background and static tissue are grey. **C,** Color flow MR image obtained by encoding the phase (flow) data from **B** and superimposing it on the magnitude (static tissue) data from **A.** Magnitude and phase thresholds were used to set the priority between color and grey scale. Blue represents flow towards the right (e.g., right portal vein branches), and red represents flow towards the left (e.g., left portal vein and middle and right hepatic veins). Paler shades of color indicate faster flow along the left-to-right axis. Helical flow in the inferior vena cava resulting from renal vein inflow causes a split-color appearance (see Color Plate I).

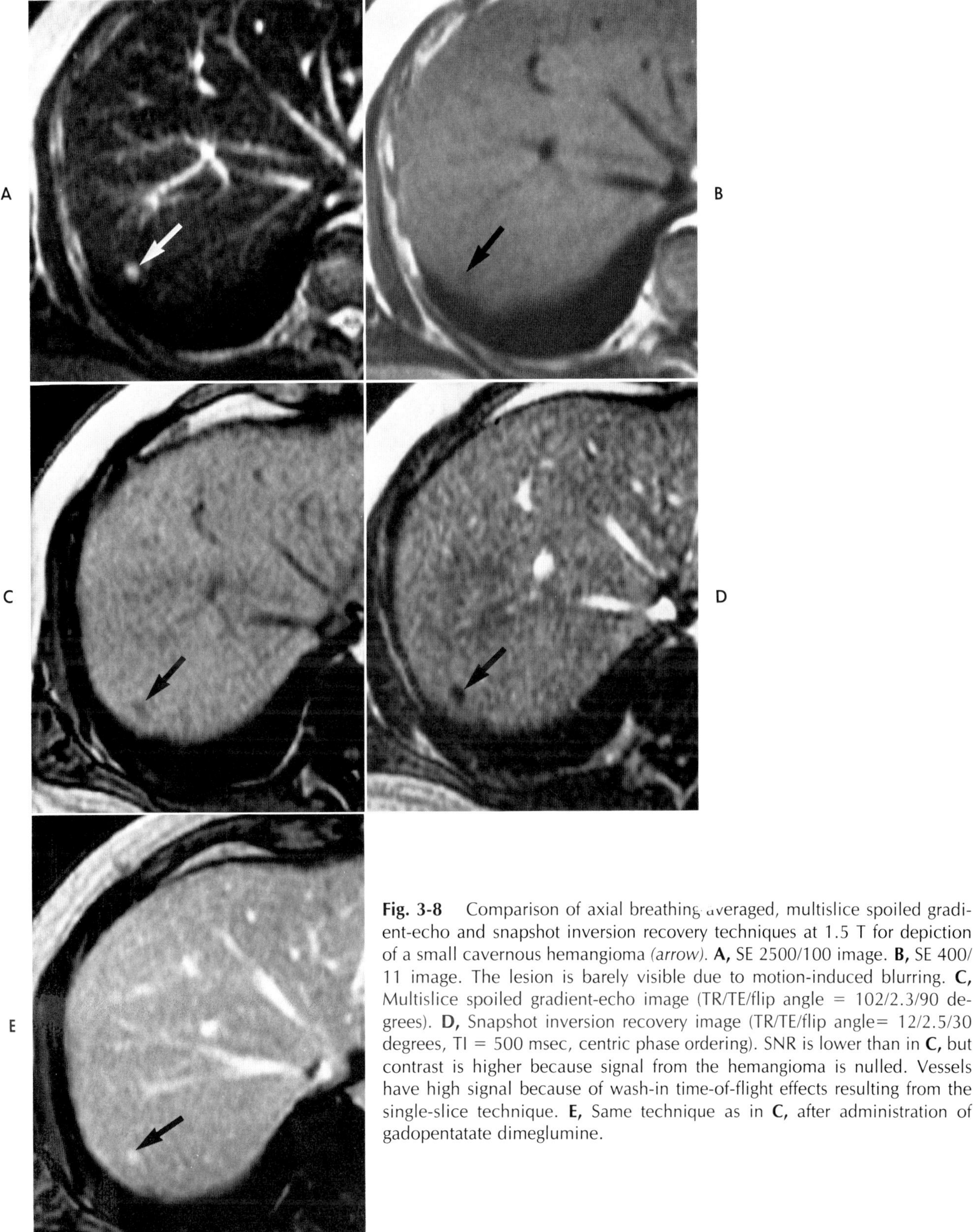

Fig. 3-8   Comparison of axial breathing averaged, multislice spoiled gradient-echo and snapshot inversion recovery techniques at 1.5 T for depiction of a small cavernous hemangioma *(arrow).* **A,** SE 2500/100 image. **B,** SE 400/11 image. The lesion is barely visible due to motion-induced blurring. **C,** Multislice spoiled gradient-echo image (TR/TE/flip angle = 102/2.3/90 degrees). **D,** Snapshot inversion recovery image (TR/TE/flip angle= 12/2.5/30 degrees, TI = 500 msec, centric phase ordering). SNR is lower than in **C,** but contrast is higher because signal from the hemangioma is nulled. Vessels have high signal because of wash-in time-of-flight effects resulting from the single-slice technique. **E,** Same technique as in **C,** after administration of gadopentatate dimeglumine.

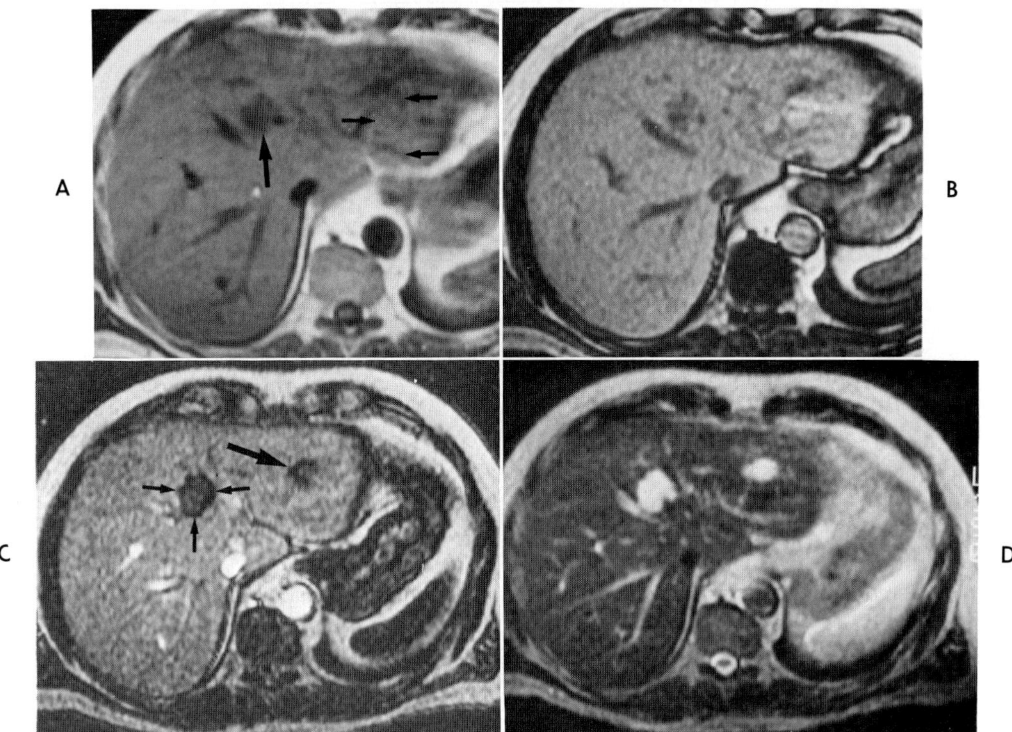

Fig. 3-9 Decreased pulsation artifact with ultrashort TR technique at 1.5 T, improving depiction of a cavernous hemangioma. **A,** SE 400/12 image. A lesion *(arrow)* is depicted in the medial segment of the right lobe. Pulsation artifact *(small arrows)* is minimal due to saturation above the imaging volume. **B,** Multislice spoiled gradient-echo image (TR/TE/flip angle = 102/2.3/90 degrees). The lesion is less conspicuous due to partial volume artifact; it was more conspicuous on the adjacent section (not shown). Pulsation artifact is more severe. **C,** Snapshot inversion recovery image (TR/TE/flip angle = 12/2.5/30 degrees, TI = 500 msec, centric phase ordering). Note the bounce-point signal void at the periphery of the lesion *(small arrows)*, indicating a long T1 that has prevented magnetization from reaching the null point of the inversion recovery curve. A second lesion in the lateral segment is obvious because of the lack of pulsation artifact. The lesion can be seen in retrospect in **A** and **B** but was partially obscured by pulsation artifact. **D,** SE 2500/100 image. Both lesions are obvious.

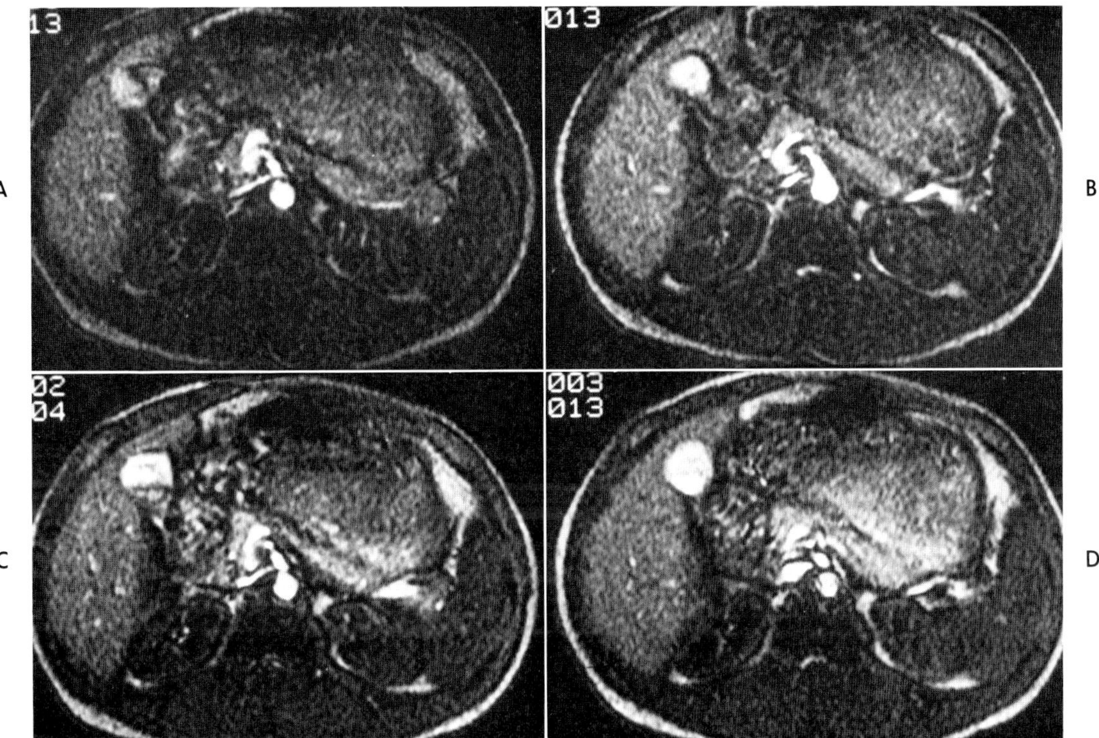

Fig. 3-10 Demonstration of minimal effect of excitation flip angle on tissue contrast in snapshot inversion recovery images at 1.5 T. TR/TE/TI = 8/2.1/76 msec, sequential view order. **A,** Flip angle = 20 degrees. **B,** Flip angle = 30 degrees. SNR is slightly better than in **A.** **C,** Flip angle = 40 degrees. **D,** Flip angle = 50 degrees. Contrast is determined primarily by TI and view order.

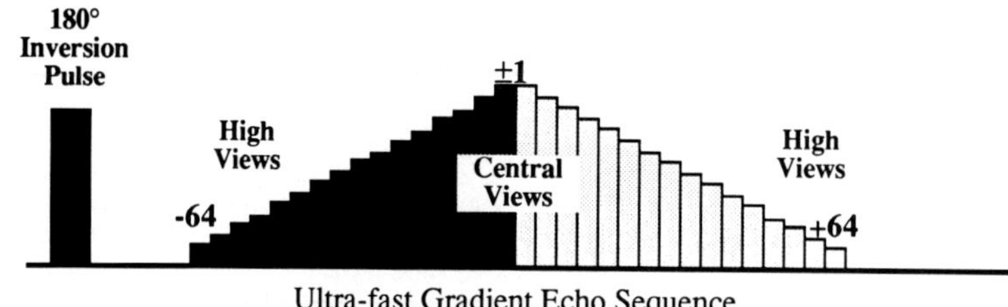

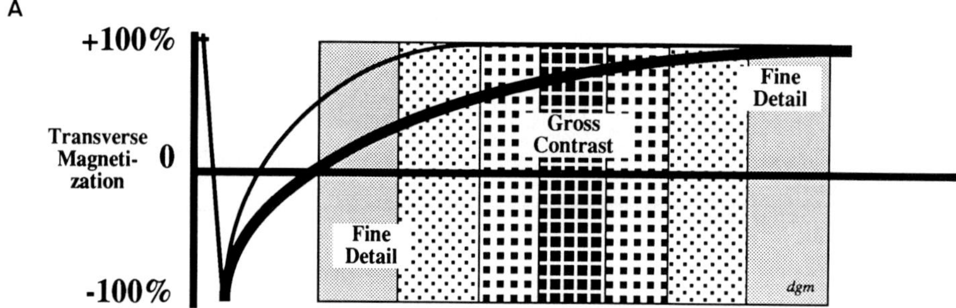

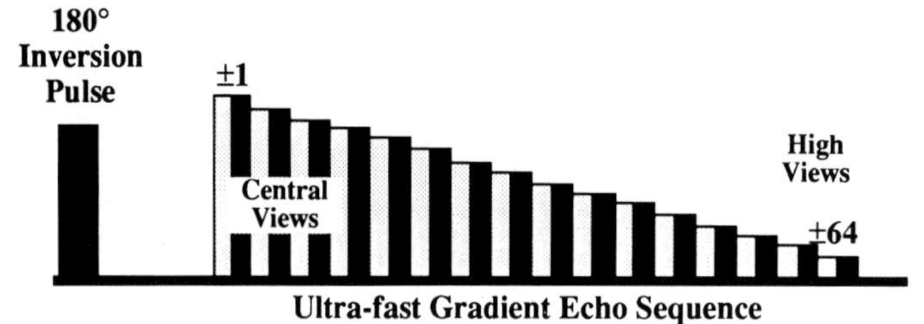

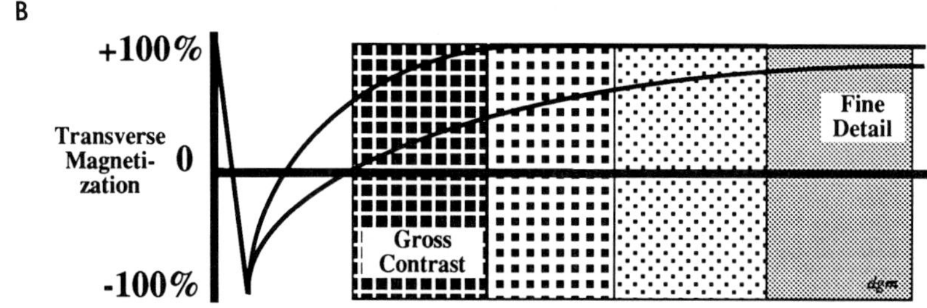

Fig. 3-11 Diagrammatic representation of the importance of view order for snapshot inversion recovery techniques. **A,** With sequential phase order, strong phase-encoding gradients are used to acquire high-order views at the beginning and at the end of the sequence. These views contribute to fine detail but have little effect on image contrast. Gross contrast is determined primarily by the central views, where the phase-encode gradient is weakest. In this example, there may be little contrast between tissues with short *(top curve)* and long *(bottom curve)* relaxation times, since the effective TI, determined by the timing of the central views, is too long. **B,** With centric view order, the central views are acquired first, so that the effective TI approximates the time between the 180 degree inversion pulse and the beginning of the gradient-echo sequence. In this example the tissue with short T1 *(top curve)* has high signal, whereas signal is nulled for the tissue with long T1 *(bottom curve)*.

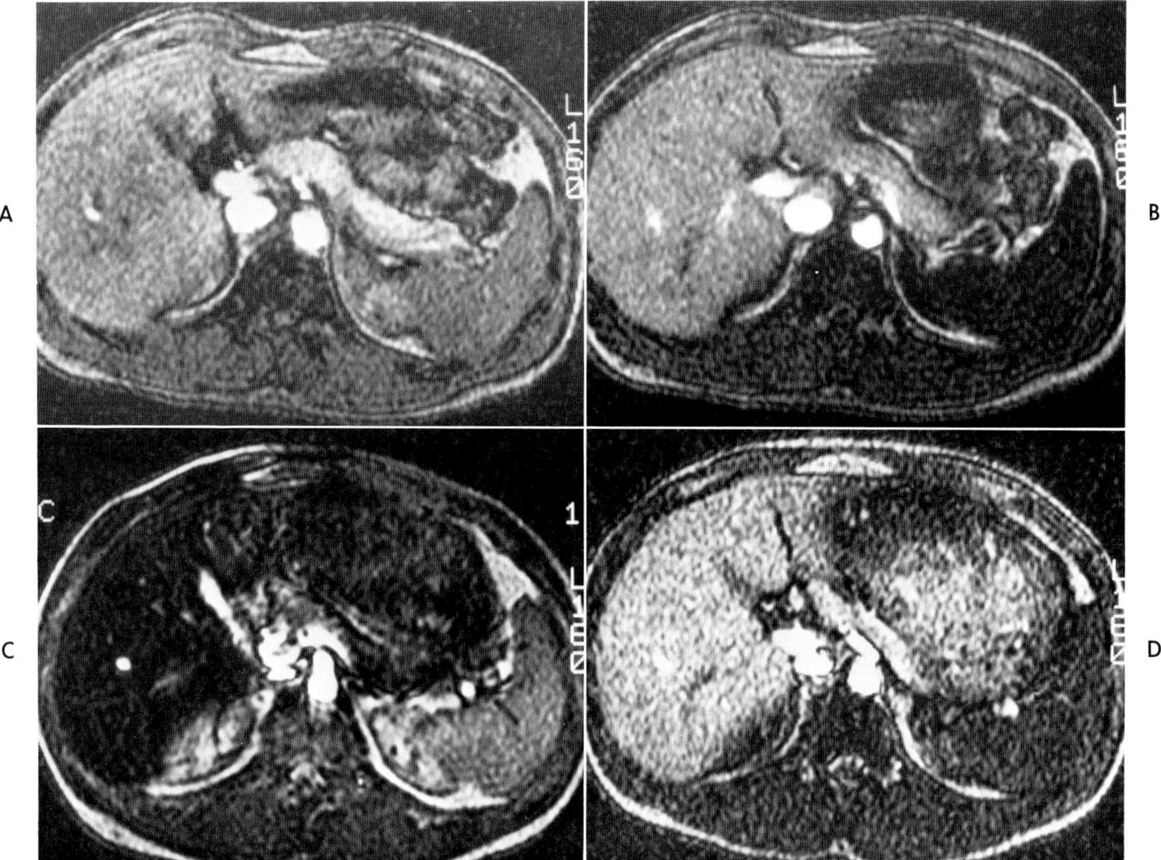

Fig. 3-12 Snapshot inversion recovery images at 1.5 T, demonstrating the importance to tissue contrast of TI and phase-encode view order (same subject as in 3-10). **A,** TI = 500 msec, sequential view order. The central phase-encode views occur long after the 180-degree inversion pulse, so the effective TI is approximately a second. Therefore there is little tissue contrast. **B,** TI = 500 msec, centric view order. The effective TI now approximates 500 msec, resulting in nulling of spleen signal. **C,** TI = 250 msec, centric view order. Hepatic signal is now nulled relative to spleen and, presumably, liver metastases. **D,** TI = 76 msec, sequential view order. The effective TI is approximately 600 msec, so tissue contrast is similar to that seen in **B.** SNR is lower because a higher sampling rate was used to minimize TE. Imaging time has been reduced from 12 to 8 seconds for acquisition of 7 sections because of the reduced TI.

As with conventional inversion recovery technique, contrast depends heavily on the TI, which is usually defined as the time between the inversion pulse and initiation of the rapid gradient-echo sequence. Excitation flip angle, an important parameter for other gradient-echo techniques, has little effect on tissue contrast (see Fig. 3-10). Snapshot inversion recovery techniques are different from conventional inversion recovery techniques in that the order in which the phase-encoding views are acquired determines the "effective" TI and therefore the resulting contrast (see Figs. 3-11 and 3-12). This is because tissue contrast depends primarily on the central phase-encoding views (those with weak phase-encoding gradients), whereas the higher order views determine fine detail and resolution. The effective TI therefore approximates the time between the inversion pulse and the central views, which occur at the middle of the acquisition when views are acquired sequentially. With centric view order, however, the central views are acquired first, so the effective TI approximates the true TI.[69,70,215] Centric view order is necessary to achieve an effective TI short enough to null the signal of tissues with short T1 relaxation times, such as liver and fat.

Short TR snapshot T2-weighted images can also be produced by preceding the gradient-echo sequence with a preparatory sequence consisting of successive 90-, 180-, and 90-degree pulses. SNR and resolution of these images tend to be suboptimal.

Multislice magnetization-prepared sequences have also been developed. This involves segmenting the acquisition, such as by acquiring four sets of 32 views each as part of a multislice technique.[69,114] This technique appears especially promising for abdominal imaging, reducing reconstruction artifacts and allowing further flexibility of contrast, resolution, and SNR. However, motion artifacts, such as from pulsatile flow, are more prominent.

MULTIPLE PHASE-ENCODING VIEWS PER EXCITATION

Multiple phase-encoding views per excitation can be acquired via gradient oscillations, such as with echo planar and its variants. These images can be obtained within milliseconds and can be extremely T2 and T2* dependent. Echo-planar techniques involve obtaining multiple phase-encoding views after a single excitation pulse (Fig. 3-13).[396,416,463,505] T1 contrast can be depicted effectively by preceding the echo-planar acquisition with an inversion pulse, but some contamination by T2 contrast is inevitable because TE cannot be short.

It is possible to obtain T2-weighted images with breath-holding if multiple spin-echo images are acquired after each excitation pulse (Figs. 1-8 and 3-14) (see Chapter 1, T2-Weighted Images).

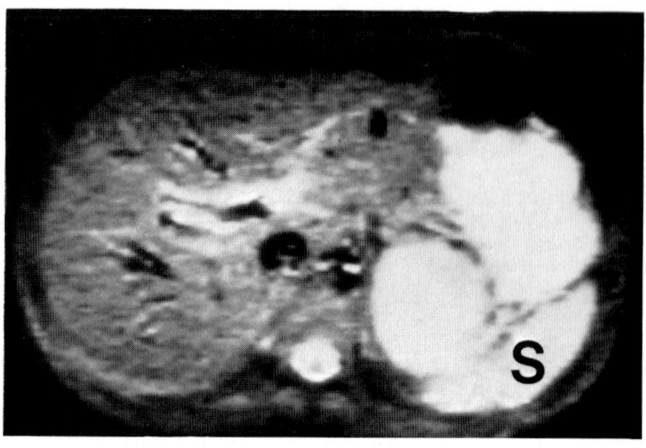

Fig. 3-13 Single shot echo-planar image. TR is infinite because there were no repetitions. TE is 26 msec. Twenty-one images were acquired in 6 seconds, using a matrix of 128 × 128 and fat suppression. *S* = spleen. (Courtesy M Cohen, S Saini, and P Hahn.)

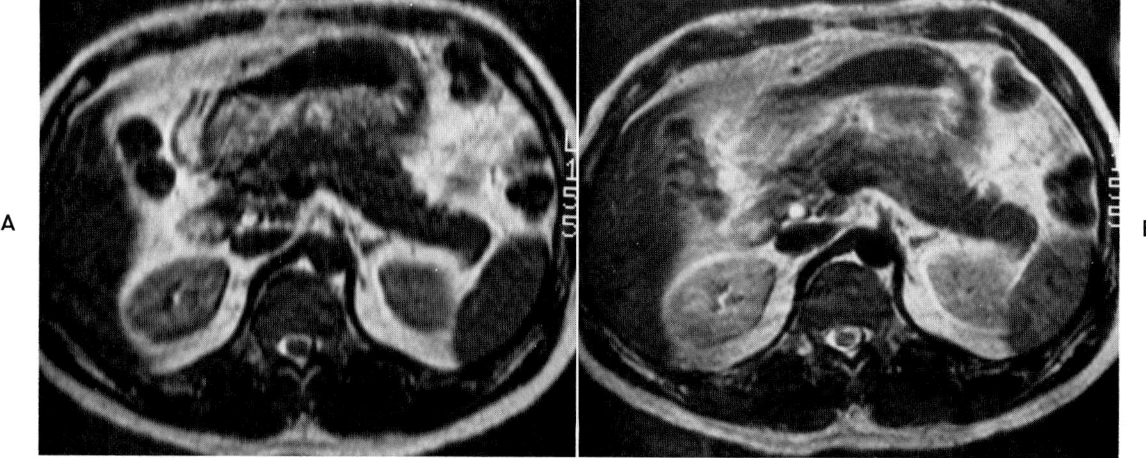

Fig. 3-14 T2-weighted images acquired during suspended respiration using conjugate spin-echo train (fast spin echo) technique, with a train of 16 echoes. **A,** SE 2500/102 image of the pancreas. Eight such images were acquired during a 31-second suspended respiration, using a 256 × 128 matrix and the average of one signal. *Arrow* = common bile duct. **B,** SE 4000/102 image (256 × 256, four signal averages; 13 images in 4:17 [m:s]). SNR and resolution are improved, and the common bile duct has higher signal intensity because of the higher TR.

Field Strength

Initially, the most successful results of hepatic MRI were reported using a mid field system (0.6 T).[500,501] This is consistent with SNR limitations at lower field and decreased T1 contrast and increased motion-induced artifact at higher field.

Recent hardware and software improvements allow effective imaging of the liver at field strengths ranging from 0.02 to 1.5 T. At low field, SNR has been improved by advances in magnet and coil design and by optimizing the bandwidth of analog-to-digital sampling (Figs. 4-1 and 4-2). At high field, improved suppression of motion-induced artifacts now allows high-quality T2-weighted images to be obtained routinely.[352,353] Effective T1 weighting at 1.5 T can also be achieved using shorter TE[358] or inversion recovery[430] techniques. Studies comparing MRI at field strengths of 0.5 T with 1.5 T for detection of liver lesions have shown no significant differences.[431,506] Field strength remains an important issue, however, since the optimum imaging technique varies with field strength.*

---

*204, 352, 431, 506, 608

LOW FIELD AND MID FIELD

Most early research emphasized the value of T2-weighted sequences for the detection of liver metastases, even at low field and mid field, because of manufacturer limitations in achieving the short TE necessary for T1-weighted spin-echo imaging.[94,166,364] In addition to using suboptimal TR and TE for T1-weighted images, these studies were biased by using scan times as long as 18 minutes for T2-weighted sequences but only 5 minutes for T1-weighted images. Since SNR and image quality are directly related to scan time, such comparisons are invalid.

For the detection of liver metastases, T1 contrast is usually greater than T2 contrast at 0.35 to 0.6 T.[200,206,430,500] However, T2-weighted images remain essential for characterizing focal liver lesions.[49,493,607]

HIGH FIELD

Until recently, consistently effective high-field hepatic MR imaging was not possible. One disadvantage of high field is the decreased effect of binding of water to macromolecules on reducing T1 relaxation time.

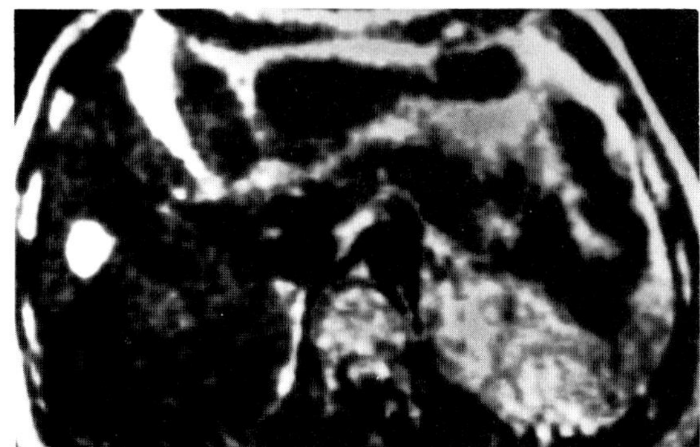

Fig. 4-1 Axial SE 2000/105 MR images of a cavernous hemangioma *(arrow)* at 0.02 T using two signal averages. (Courtesy Massimiliano D'Erme.)

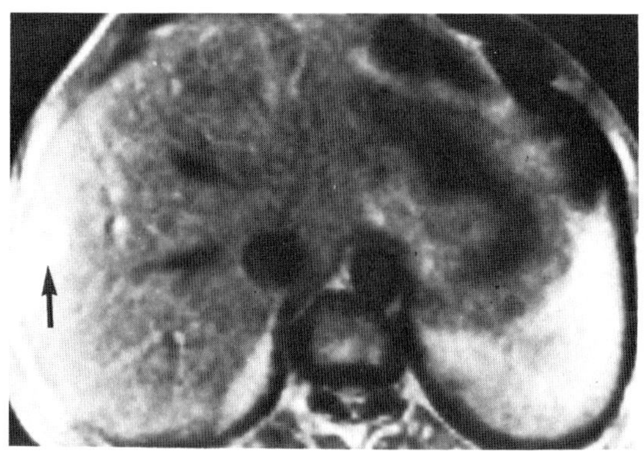

Fig. 4-2 Axial MR image of a metastasis from adenocarcinoma at 0.02 T using two signal averages (SE 2000/30), depicted as a ring lesion at the periphery of the right lobe *(arrow)*. (Courtesy Massimiliano D'Erme.)

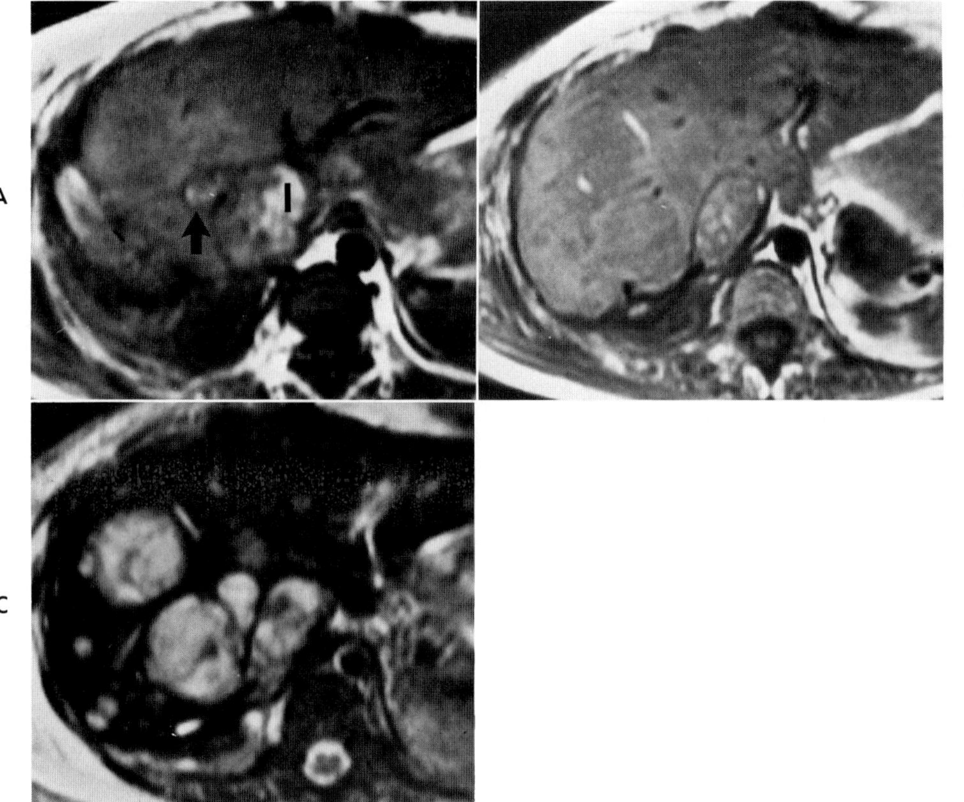

Fig. 4-3 Limitation of T1-weighted images with TE = 20 msec at 1.5 T in a patient with metastases and inferior vena cava thrombus from adrenal carcinoma. **A,** Axial SE 600/20 image at the level of the right hepatic vein origin shows thrombus in the inferior vena cava *(I)* extending into the right hepatic vein *(arrow),* but no hepatic lesions are identified. **B,** Axial image caudad to **A** reveals heterogeneity of the right lobe, suggesting hepatic metastases. **C,** Axial T2-weighted (SE 2800/100) image corresponding to **B,** depicting numerous heterogeneous, well-defined lesions, in addition to the thrombus in the inferior vena cava.

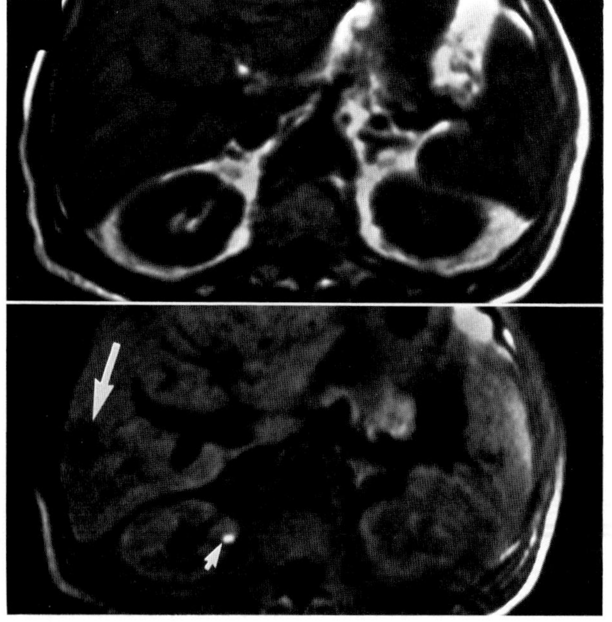

Fig. 4-4 Improved lesion conspicuity on T1-weighted images (SE 400/20) at 1.5 T by fat suppression. A metastasis is obscured by ghost artifact from moving fat *(top),* but the lesion *(large arrow)* and the hyperintense renal cyst *(small arrow)* are obvious with fat suppression. (From Mitchell, D.G., Vinitski, S., Saponaro, S., et al.: Radiology 178:67-71, 1991.)

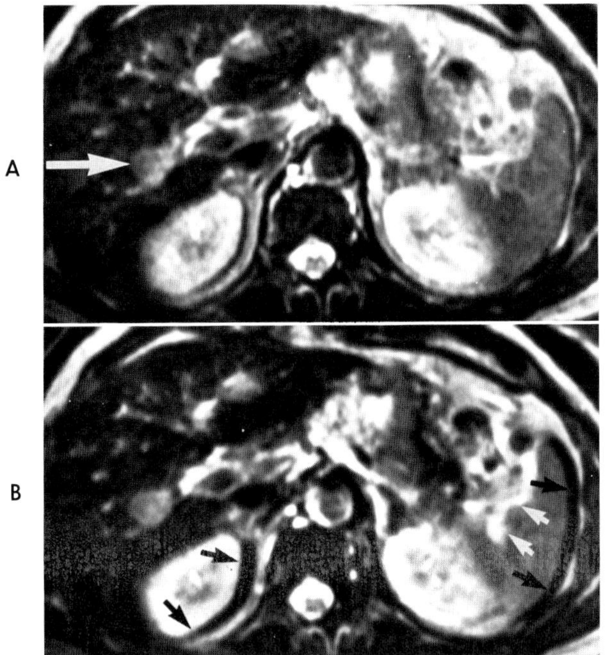

Fig. 4-5 Composite axial MR image (SE 2500/100) showing the effects of reducing sampling bandwidth at 1.5 T. **A,** 32 kHz (manufacturers standard). **B,** 8 kHz. The lesion *(large arrow)* is obvious with both techniques. Although SNR is better at 8 kHz **(B),** chemical shift artifact *(small arrows)* is more severe. (From Mitchell, D.G., Vinitski, S., Rifkin, M.D., et al.: AJR 153:419-425, 1989.)

Thus T1 relaxation for many tissues is prolonged as field strength increases.[153,346] More importantly, T1 is more prolonged for tissues with a large intracellular surface area, such as normal liver, than for tissues rich in free water, such as liver lesions. Therefore T1 contrast between liver and lesion decreases as field strength increases. Thus even with multiple averages, T1-weighted images have generally been inferior to T2-weighted images at 1.0 and 1.5 T when TE is 20 msec or longer (Fig. 4-3).[140,400,431,506] Some malignancies, however, may be seen better even with TE of 20 msec.

Effective T1 contrast can be achieved at 1.5 T. Inversion recovery images with intermediate or short TI have contrast between liver and lesion similar to or better than that of T2-weighted images.[400,431,506] T1-weighted spin-echo images can also be improved by minimizing TE. In one study, reducing TE from 20 msec to 12 msec improved CNR and lesions became more conspicuous (see Fig. 1-1).[358] Similarly, T1-weighted gradient-echo images with TE of 5 msec, acquired at 1.5 T during breath-holding, can achieve similar contrast as T2-weighted spin-echo images.[464] T1 contrast can be improved further by suppressing signal from fat (Fig. 4-4), which improves the dynamic range for comparing liver and lesion and reduces the artifact from moving fat and from truncation.[358,478] In patients with fatty liver, however, fat suppression may obscure lesions.

T2 contrast between liver and lesion is greater at high field than at mid field, primarily because the T2 of normal liver is shorter.[29] This was not expected theoreti-

cally, since T2 relaxation times are generally independent of field strength. The increased contrast between liver and lesion, as well as the shorter estimates of hepatic T2 relaxation, might be due to diffusion of water molecules in the region of hepatic stores of iron or other paramagnetic substances.

Another advantage of high field systems regarding T2-weighted images is higher SNR. Whereas T2-weighted images often have unacceptable SNR at lower field strengths, high field systems allow the use of longer TE while maintaining adequate SNR. In fact, because thick slices (e.g., 7 mm or more) and large field of view (e.g., 32 cm or more) are needed to cover the entire liver, and at least two signals are typically averaged to suppress motion artifact, there is usually more SNR than needed, even with long TE. Thus reducing the sampling bandwidth is usually not recommended for high field MR imaging of the liver (Fig. 4-5).

The major limitation of high field MRI of the abdomen has been the severity of motion-induced artifact.[614] This is probably because stronger gradients are used for position encoding, increasing the magnitude of phase errors and thus the prominence of ghosts. Additionally, prolongation of T1 is less for fat than for most other tissues,[242,346] causing ghosts from adipose tissue to have higher signal relative to other tissues at high field. Fortunately, motion-artifact suppression techniques (see Chapter 2) allow reproducible high-quality images to be obtained. Successful imaging of the liver at 1.5 T depends on maximal suppression of motion artifact.[352]

Chemical Shift Techniques

SPECTROSCOPY

MR spectroscopy is based on the chemical shift between nuclei, depending on their magnetic environment. Spectroscopic techniques can reveal valuable chemical information noninvasively. Some preliminary results suggest that spectroscopy may be potentially important for evaluating hepatic pathophysiology.[27,270,335]

Most initial spectroscopic research has involved measurement of relative concentrations of phosphorus metabolites. In healthy volunteers, increased phosphomonoesters and decreased inorganic phosphate and adenosine triphosphate vary linearly with dose of intravenous fructose.[536] Metabolic alterations have been noted from therapy for a variety of hepatic neoplasms.[334] High phosphomonoester levels have been noted in patients with Caroli's disease, Budd-Chiari syndrome, sclerosing cholangitis, and alcoholic hepatitis, probably because of relatively high concentrations of phosphorylethanolamine and/or phosphorylcholine from structural damage. Hepatic metabolite concentrations were noted to be decreased by up to 50% in alcoholic hepatitis and cirrhosis, presumably because of decreased hepatic function, although metabolite ratios were not altered.[333] Hepatic intracellular pH was also noted to be more acidic in alcoholic cirrhosis and more alkaline in alcoholic hepatitis. Phosphorus spectroscopy may also be useful for detecting damage to donor livers before transplantation.[124,375,446]

CHEMICAL SHIFT IMAGING

Chemical shift imaging techniques take advantage of the difference in resonant frequency (chemical shift) between triglyceride and water protons. This shift is approximately 3.5 ppm, or 230 Hz for 1.5 T and 93 Hz for 0.6T.

Opposed-Phase Images

Opposed-phase images can be obtained by changing the timing of the 180-degree pulse so that it no longer occurs at the center of the gradient refocused echo time.[99] By so doing, the refocusing of transverse magnetization induced by the 180-degree pulse is incomplete, causing the phases of triglyceride and water magnetization to be 180-degrees out of phase with each

other when the echo is formed. Pixel brightness is thus the net difference between triglyceride and water magnetization (Figs. 5-1 and 5-2).

The phases of water and triglyceride are also opposed on gradient-echo images with appropriate TE. Since there is no 180-degree refocusing pulse, the water and triglyceride phases cycle in and out with respect to each other as TE increases.[581] For instance, at 1.5 T, TE of approximately 2.1, 6.3, and 10.5 msec yields opposed-phase images, whereas TE of approximately 4.2, 8.4, and 12.6 msec yields in-phase images. The difference

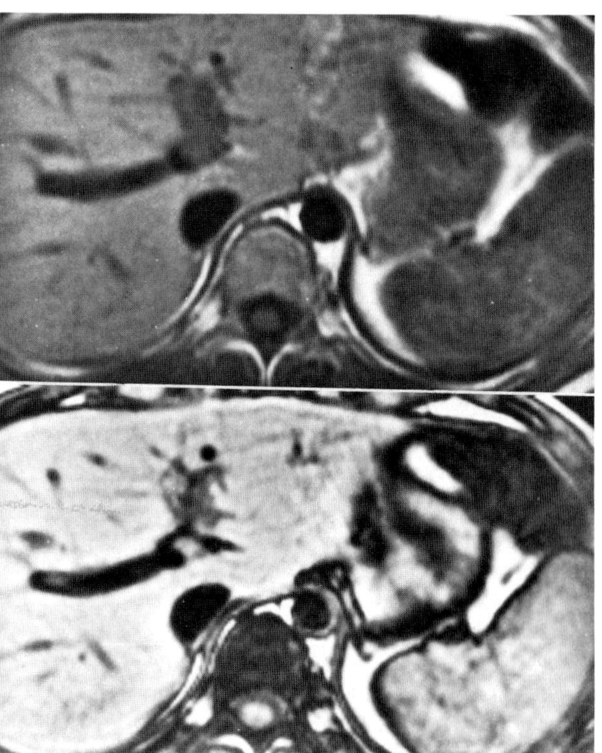

Fig. 5-1 Composite in-phase (**A;** 400/12) and opposed-phase (**B;** 400/14) SE image at 1.5 T in a normal volunteer. On these T1-weighted images, liver is more intense than spleen with in-phase (**A**) and opposed-phase (**B**) techniques, indicating that there is little if any hepatic fat.

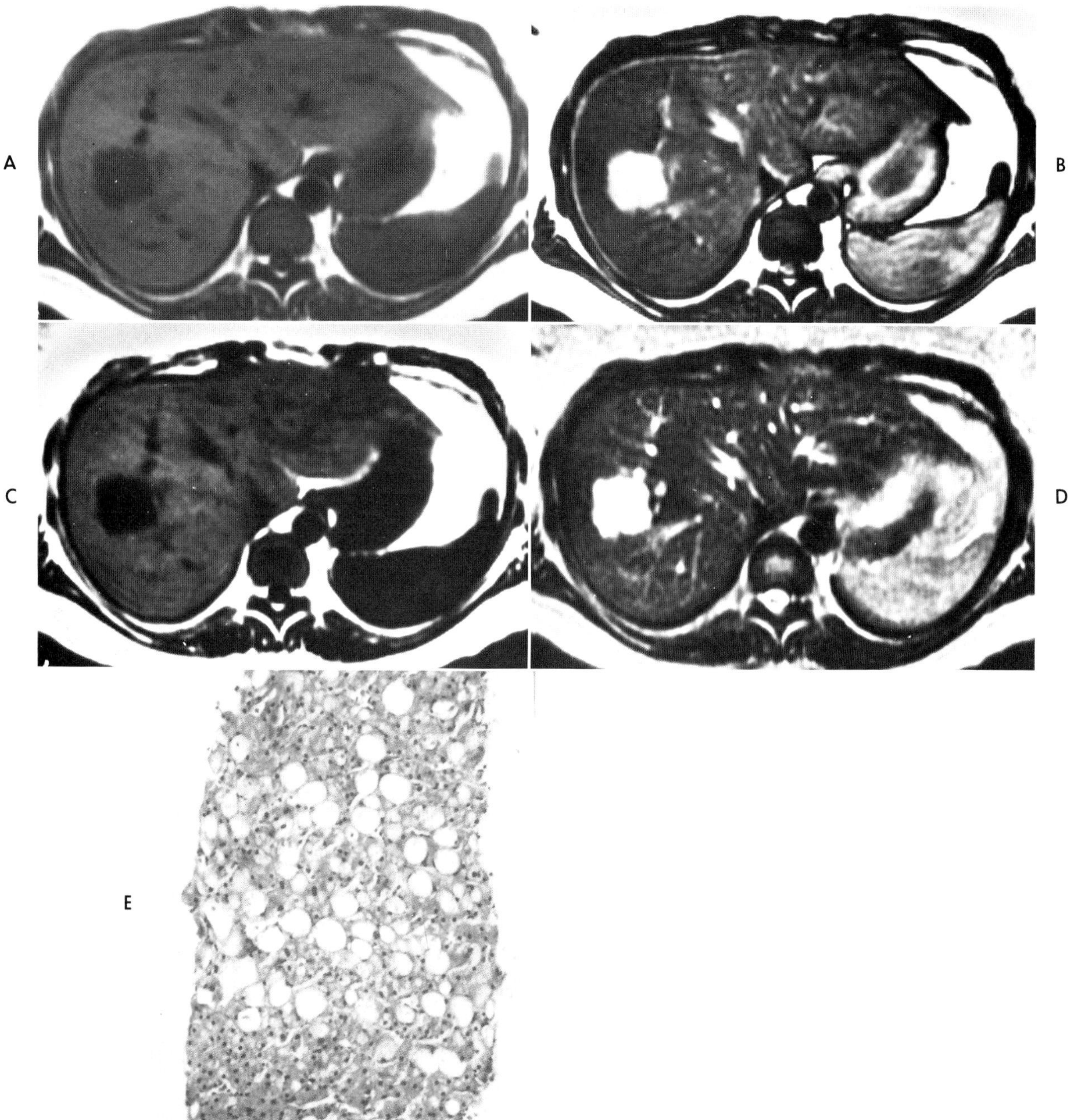

Fig. 5-2   Severe fatty infiltration in a patient with a presumed cavernous hemangioma at 1.5 T. **A,** In-phase SE 500/20 image reveals a hyperintense liver with a low-intensity lesion in the anterior segment of the right lobe. **B,** Corresponding opposed-phase image (400/22) reveals a dramatic decrease in relative hepatic signal, so that the liver is markedly less intense than both spleen and the lesion in spite of similar TR and TE. **C,** Corresponding water-suppressed image (500/20) shows absent signal in the spleen and liver lesion but significant hepatic fat signal. **D,** Corresponding T2-weighted image (SE 2500/100) shows normal relative intensity of the liver. The lobulated hyperintense lesion is most consistent with hemangioma. **E,** Histologic section (H & E) demonstrating severe fatty infiltration.

between in-phase and opposed-phase images is greater at short TE (see Fig. 3-2).

Normal liver tissue contains less than 1% triglyceride by weight. Membrane lipids, which constitute 5% to 10% of the tissue weight, do not contribute significant signal to MR images. Thus liver and other tissues whose signal is entirely from water protons, such as cancer and spleen, show no difference in signal intensity between in-phase (conventional) and opposed-phase images (see Fig. 5-1). The signal of fatty liver, however, decreases on opposed-phase images relative to normal liver and spleen or liver lesions (Fig. 5-2).*

The effect of pulse sequence timing parameters (TR, TI, and TE) on contrast in opposed-phase images is independent of the effects of chemical shift–induced contrast. On T2-weighted opposed-phase images, cancer-liver contrast is additive, since both the T2 relaxation time difference and the MR-observable fat content difference tend to decrease liver signal intensity relative to cancer (Fig. 5-3).

T2-weighted opposed-phase images equal or outperform T2-weighted conventional images in patients with

normal and fatty livers, respectively (see Table 1-1, p. 4). Thus opposed-phase T2-weighted images can be valuable in screening for hepatic metastases, because fatty infiltration is common in these patients. Among patients with metastatic cancer, 70% show greater CNR on opposed-phase than on in-phase T2-weighted images.[276,450,502] Since triglyceride accumulates in liver but not cancer, triglyceride can be exploited as if it were a contrast agent. Hepatocellular carcinomas occasionally accumulate fat, however, so the opposed-phase technique reduces contrast between liver and some hepatocellular carcinomas on T2-weighted images.

T1-weighted opposed-phase images show loss of cancer-liver contrast, since hepatocellular fat decreases liver signal intensity, competing with the T1 relaxation time difference between cancer and liver (see Fig. 5-3). Therefore T1-weighted pulse sequences should not be combined with the opposed-phase technique for lesion detection, since this tends to obscure liver cancer (see Table 1-1, p. 4).

T1-weighted opposed-phase images are highly effective for reliable diagnosis or exclusion of focal and diffuse fatty liver.[280,348,468] Because fatty liver can interfere with detection of lesions or cirrhosis by other mo-

---

*198, 276, 280, 348, 450, 502

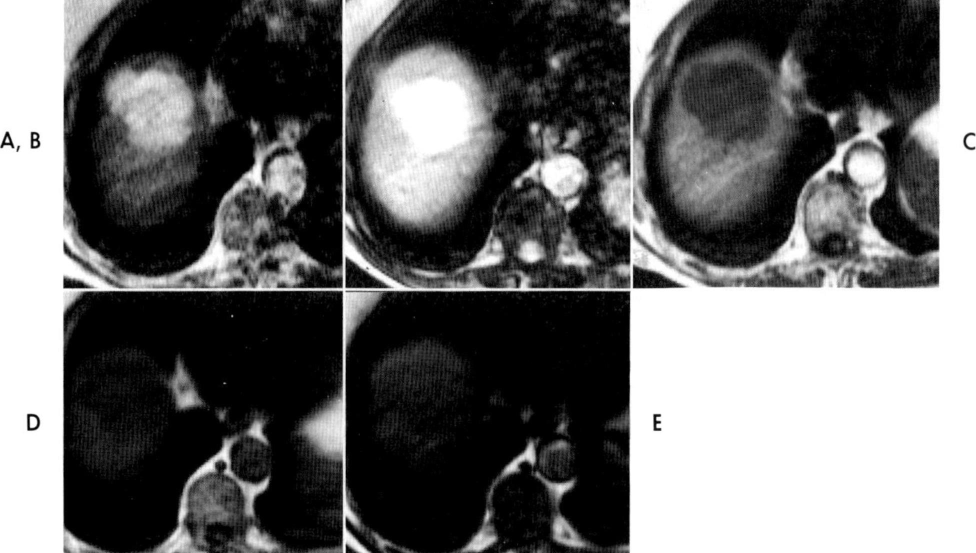

Fig. 5-3 Colon adenocarcinoma metastatic to the liver at 0.6 T. **A,** SE 2000/60/2 image shows a lesion as high signal. **B,** Opposed-phase SE 2000/60/2 shows improved CNR. **C,** SE 260/18/12 (7-minute scan time) image of the liver and spleen shows excellent anatomic resolution because of a large SNR and suppression of motion artifacts by signal averaging. **D,** SE 260/30/8 (4.7-minute) sequence shows poorer anatomic resolution because of a reduction in SNR and increase in ghosting, attributable to the use of a longer echo delay (TE) and fewer data acquisitions than in **C.** CNR is reduced, reflecting the loss of T1-dependent contrast (or introduction of T2-dependent contrast) by lengthening the TE to 30 msec. **E,** Opposed-phase image shows a loss in CNR relative to **D.** Since the opposed-phase image decreases the signal intensity of fatty liver tissue but does not change the signal intensity of cancer, CNR is decreased in comparison to the conventional in-phase image **(D).**

dalities, opposed-phase T1-weighted images can be a valuable adjunct to conventional MR images. Opposed-phase images are most effective if they are compared with conventional in-phase images acquired with identical TR and TE.

Fat Suppression

The chemical shift between fat and water can also be used to decrease or eliminate the signal from fat.* Chemical shift selective fat suppression must be distinguished from short tau inversion recovery (STIR). In STIR images, fat is suppressed because of its short T1, rather than its chemical shift relative to water.

The benefits of fat suppression include reduced motion artifact and improved dynamic range, both of which can increase contrast between liver and lesion (Fig. 4-4).[358,478] By decreasing the contrast at borders between fat and low signal structures, truncation artifacts may also be reduced. Fat suppression appears especially beneficial for T1-weighted images of the pancreas (Fig. 5-4). For T2-weighted images, fat suppression improves the contrast of bowel and most pathology relative to fat.[357] As with opposed-phase T1-weighted images, however, fat suppression may obscure lesions on T1-weighted images in patients with fatty livers.

---

*141, 254, 443, 517, 518

Although fatty liver may be detected by comparing conventional with fat suppressed images, opposed-phase images are more sensitive and reliable for this purpose.[348] On opposed-phase images, hepatic lipid eliminates an equal amount of signal from water protons. In fat suppressed images, however, lipid signal is simply reduced, without effecting the signal of hepatic water. Additionally, opposed-phase images are less vulnerable to magnetic field heterogeneity than fat-saturation images (see Chapter 14).

Selective radiofrequency presaturation of triglyceride magnetization is a commonly used technique for chemical shift selective fat suppression.[357] This is accomplished by exciting triglyceride protons by a frequency selective pulse and then spoiling the resulting transverse magnetization, usually by dephasing gradients. The remaining magnetization, which is primarily from water protons, is then excited to produce the image.

Chemical shift presaturation is vulnerable to heterogeneity of the main magnetic field, since this alters the resonant frequency of the lipid protons. Thus the saturation pulse may match the resonant frequency of triglyceride at some portions of the volume of interest but not at others. Even worse, magnetic field heterogeneity may result in undesired water suppression in some regions, obscuring important information.[357] These suboptimal results are usually most evident at the periphery of the

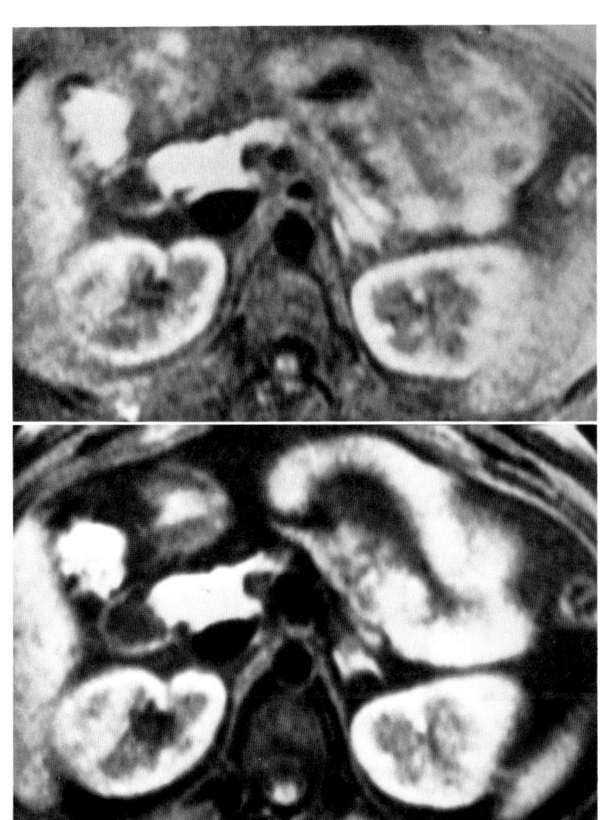

Fig. 5-4 Improved fat saturation at 1.5 T by combination with opposed-phase technique (TR/TE = 400/14 msec). **A,** In-phase image reveals moderate suppression of lipid signal, which has intensity similar to that of muscle and renal medulla. **B,** Same parameters with opposed-phase technique. Phase cancellation between triglyceride and olefinic acid have reduced the signal intensity of fat so that it is now a virtual signal void. Note the high signal intensity of the pancreas.

field of view and at bottom or top slices of multislice sequences. Recently, a three-point technique has been developed to correct for field homogeneity, using three measurements with phase shifts of 0, π, and $-\pi$.[167]

Lipid signal may also be suppressed by real-time subtraction of raw data from in-phase and opposed-phase images,[518] although motion artifact suppression is difficult to implement with this technique. The presaturation and real-time subtraction techniques can be combined to achieve better fat suppression than with either technique alone.[517] Another useful combination technique involves presaturation before acquisition of an opposed-phase image. Fat suppression on opposed-phase fat-saturated images is greater than on in-phase fat-saturated images (see Fig. 5-4).[65,289,358] This is presumably because the phases of lipids with different resonance frequency, such as olefinic acid and incompletely suppressed triglyceride, are opposed.

Hepatic Contrast Agents

Exogenous pharmaceutic compounds that change MR signal intensity by altering T1 and/or T2 relaxation times have great potential for improving diagnosis of focal and diffuse hepatic disease. MRI contrast agents can be used to improve contrast for lesions versus liver and vessels and thus allow detection of smaller lesions, simplify the MR examination, improve patient throughput, and reduce cost. It is also hoped that pharmaceutics will allow assessment of hepatobiliary and reticuloendothelial function.[613] These potential gains must be balanced against added cost, inconvenience, and risk of drug administration.[610,611]

EXTRACELLULAR SPACE AGENTS

Extracellular space agents, such as gadopentetate dimeglumine (gadolinium[Gd]-DTPA) and gadoteridol, initially are distributed within the intravascular compartment and rapidly diffuse throughout the interstitial extravascular space, analogous to water soluble iodinated contrast agents (Fig. 6-1).* As a result of this nonspecific vascular and interstitial distribution, gadopentetate dimeglumine tends to obscure liver metastases on conventional SE images (Fig. 6-1).[59] This occurs because most tumors have a large extracellular space and increased capillary permeability, resulting in greater accumulation of gadopentetate dimeglumine in tumor tissue than in surrounding liver. Iodinated agents have a similar biodistribution and show similar contrast equilibration into the interstitial compartment of the tumor, resulting in a net loss in image contrast on enhanced liver CT.

Extracellular agents are most effective for enhancing contrast between liver and tumor when images are obtained within 2 minutes of administration.† Fast pulse sequences are necessary for effective use of gadopentetate dimeglumine to detect hepatic lesions (Fig. 6-2). In most cases the enhancement pattern with gadopentetate dimeglumine matches that seen with CT. Initially, the tumor enhances most at its periphery. After a longer delay, the tumor "fills in" as contrast agent accumulates within the interstitial space of the tumor. As with CT,

nonspecific contrast material is more effective if images are obtained rapidly after injection into the superior mesenteric or splenic arteries for arterial portography.[406]

Dynamic scanning after injection of gadopentetate dimeglumine may help differentiate hemangiomas from other lesions (Figs. 6-3 and Chapter 10, Cavernous Hemangioma). Most hemangiomas enhance slowly. At 15 minutes, hemangiomas usually remain more intense than liver, a finding unusual for any other lesion.

Delayed CT scans (e.g., 4 hours after contrast) are useful for detecting liver lesions, since 3% to 5% of a dose of iodinated contrast agents is excreted through the biliary system.[30] Gadopentetate dimeglumine is not taken up significantly by hepatocytes, however, so contrast between liver and lesion is not improved on delayed MR images.[380]

TARGETED AGENTS

The major disadvantage of extracellular or blood pool agents is their lack of specificity for hepatic parenchyma or tumors (Fig. 6-4) (see also Color Plate II). Agents that accumulate preferentially within hepatocytes, bile, or Kupffer cells are currently undergoing clinical investigation.

Hepatocyte Agents

Hepatocyte agents, such as Mn-DPDP, Fe-EHPG, Fe-HBED, and Gd-BOPTA, appear to be delivered preferentially to hepatocytes via cell surface receptors.* Selective enhancement of normal liver tissue can improve depiction of focal lesions and may allow evaluation of regional hepatic function (Fig. 6-5). These agents and/or their metabolites are excreted and concentrated in bile. In the presence of biliary obstruction the uptake and excretion of these agents may be reduced. Nevertheless, hepatobiliary agents increase hepatic parenchymal intensity and enhance the detection of lesions even in the presence of biliary obstruction[275] or severe hepatocellular dysfunction (e.g., hepatitis).[528]

"Negative" hepatocellular contrast can be achieved by targeting iron oxide particles to hepatocyte receptors, decreasing hepatic signal intensity.[245,427-429,589] Reticu-

---

*59, 455, 459, 583, 612
†84, 113, 192, 244, 307, 343, 459, 472

*121, 175, 212, 273, 287, 377, 482

35

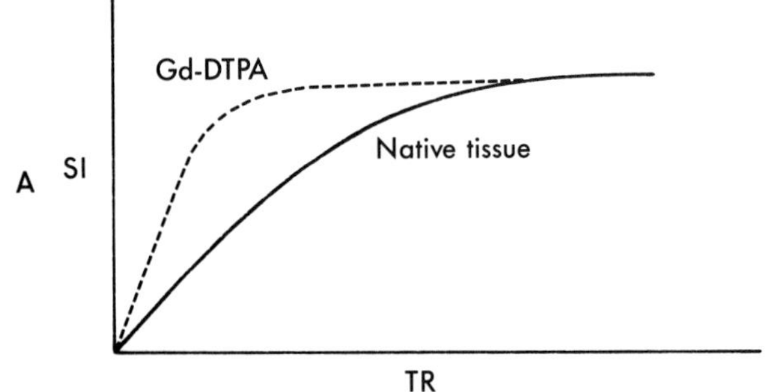

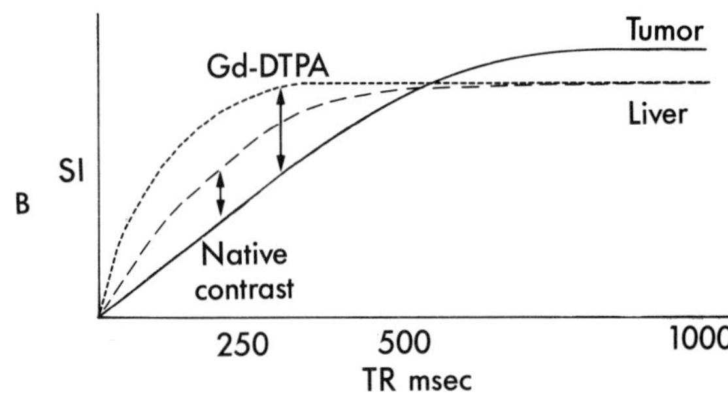

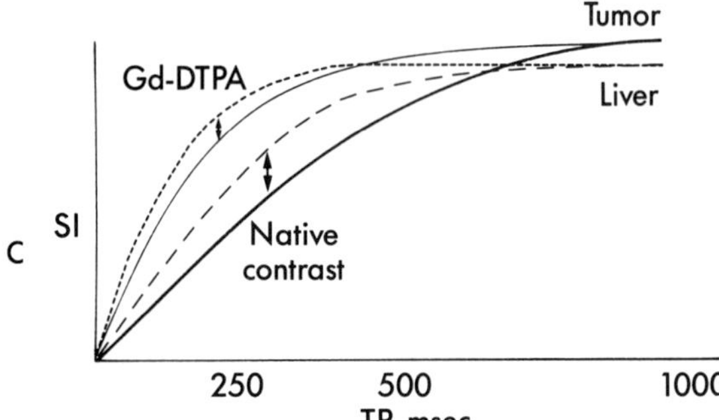

Fig. 6-1   A, Paramagnetic enhancement of T1 relaxation shows the greatest increase in signal intensity relative to native tissue at short TR. At long TR (greater than 1000 msec), tissue T1 differences contribute less to image contrast, since sufficient time exists between repetitions for recovery of magnetization. In general, short repetition times and short echo delays are required to maximize T1-dependent contrast when spin-echo sequences are used. **B,** Tumor tissue shows a lower signal intensity than liver on T1-weighted short TR spin-echo images. Spin density or T2-weighted images acquired using long TR show tumor to have a greater signal intensity than liver. Ideally, a contrast agent would selectively enhance only one of the two tissues (liver) to maximally increase image contrast. Such selective enhancement occurs only transiently after bolus administration of Gd-DTPA. **C,** Since nonspecific intravascular contrast agents such as Gd-DTPA enhance both tumor and liver, the net improvement in image contrast (tumor-liver signal difference) is limited. In fact, at delayed time points after infusion of Gd-DTPA, the tumor may enhance more than adjacent liver, resulting in a net loss of tumor-liver contrast. The major value of tissue-specific biliary agents is to satisfy the conditions of **B** over a long period of time, allowing more optimal conditions for im-

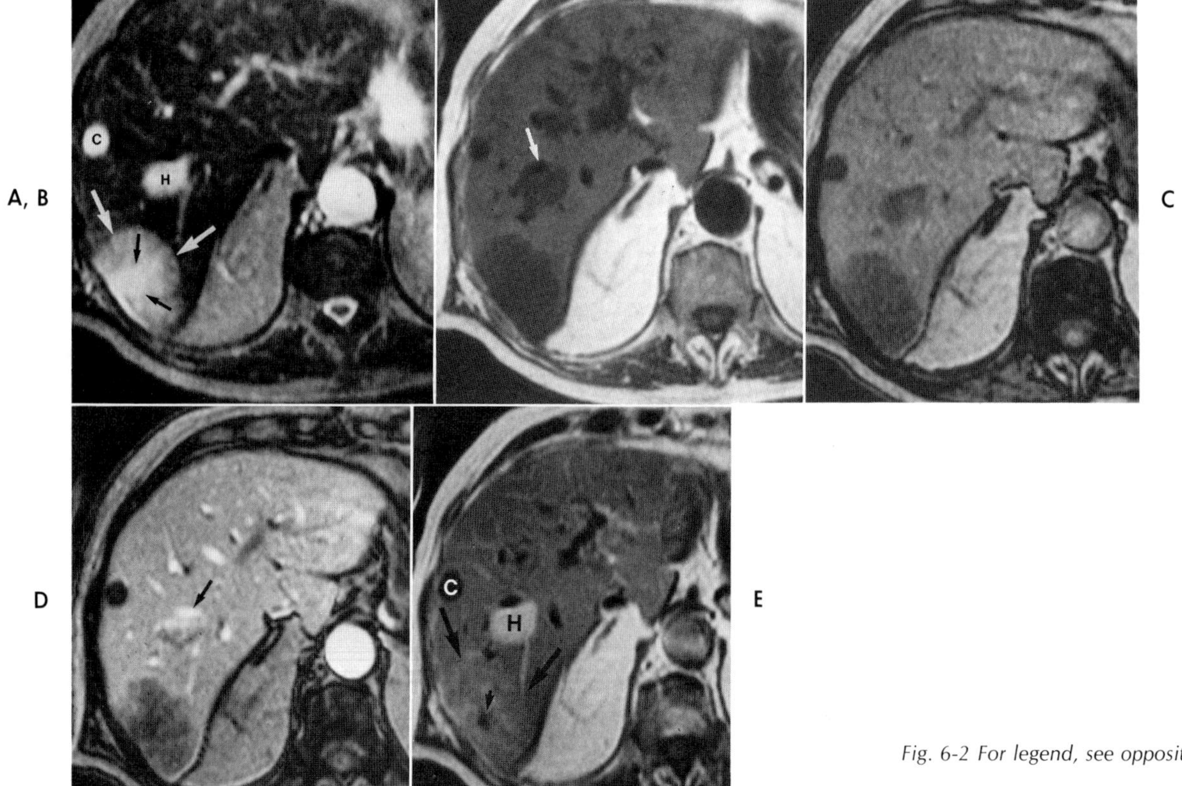

Fig. 6-2 For legend, see opposite page.

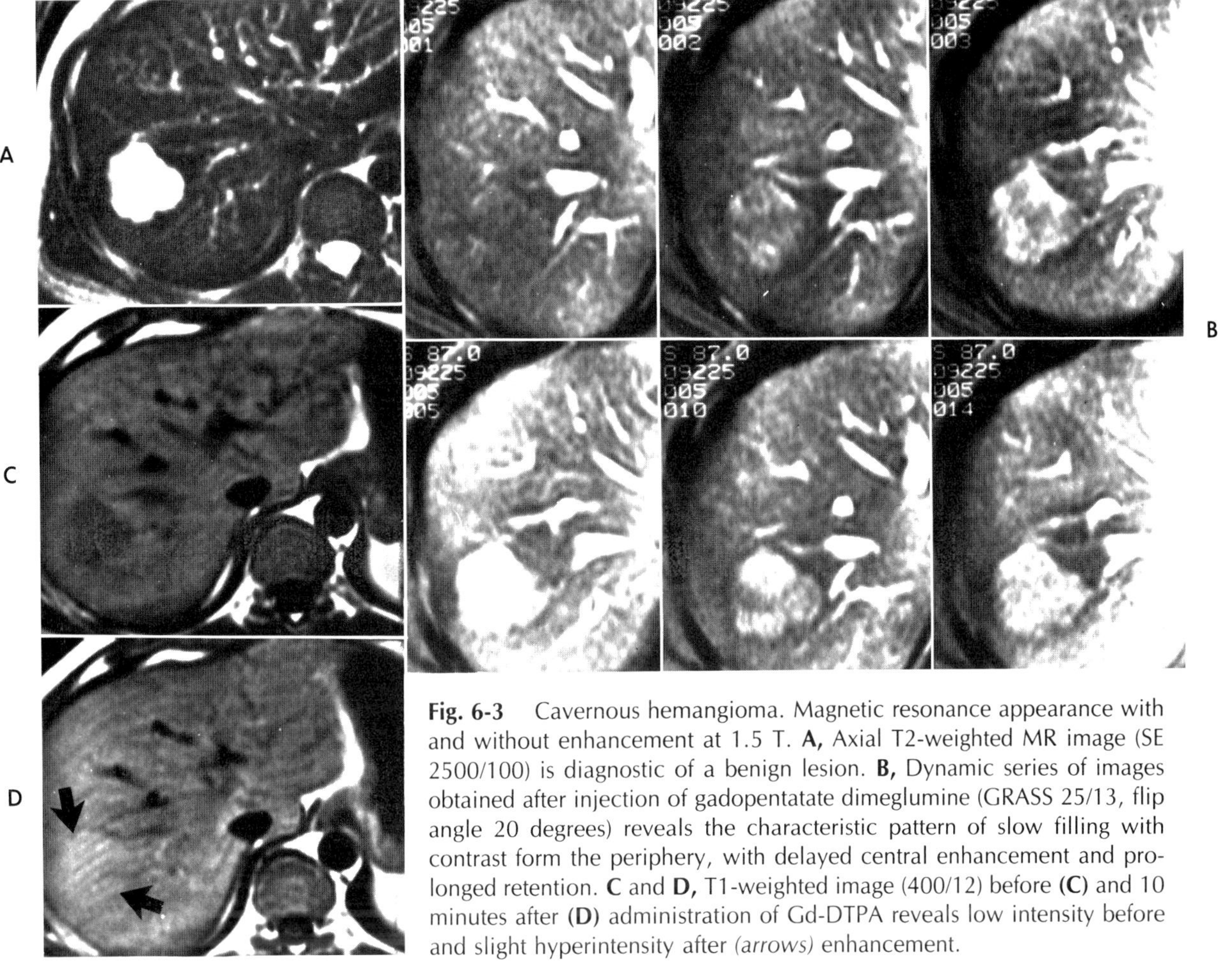

Fig. 6-3 Cavernous hemangioma. Magnetic resonance appearance with and without enhancement at 1.5 T. **A,** Axial T2-weighted MR image (SE 2500/100) is diagnostic of a benign lesion. **B,** Dynamic series of images obtained after injection of gadopentatate dimeglumine (GRASS 25/13, flip angle 20 degrees) reveals the characteristic pattern of slow filling with contrast form the periphery, with delayed central enhancement and prolonged retention. **C** and **D,** T1-weighted image (400/12) before **(C)** and 10 minutes after **(D)** administration of Gd-DTPA reveals low intensity before and slight hyperintensity after *(arrows)* enhancement.

Fig. 6-2 Metastasis, hemangioma, and cyst at the same level, before and after enhancement with gadoteridol (ProHance; Squibb), a gadolinium chelate with nonspecific extracellular biodistribution similar to that of gadopentetate dimeglumine. **A,** SE 3000/100 image reveals three lesions in the right hepatic lobe. The brightest is a cyst *(C)* and the hemangioma *(H)* is slightly less intense. The largest lesion, a metastasis *(white arrows)*, is heterogeneous except for high signal central necrosis *(black arrows)*. **B,** SE 400/12 image. Note the vascular signal void anterior to the hemangioma *(arrow)*. **C,** T1-weighted gradient-echo image (TR/TE/flip angle = 102/2.3/90 degrees), 12 images obtained in 14 seconds during suspended respiration. **D,** As in **C,** less than 1 minute after administration of gadoteridol. All three lesions are conspicuous. Note enhancement of the vessel anterior to the hemangioma *(arrow)*. **E,** SE400/12 image, 15 minutes after contrast administration. The metastasis *(large arrows)* is nearly isointense with liver, except for the central low intensity necrosis *(small arrow)*. The hemangioma *(H)* is hyperintense, whereas the cyst *(C)* has not enhanced.

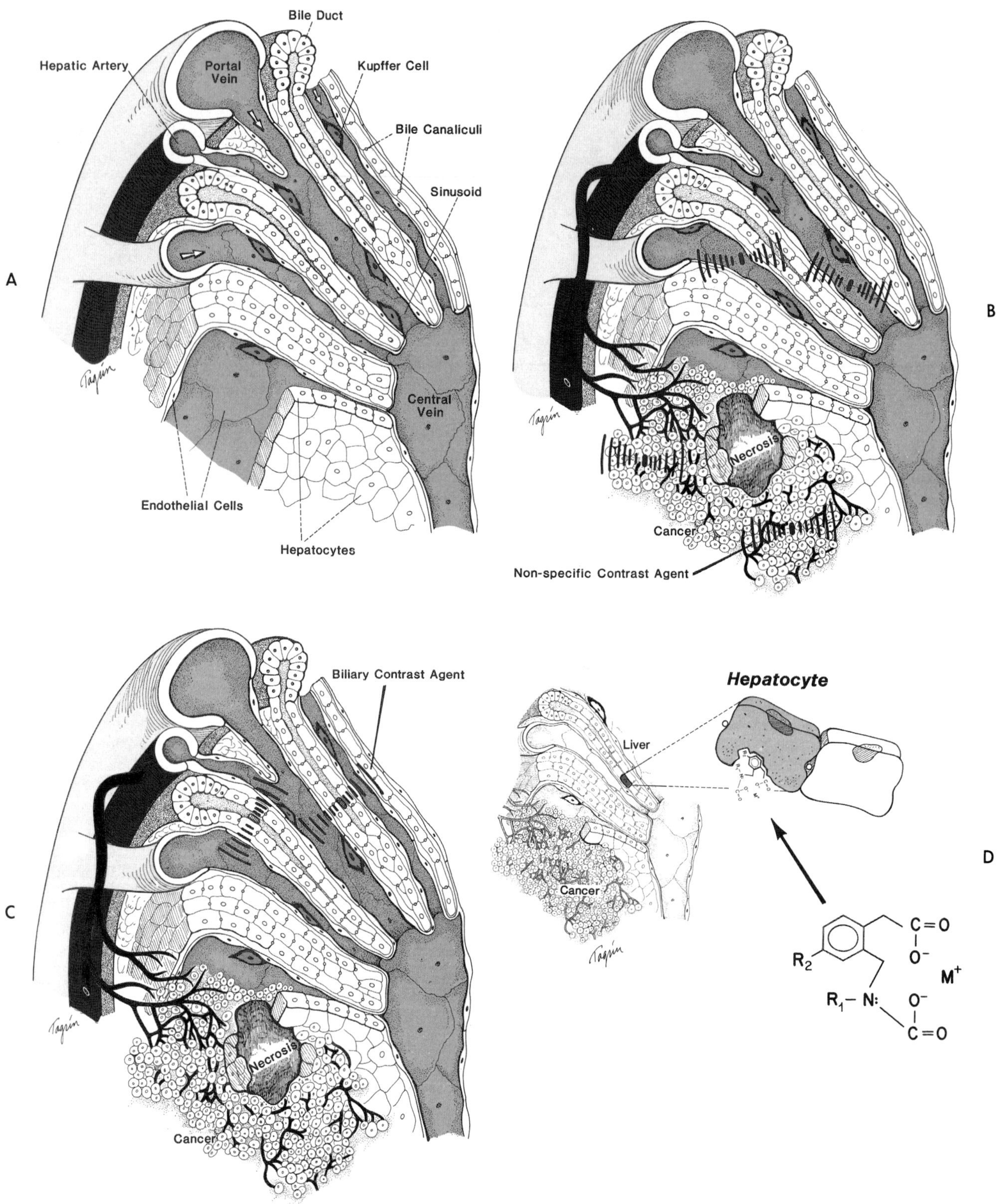

Fig. 6-4 For legend, see opposite page.

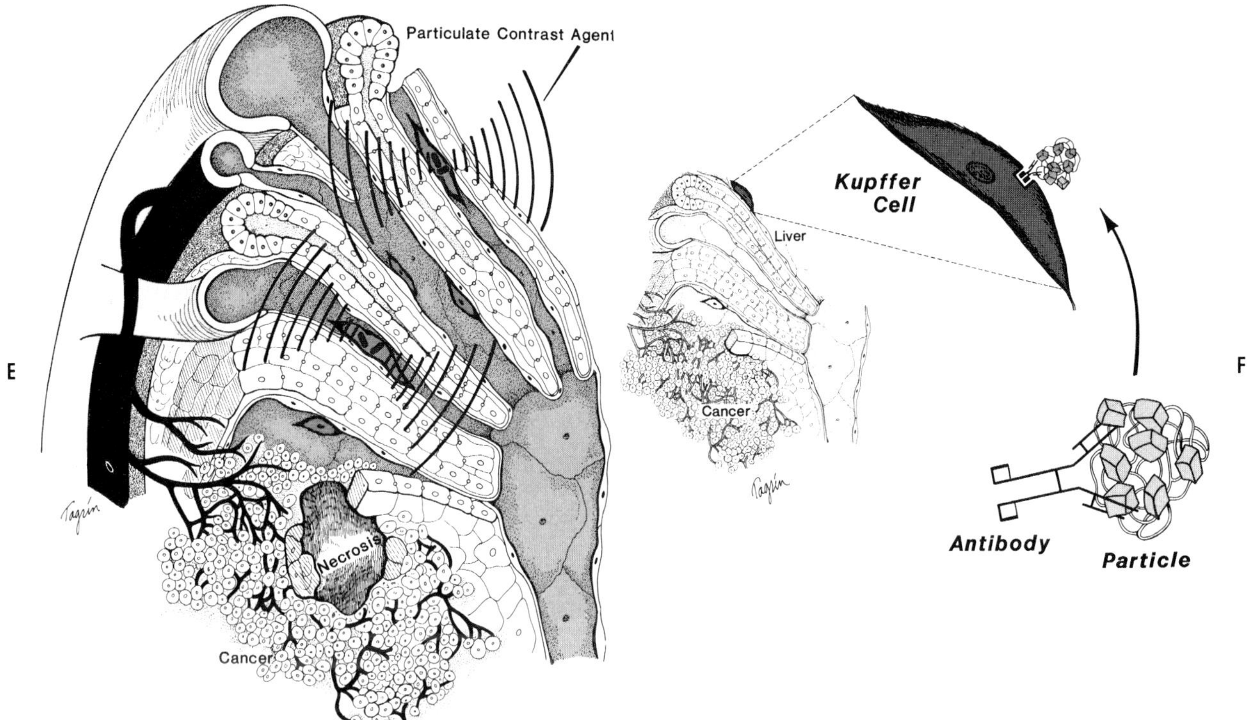

Fig. 6-4 Functional hepatic anatomy and its implications for specific and nonspecific contrast media. **A,** Normal lobular hepatic anatomy showing major structures and cell types. **B,** Cancer is shown with peripheral vascular supply and central necrosis. Nonspecific extracellular contrast agents distributed to enhance both normal liver and perfused cancer tissue. **C,** Hepatobiliary contrast agents are taken up by hepatocyte and excreted into bile ducts. After the contrast agent has been cleared from the bloodstream, selective enhancement is seen in normal liver tissue. **D,** Schematic drawing of low molecular weight paramagnetic complex targeted to a hepatic cell surface receptor or transport protein. $M+$ represents a paramagnetic metal ion (e.g., gadolinium, iron, or manganese). The ligand-metal complex shown is schematically representative of Fe-EHPG, Mn-DPDP, and Gd-BOPTA. **E,** Reticuloendothelial (particulate) contrast agents are phagocytosed by Kupffer cells lining the hepatic sinusoids. These cells may ingest more than one particle, and superparamagnetic materials have large effects on tissue proton relaxation. Since there is no phagocytosis by cancer cells, selective enhancement of liver tissue is seen. **F,** Model of phagocytosis. A composite particle circulating in the bloodstream is recognized as foreign, coated with antibodies or other opsonins and internalized by macrophages such as hepatic Kupffer cells (see also color Plate II).

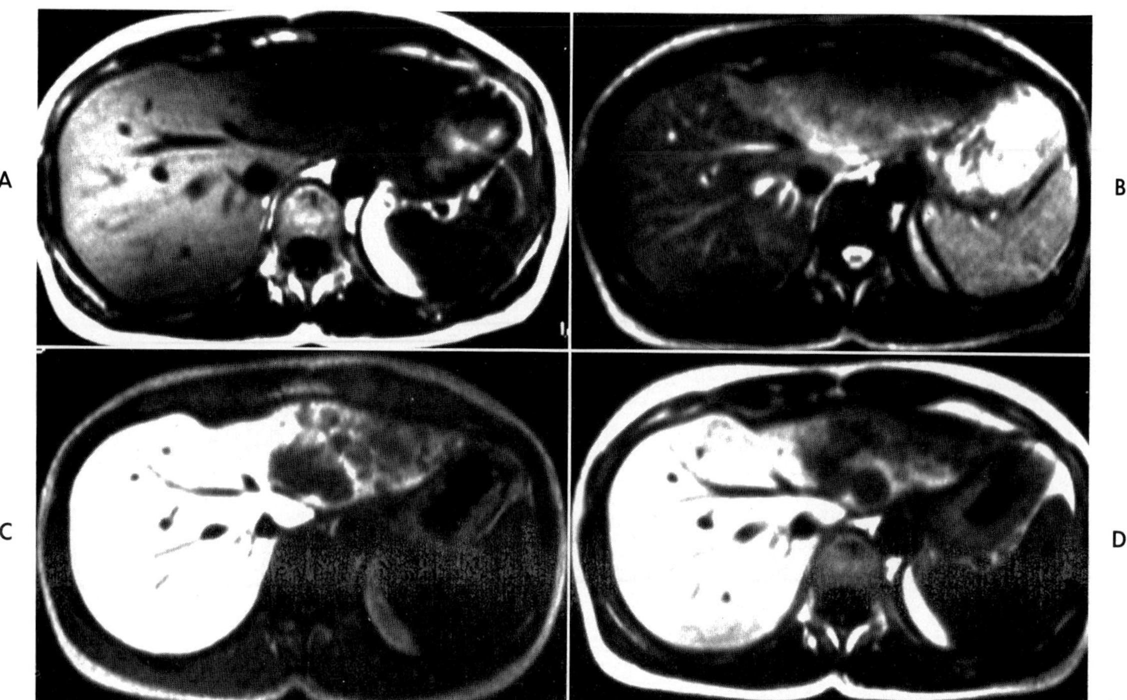

Fig. 6-5. Improved depiction of hepatocellular carcinoma after enhancement with Mn-DPDP at 1.5 T. **A,** Precontrast T1-weighted image (SE 500/15). A diffuse low–signal-intensity abnormality is seen involving the left hepatic lobe. **B,** T2-weighted SE 2000/70 precontrast image of the same patient. A diffuse, hyperintense abnormality involves the left hepatic lobe. The area of abnormality appears slightly larger on this T2-weighted image than the T1-weighted image, consistent with a component of edema. **C,** Approximately 30 minutes after intravenous infusion of Mn-DPDP, 10 mmol/kg, the SE/500/15 image now reveals multiple nodules in the left hepatic lobe. These discreet spherical lesions are distinguished from edema in the surrounding, residual noncancerous liver tissue. **D,** T1-weighted gradient-echo sequence (100/6, flip angle 60 degrees) shows selective contrast enhancement of normal liver and clinical findings similar to the spin-echo technique. Note the dramatic increase in signal intensity of normal liver tissue, increasing the SNR, anatomic resolution, and diagnostic confidence. (Courtesy E. Rummeny.)

loendothelial tissues such as the spleen and bone marrow are less affected by agents such as these.

Particulate Agents

Particulate agents are removed from the bloodstream by the reticuloendothelial system. Since 80% of reticuloendothelial cells are located in the liver, these agents can be targeted to functioning liver and will be excluded from neoplastic lesions. Superparamagnetic crystalline iron oxides have up to 100 times greater magnetic susceptibility than paramagnetic preparations per unit weight.* In liver tissue the T2 relaxivity of iron oxide is approximately 10 times greater than the T1 relaxivity of gadopentetate dimeglumine. Pulse sequences sensitive to T2 and T2* relaxation (long TR/long TE spin-echo and most gradient-echo techniques) are particularly useful in conjunction with superparamagnetic contrast agents.[147,499,538,549]

Tumors lack phagocytic activity and therefore do not take up iron oxide particles.[461,499] The signal intensity of a tumor is thus unchanged, whereas surrounding liver shows a dramatic loss of signal intensity (Figs. 6-6 and 6-7).[148,253,310,462] Although uptake of iron oxide may be decreased in cirrhotic livers, experimental results suggest that iron oxide should be effective in improving contrast between tumors and cirrhotic liver.[81]

Depending on their size, iron oxide particles remain in circulation for several minutes and are then stable in the liver for several hours. In general, larger particles are taken up more rapidly and to a greater extent by the liver.[412] During this time, iron oxide remains in the

---

* 126, 132, 195, 246, 301-303, 562

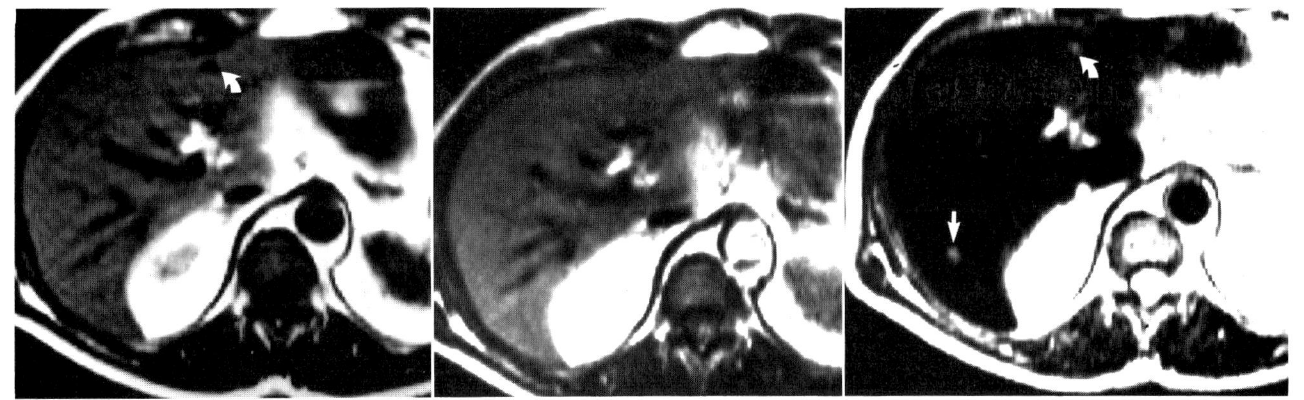

Fig. 6-6   Metastatic colonic cancer at 0.6 T. **A,** SE 260/14 MR image obtained before iron oxide injection shows one lesion *(curved arrow)* in left lobe of liver. **B,** SE 1500/40 MR image obtained before iron oxide injection. Lesion in left lobe of liver not visible. **C,** SE 1500/40 MR image obtained after injection of 20 μmol Fe/kg of AMI-25. Lesion in left lobe *(curved arrow)* confirmed; additional lesion *(straight arrow)* visible in right lobe. (From Fretz, C.J., Stark, D.D., Metz, C.E., et al: AJR 763-770, 1990.)

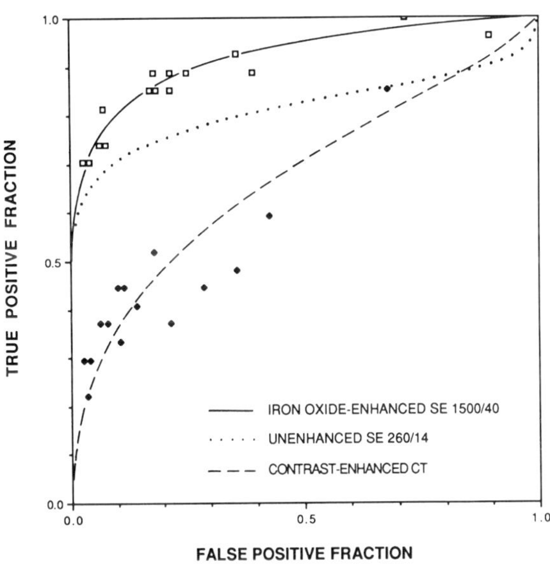

Fig. 6-7   Composite receiver-operating–characteristic (ROC) curves indicate relative accuracies with which focal hepatic lesions are detected by contrast-enhanced CT, unenhanced MR (SE 260/14), and iron oxide-enhanced MR (SE 500/40) at 0.6 T. Plotted data points represent specific ROC points of each reader for iron oxide-enhanced MR *(squares)* and contrast-enhanced CT *(diamonds)*. (From Fretz, C.J., Stark, D.D., Metz, C.E., et al.: AJR 155:763-770, 1990.)

Kupffer cells of normal liver parenchyma without significant redistribution. This temporal stability may be desirable in clinical practice, since careful coordination of drug administration and the time of scanning is not required. The iron particles are metabolized and cleared from the liver within a few days and incorporated into red blood cells.[411,460]

The hepatic concentration of iron oxide is greatest if enough time elapses after injection for most of the agent to be cleared from the blood. On these images, blood vessels may be depicted as bright structures relative to low-signal liver, especially if gradient moment nulling is used to reduce motion artifact. These bright blood vessels may therefore mimic bright liver lesions. Images obtained within 10 minutes after injection of iron oxide particles, before the agent is cleared from the blood, may be preferable to delayed images because vessels have low signal.[188]

The diagnosis of cavernous hemangiomas may also be complicated by the use of iron oxide particles. Since particles circulate in the bloodstream, vascular lesions may contain enough particles so that their intensity decreases, appearing similar in some cases to metastases.[188] Furthermore, the liver cannot be used to assess the relative signal intensity of the suspect lesion. To diagnose hemangiomas, it may be necessary to obtain a set of T2-weighted images before administration of iron oxide particles. Alternatively, a dynamic blood pool study with immediate and delayed images can be performed.

Pulse sequence selection for iron oxide enhancement is simplified because of the potent and selective T2 relaxation enhancement, which essentially eliminates signal from normal liver tissue. Intermediate or T2-weighted pulse sequences with timing parameters in the range of SE 500/30 to SE 2000/60 are similarly effective. In clinical practice a TE of approximately 30 msec may be useful, with TR chosen based on the number of sections necessary to cover the liver.

Although preclinical (animal) investigations suggested that iron oxide particles would be safe,[14] hypotension and other adverse reactions were reported in the first clinical trials.[499] Alternative preparations are currently being investigated.

It is possible that combination with other agents may allow the use of a lower dose of iron oxide. Such "dual-contrast" techniques can improve contrast between liver and lesion beyond what might be achieved by a low dose of either agent alone. For example, superparamagnetic agents, which reduce the signal of normal liver tissue, might be combined with gadopentetate dimeglumine, which increases the signal intensity of hepatic metastases.[590]

Particulate contrast agents can be created by incorporating either paramagnetic or superparamagnetic agents within liposomes.* As with other particulates, their serum half-life and biodistribution depends primarily on their size.

PANCREAS AND SPLEEN

The pancreas and spleen are usually more vascular than common adenocarcinomas. Therefore administration of nonspecific agents (e.g., Gd-DTPA and gadoteridol) enhances the pancreas[73] and spleen[340,458] more than the tumor if images are obtained before equilibration into the interstitial compartment of the tumor. Enhancement of the spleen is often heterogeneous within the first minute after injection (Fig. 6-8), a finding that should not be mistaken for multifocal pathology.[340] Splenic enhancement is homogeneous thereafter.

For unknown reasons, Mn-DPDP appears to enhance the pancreas.[159] This agent may therefore be useful for improving detection of pancreatic carcinoma.

Particulate contrast agents are especially effective for selective enhancement of the spleen. In patients with focal splenic tumors, administration of iron oxide decreases the intensity of normal splenic tissue, increasing tumor-spleen contrast.[588] This technique permits demonstration of lesions invisible on conventional MR images (Figs. 6-9 and 6-10).

---

*174, 247, 412, 544, 555-558

In patients with diffuse infiltration by lymphoma, abnormal neoplastic tissue with diminished or absent phagocytic capacity reduces the number of particles taken up per unit volume of spleen. The signal loss after administration of iron oxide is therefore less in infiltrated spleens than in normal spleens. This is different from splenomegaly due to passive congestion, where phagocytic capacity is maintained. In a small series, postcontrast SNR permitted separation of patients with lymphomatous and benign splenomegaly (Fig. 6-11).[586]

The iron oxide preparation that has been used in most clinical trials has a median particle diameter of 70 nm and is taken up in the liver more than the spleen by a ratio of 83% to 6%.[586] The dose of 40 μmol/kg that has been effective in demonstrating splenic pathology is twice the dose needed for the liver. Whether this will limit applications in the spleen of iron oxide contrast agents is not yet known.

ORAL AGENTS

Oral agents can be administered to improve delineation of the bowel. Additionally, distension of the stom-

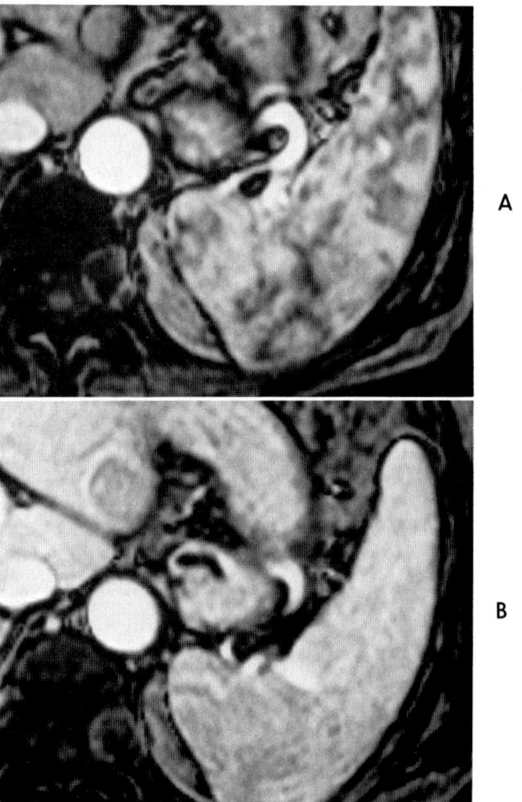

Fig. 6-8 **A,** Heterogeneous enhancement of the spleen immediately after injection of 0.3 mmol/kg of gadoteridol at 1.5 T on spoiled gradient-echo image (TR/TE/flip angle = 140/2.3/90 degrees). **B,** The spleen appears homogeneous on images acquired 20 seconds later.

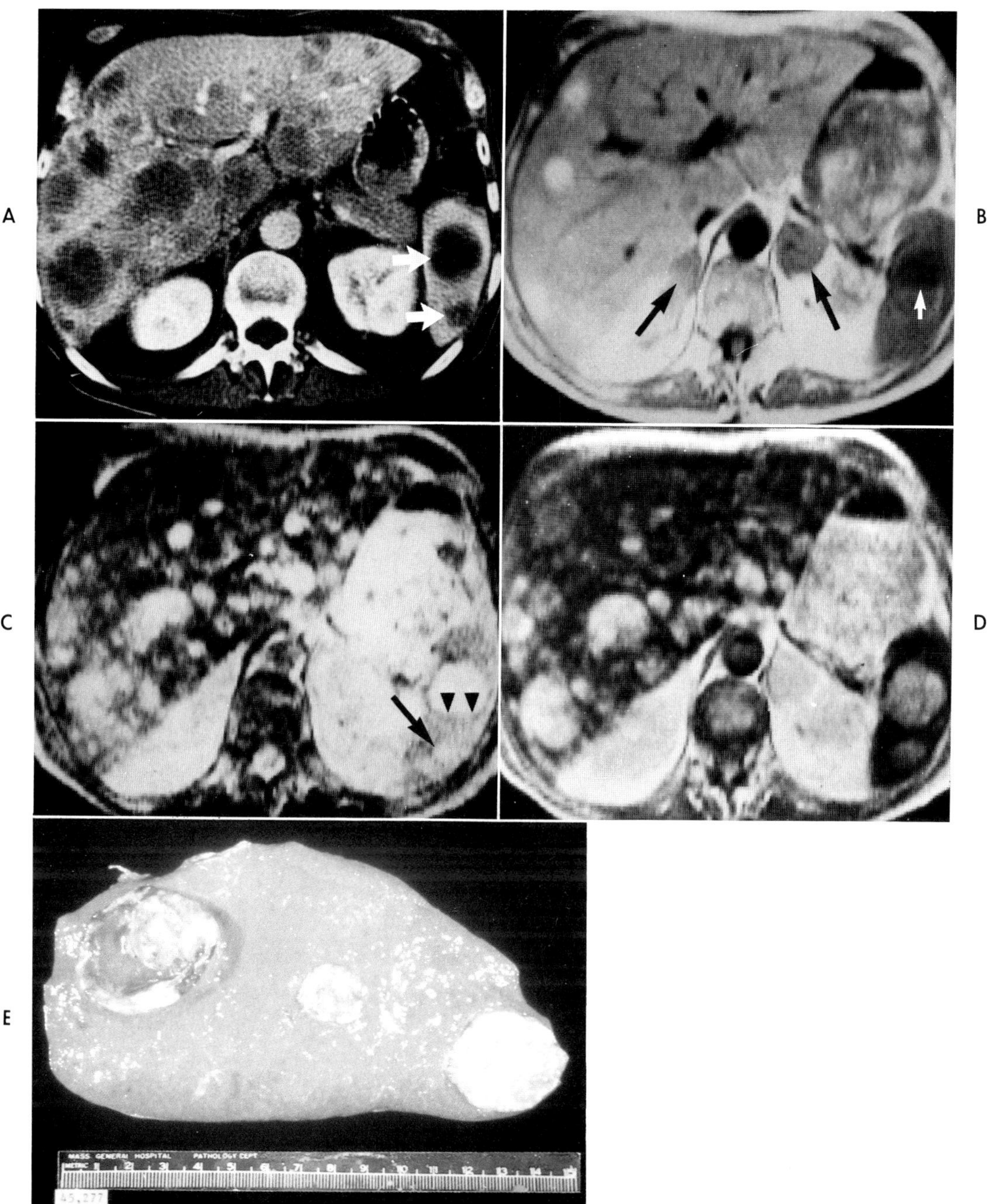

Fig. 6-9 Melanotic melanoma metastatic to spleen, liver, and adrenal glands. **A,** CT shows multiple focal lesions in the liver. Two lesions are visible in the spleen *(arrows).* **B,** T1-weighted axial MR image (SE 350/21) shows two hyperintense lesions in the liver. Many other liver lesions are isointense and not visible. There are bilateral adrenal masses *(arrows),* confirmed on a CT image cephalad to **A.** One of the lesions in the spleen is visible and has a fluid-fluid level *(small arrows).* The other lesion is not visible. **C,** Corresponding heavily T2-weighted image (SE 2350/120) confirms multiple hepatic lesions, and begins to resolve second lesion in the spleen *(arrow).* Because of diamagnetic T2 shortening caused by debris in the dependent part of the larger splenic metastasis, the supernatant fluid has a higher signal intensity than the dependent layer on the T2-weighted image *(arrowheads).* **D,** Approximately 1 hour after injection of the particulate superparamagnetic iron oxide contrast agent AMI-25, the SE 1500/40 pulse sequence becomes a heavily T2-weighted sequence. Conspicuity of multiple liver lesions is markedly improved; and both splenic lesions are demonstrated clearly. At autopsy, liver lesions were intensely melanotic. Associated T1 shortening makes some of the liver lesions hyperintense, even on T1-weighted images. Lesser degrees of T1 shortening produces isointensity. **E,** Spleen—pathologic specimen.

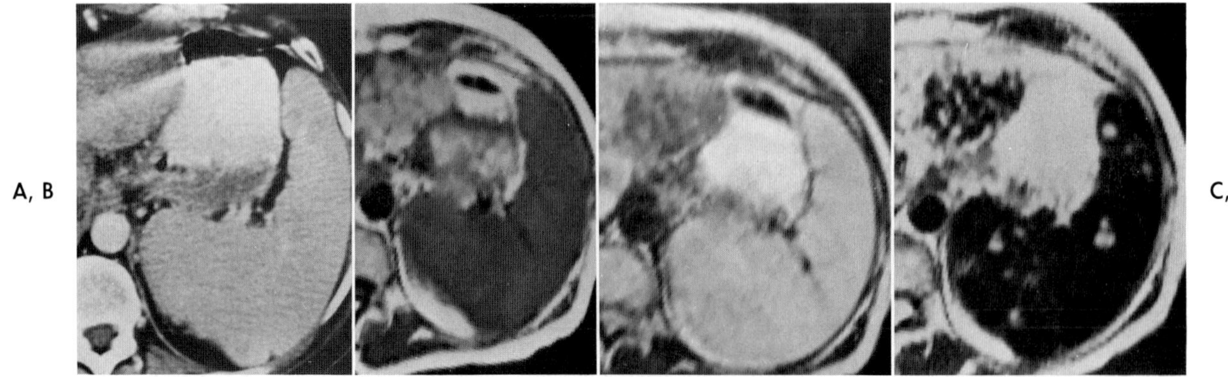

Fig. 6-10 Enhanced detection of multiple splenic breast cancer metastases. **A,** Contrast CT shows no definite splenic lesion. **B** and **C,** Axial T1- and T2-weighted MR images (0.6 T) also fail to demonstrate a splenic abnormality. **D,** After intravenous injection of superparamagnetic iron oxide, T2-weighted image at same level as **A** to **C** shows multiple lesions not previously suspected. (From Weissleder, R., Hahn, P.F., Stark, D.D., et al.: Radiology 169:399-403, 1988.)

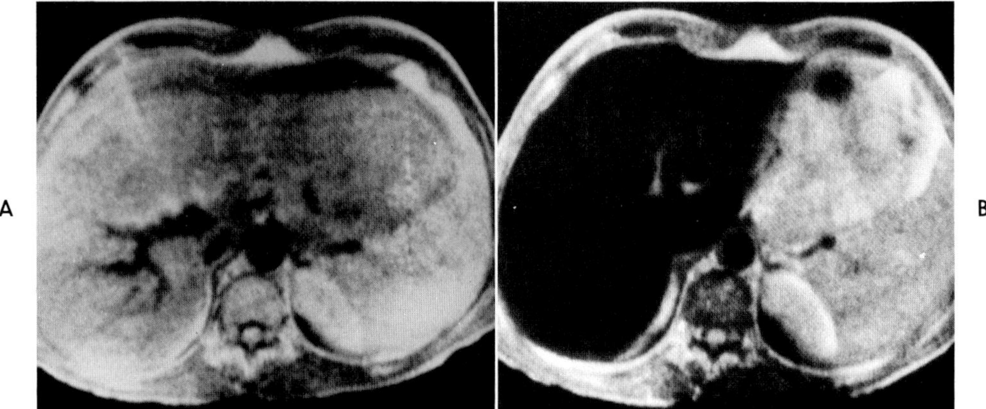

Fig. 6-11 Enhanced detection of splenic lymphoma. **A,** SE 1500/42 image at 0.3 T shows normal splenic configuration and signal intensity. **B,** Same pulse sequence after administration of 40 μmol/kg of superparamagnetic iron oxide (AMI-25) shows marked hepatic signal loss. Diffuse infiltration by Hodgkin disease prevents iron particle phagocytosis by the spleen, resulting in very little signal decrement compared with the unenhanced image. In benign splenomegaly, phagocytosis is preserved, resulting in marked splenic signal loss. (From Weissleder, R., Elizondo, G., Stark, D.D., et al.: AJR 152:175-180, 1989.)

ach displaces the small bowel inferiorly, improving visualization of the pancreatic body and tail.[510] As with agents administered intravenously, oral agents can increase or decrease the signal intensity of bowel lumen, depending on the agent and pulse sequence. The greatest problem in the development of oral contrast is to design a safe and palatable agent that resists dilution in the small bowel and concentration in the colon or that is effective over an extremely broad range of concentrations.

Iron oxide agents shorten T2 or T2,* decreasing the signal intensity of bowel lumen.[185,186,296,437] Signal intensity can also be decreased by clay (e.g., Kaopectate; Upjohn; Kalamazoo, MI)[290,356] or barium,[286,315,442] which shorten T2 by binding water (Fig. 6-12). Agents with low proton density, such as perfluorocarbons, decrease lumen signal by displacing water.[326,327,449] Other agents, such as gadopentetate dimeglumine,[250] iron solutions,[597] lipid-rich food supplements,[160] paramagnetic oil emulsions,[285] and sucrose polyester,[19] increase the signal intensity of bowel lumen on T1-weighted pulse sequences. One must be aware that the

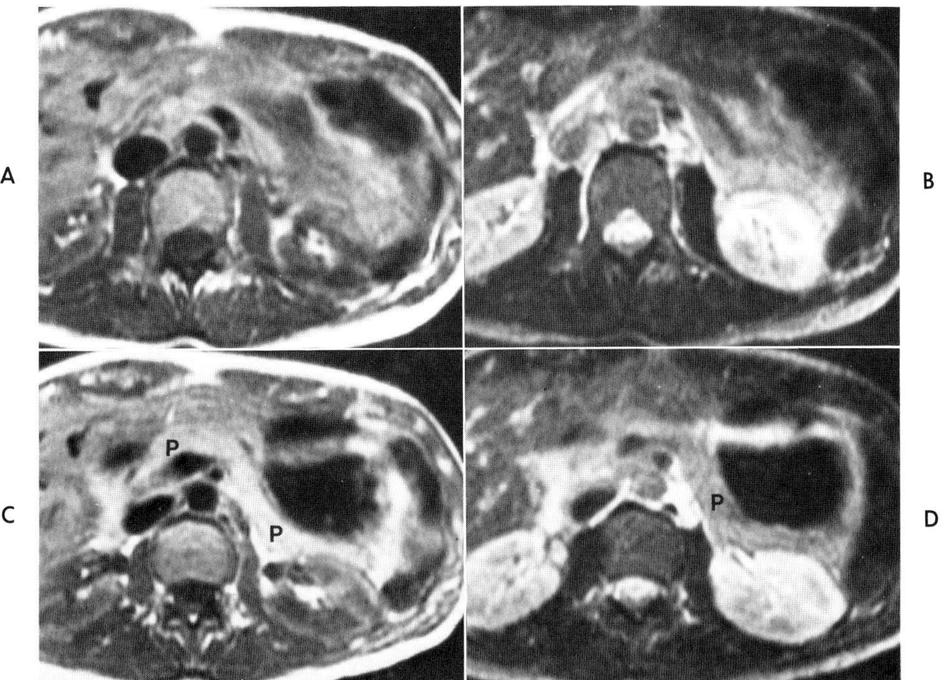

Fig. 6-12   SE 400/14 and SE 2500/100 images at 1.5 T before (**A** and **B**) and approximately 30 minutes after (**C** and **D**) ingestion of 16 oz of Kaopectate (attapulgite). Except for a thin layer on top, the gastric lumen has low signal on both T1- and T2-weighted images after ingestion, improving depiction of the pancreatic body and tail *(P)*. (From Mitchell, D.G., Vinitski, S., Haidet, K., and Rifkin, M.D.: Radiology 181:475-480, 1991.)

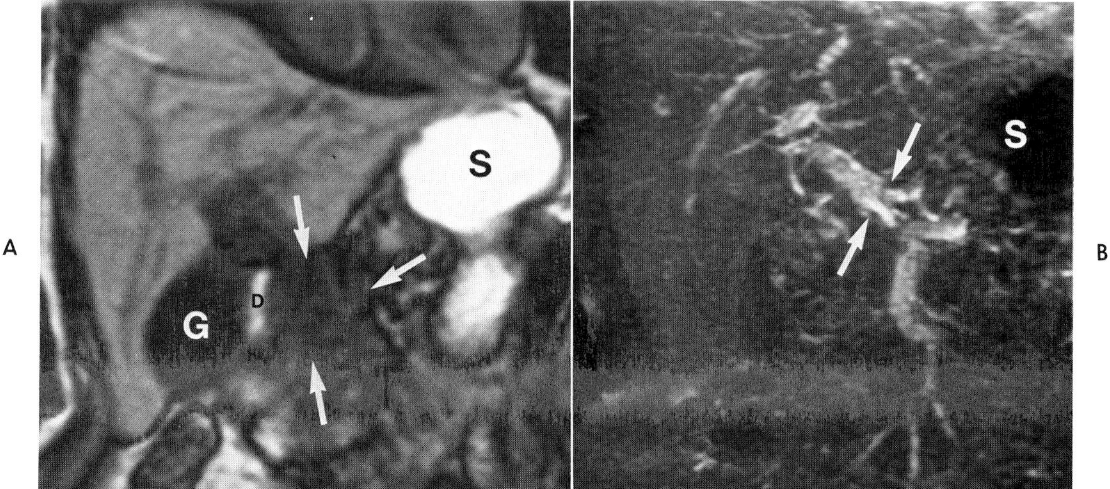

Fig. 6-13   Kaopectate for oral contrast on gradient echo images at 1.5 T, in a patient with pancreatic carcinoma. **A,** Coronal 101/2.3 image (flip angle = 90 degrees). A low signal mass in the pancreatic head *(arrows)* compresses the duodenum *(D)*. Kaopectate within the duodenum and stomach *(S)* have high-signal intensity. G = gallbladder. **B,** Coronal composite MR angiographic slab (27/7.4; flip angle = 20 degrees). There is no interference form high-signal fluid in bowel. S = stomach. The mass encases the portal vein *(arrows)*.

safety for oral administration of experimental preparations of gadopentetate dimeglumine has not yet been documented.

Nontoxic polymers, such as polyethylene glycol and cellulose, restrict the motion of water molecules, thus enhancing both T1 and T2 relaxation. When paramagnetic or superparamagnetic agents are codispersed with polymers, their relaxivity is enhanced, reducing the concentration of magnetic agents necessary for the desired effect.[274,543]

The choice between increasing the signal of intestinal contents ("positive contrast") or suppressing it ("negative contrast") may depend on the pulse sequence selected to image the abdomen.[61] On T2-weighted images, negative contrast is preferable, since this decreases artifact from bowel motion and prevents confusion between high-signal pathology and bowel. Similarly, contrast between bowel and blood vessels is improved in "bright blood" gradient-echo techniques when bowel signal is reduced.

On images with fat suppression, negative contrast may produce a "double-contrast" effect, improving depiction of the bowel wall. Additionally, suppressing the signal of the bowel and fat reduces artifact and optimizes dynamic range.

On T1-weighted images, low-signal bowel may mimic low-signal pathology. Therefore it may be preferable to increase the signal of intestinal contents by selecting agents that reduce T1 relaxation times for use with T1-weighted images. It is not clear whether positive or negative contrast is preferable for use with fat suppressed T1-weighted images.

Some "negative" agents, such as clay, become "positive" agents with short TE (Fig. 6-13).[356] This is because the T2-shortening effects are nulled by short TE, unmasking the T1-shortening effects. This biphasic effect, bright on T1-weighted images and dark on T2-weighted images, can be achieved by clay suspensions such as Kaopectate[356] or an appropriate concentration of paramagnetic materials.

Normal Anatomy and MRI Appearance

LIVER

Techniques for resection of hepatic malignancies, including metastases, have improved greatly in the past few years. Sensitivity for additional lesions and their localization within hepatic segments has therefore become increasingly important.* Current concepts of surgical anatomy consider the liver to be divided into eight or nine segments, each of which can be resected individually or in combination with other segments, providing enough hepatic tissue remains to preserve hepatic function.[512] Segment I is the caudate lobe. The left lobe is divided by the falciform ligament into lateral and medial segments. Segments II and III are the portions of the lateral segment that are anterior and posterior, respectively, relative to the plane of the left hepatic vein.

Segment IV is the medial segment of the left lobe. The right hepatic lobe is divided into anterior and posterior segments. Each of these two segments of the right lobe is divided into inferior (V and VI) and superior (VII) and (VIII) segments by the plane of the major branches of the right portal veins (Fig. 7-1) (see also Color Plate III). Some formalisms of hepatic anatomy divide segments II and III by a horizontal plane at the left of the left portal vein.[512]

The vascular anatomy of the liver defines cleavage planes for hepatic surgery. Hepatic arterial, portal venous, and biliary systems are adjacent to each other within intrasegmental hepatic parenchyma, whereas blood drains into hepatic veins between hepatic segments and lobes (Figs. 7-2 to 7-5). The right hepatic vein, located in the right intersegmental fissure, sepa-

*3, 304, 369, 370, 477, 508, 512

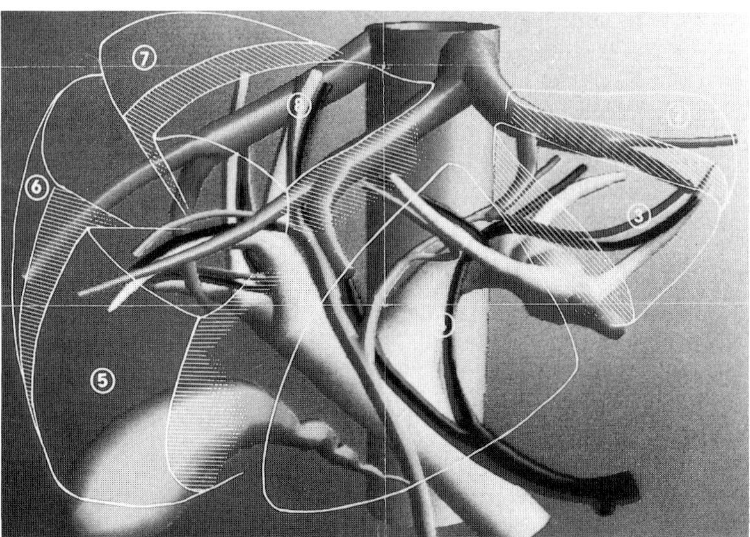

Fig. 7-1 Functional anatomy of the liver. Three-dimensional representation. Blue = systemic veins; gray = portal veins; red = hepatic arteries; green = bile ducts (see Color Plate III). (Courtesy Hepato-Biliary Surgery and Liver Transplant Unit of Hospital Paul Brousse, Villejuif, France.)

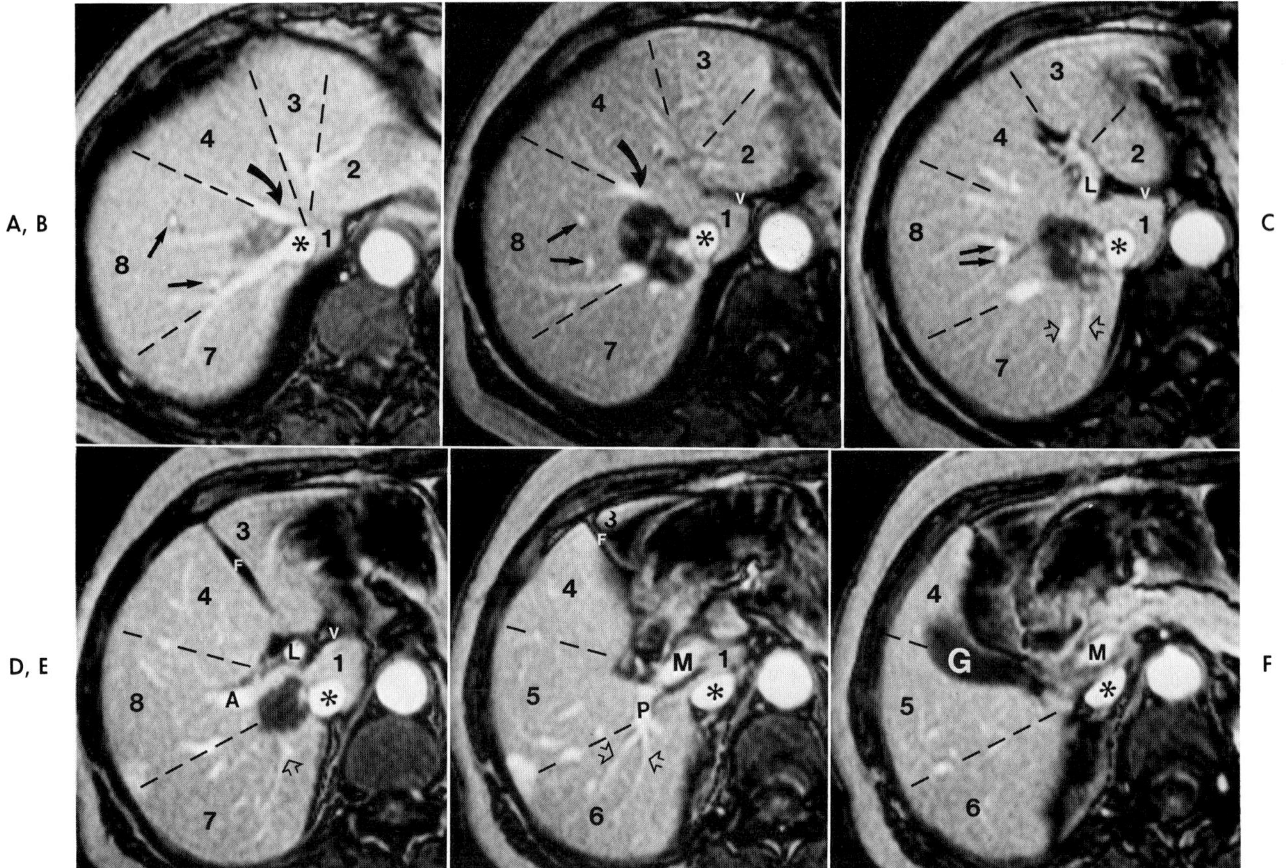

Fig. 7-2   Hepatic segmental anatomy depicted at 1.5 T, using T1-weighted gradient-echo technique (TR/TE/flip angle = 84/2.4/90 degrees) after bolus enhancement with gadopentatate dimeglumine. Six consecutive slices are illustrated, 8-mm thick with 1-mm gaps obtained as part of a 12-section acquisition during a single 12-second suspended respiration. The middle hepatic vein *(curved arrow)* divides the liver into right and left lobes, which are further divided into four sectors by the right and left hepatic veins in **A** and **B.** The left hepatic vein divides segments 2 and 3 superiorly, whereas inferiorly these segments are defined by branches of the left portal vein which perfuse them. *Straight arrows* in **A** to **C** indicate branches of the anterior right portal vein *(A)*, whereas open arrows in **C** to **E** indicate branches of the posterior right portal vein *(P)*. The ligamentum venosum *(V)* separates segment 2 from segment 1 (caudate lobe). The proximal left portal vein *(L)* and the falciform ligament *(F)* separate segment 3 from segment 4. The level of the bifurcation of the right portal vein into its anterior *(A)* and posterior *(P)* branches, located between the sections in **D** and **E,** defines the transition from the cranial segments 7 and 8 to the caudal segments 5 and 6 of the right lobe. Inferiorly, the plane of the gallbladder *(G)* parallels the middle hepatic vein and separates the left and right hepatic lobes. There are two cavernous hemangiomas, a large one involving segments 7 and 8 centrally and one located peripherally at the junction of segments 5 through 8. *Asterisk* indicates the inferior vena cava.

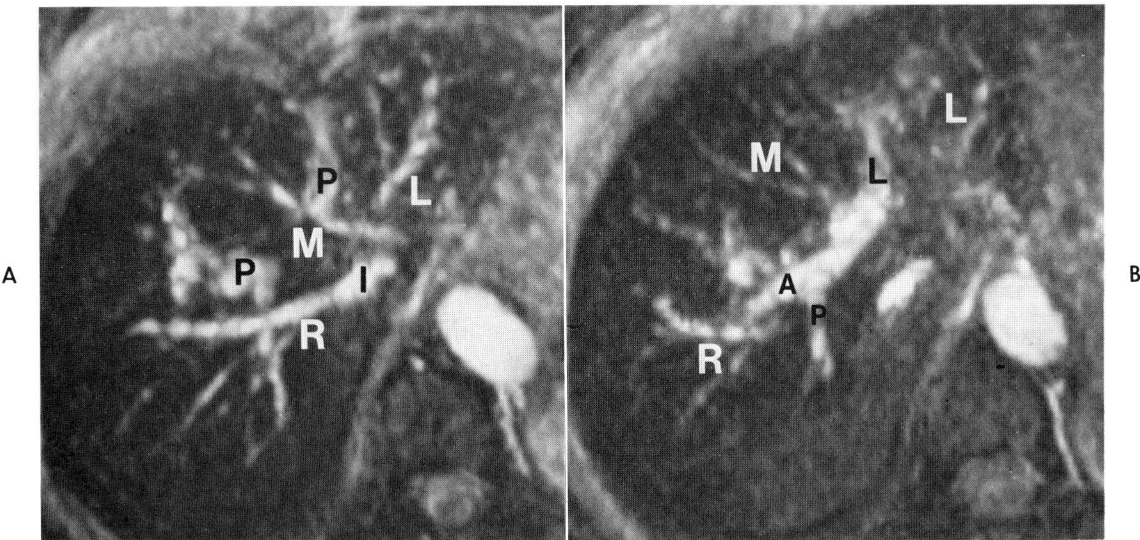

Fig. 7-3   Axial MR angiographic anatomy at 1.5 T on composite slabs that are approximately 4-cm thick. Hepatic intensity is reduced because of transfusional iron overload. There is abundant ascites. **A,** At the cephalad aspect of the liver, the right *(R)*, middle *(M)* and left *(L)* hepatic veins join the inferior vena cava *(I)*. Also note the left and right portal veins *(P)*. **B,** Inferior to **A,** note the anterior *(A)* and posterior *(P)* branches of the right portal vein and the left portal vein *(L)*. The peripheral portions of the right *(R)*, middle *(M)*, and left *(L)* hepatic veins can be seen dividing the hepatic segments.

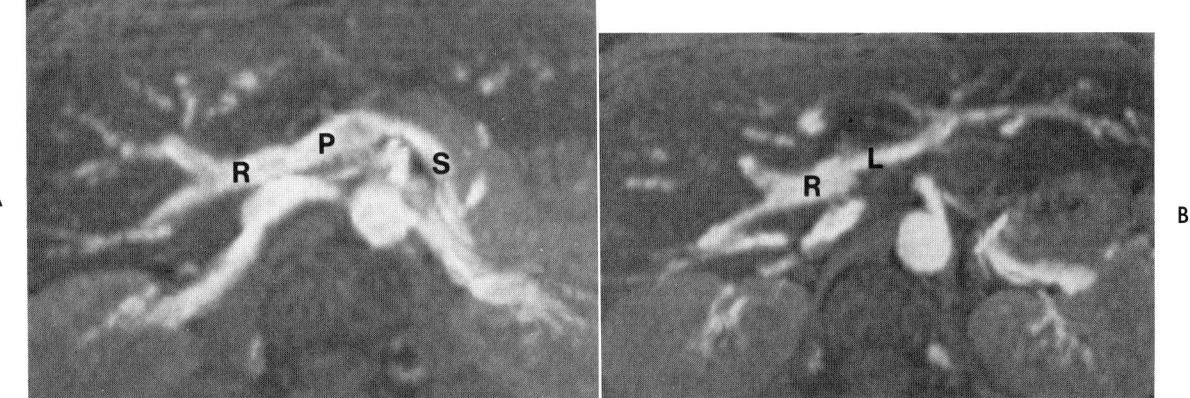

Fig. 7-4   Portal venous anatomy depicted at 1.5 T on 4-cm MR angiographic axial composite slabs. Hepatic signal intensity is reduced because of fatty liver, producing partial cancellation of water and fat signal. **A,** The splenic vein *(S)* courses to the right where it joins the superior mesenteric vein (not shown; below this plane) to form the main portal vein *(P)*. The main portal vein continues cephalad and to the right, where it gives rise the the right portal vein *(R)*, which is horizontal. **B,** On a slab cephalad but overlapping relative to **A,** the bifurcation into right *(R)* and left *(L)* portal veins is depicted. The left portal vein is cephalad to the right portal vein, accounting for its absence in **A.**

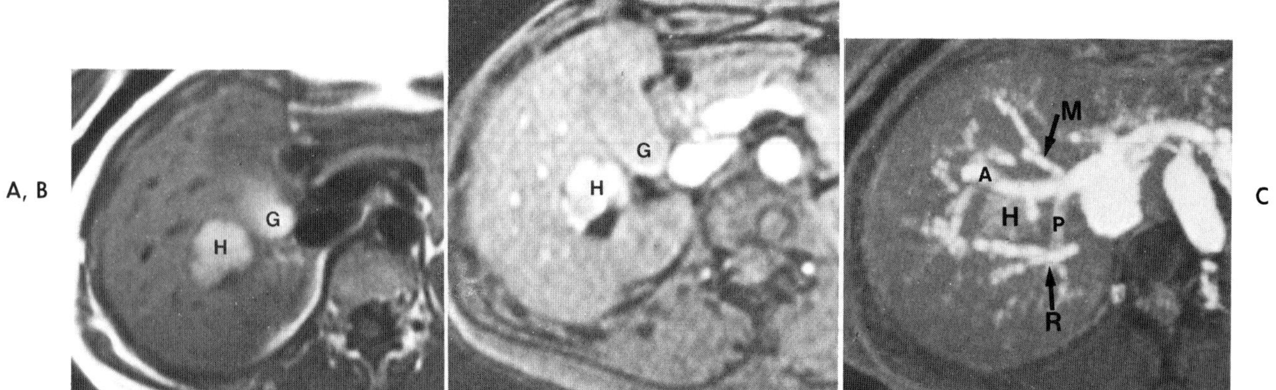

Fig. 7-5 Intrahepatic hematoma of uncertain cause in a healthy young woman. **A,** SE 400/12 image at 1.5 T depicts a high signal mass *(H)* within the right hepatic lobe. There is a posterior low-signal component. *G* = high signal concentrated gallbladder bile. **B,** Corresponding gradient-echo image (TR/TE/flip angle = 25/13/20 degrees). The lesion has a similar signal pattern. High signal persists because the T2 and T2* are relatively long, indicating that there are little if any intact red blood cells, except for the posterior low-signal component. **C,** Composite MR angiographic slab, approximately 4-cm thick. The hematoma *(H)* is located posterior to the anterior branch of the right portal vein *(A)*, between the right *(R)* and middle *(M)* hepatic veins. Thus the hematoma is centered within the anterior segment. *P* = posterior segmental portal vein.

rates the posterior and anterior segments of the right hepatic lobe. The middle hepatic vein, in the interlobar fissure, separates the right and left hepatic lobes. The left hepatic vein, within the cephalad portion of the left intersegmental fissure, separates the medial and lateral segments of the left hepatic lobe. The caudate lobe, which is perfused and drained by branches of the left and right hepatic vessels, as well as its own accessory vessels, is situated medial to the right lobe, between the inferior vena cava and the fissure for the ligamentum venosum.[100]

Portal veins are located intrasegmentally. The main portal vein branches into the left portal vein, which ascends within the left intersegmental fissure, and the right portal vein, which is horizontal. The left portal vein divides into medial and lateral segmental branches, whereas the right portal vein divides into anterior and posterior segmental branches.

A variety of landmarks define the surgical planes of the liver. The interlobar fissure is defined superiorly by the middle hepatic vein and inferiorly by a line drawn between the inferior vena cava and the gallbladder. The left intersegmental fissure is defined superiorly by the left hepatic vein and inferiorly by the left main portal vein and the falciform ligament. On occasion, the left lobe of the liver extends lateral to the spleen, where it can mimic a perisplenic collection or mass (Fig. 7-6).[423]

Transverse MR images demonstrate these major vas-

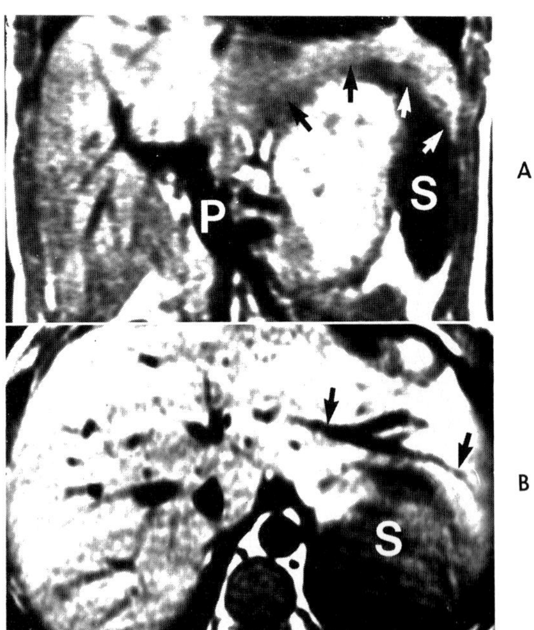

Fig. 7-6 Left lobe of liver extending lateral to the spleen. **A,** Coronal SE 400/20 image at 1.5 T at the level of the main portal vein *(P)* shows an elongated left lobe *(arrows)* extending lateral to the spleen *(S)*. **B,** Axial SE 400/12 image shows the left portal vein *(arrows)* extending lateral to the spleen *(S)*.

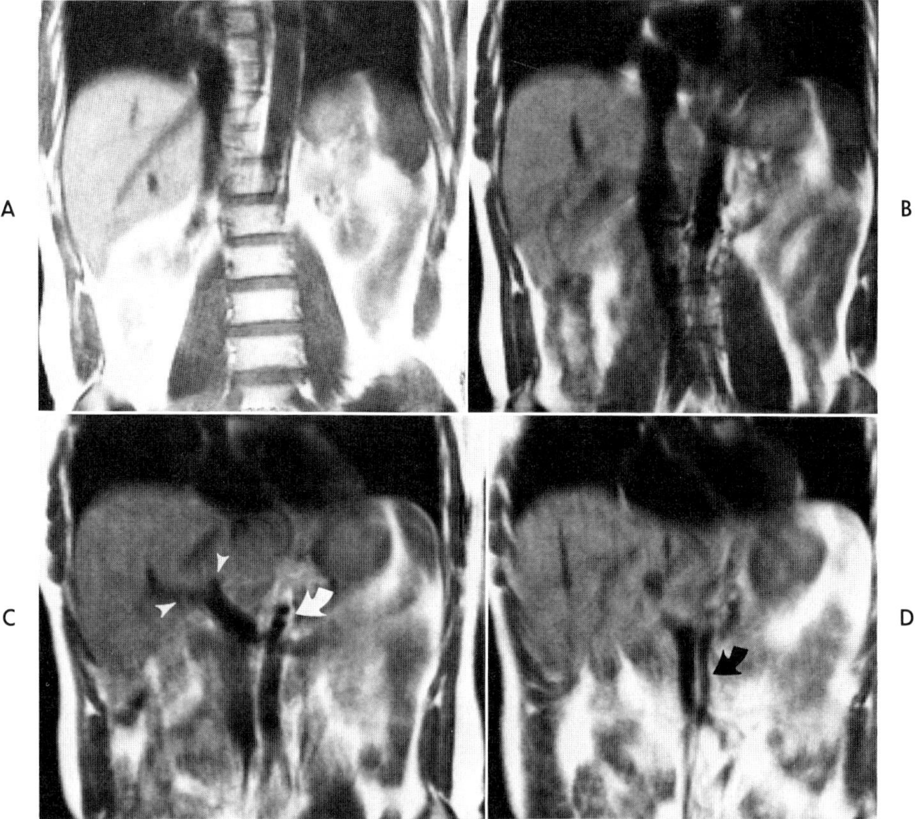

Fig. 7-7 Coronal images 0.6 T at 2-cm intervals. **A,** Anteriorly, the right hepatic vein is seen draining into the inferior vena cava. **B,** The course of the intrahepatic and retroperitoneal inferior vena cava is demonstrated. **C,** The relationship of the portal vein *(arrowheads)* to the celiac and superior mesenteric arteries *(arrow)* is well seen. Venous patency is established by the normal "flow void." **D,** Anteriorly, the superior mesenteric vein and artery *(arrow)* are seen within the intestinal mesentery, caudal to the porta hepatis.

cular structures and landmarks most consistently.[136] When patent, the major branches of the portal and hepatic veins should be identified in virtually all individuals. The hepatic artery can usually be identified, especially if flow-sensitive images are obtained. Sagittal sections often show the middle hepatic vein draining into the inferior vena cava. Coronal images demonstrate the right hepatic vein (Fig. 7-7) and central portions of other hepatic and portal veins but generally fail to visualize subsegmental branches, which are oriented oblique to this plane. The relationship of the liver to the lung base, pleural space, diaphragm, subdiaphragmatic regions, and adjacent viscera are depicted well in both the sagittal and coronal planes.

BILIARY SYSTEM

Normal intrahepatic bile ducts are not visible by MRI, unless heavily T2-weighted images with adequate spatial resolution and SNR can be achieved. The extra-

hepatic common duct and cystic duct can usually be detected if effective motion-artifact suppression and anatomic resolution are achieved (Figs. 7-8 and 7-9). The common hepatic duct is best demonstrated in obese patients where the common bile duct is visualized anterior to the main portal vein, whereas the common bile duct can be located best at the posterolateral border of the head of the pancreas, at its junction with the second portion of the duodenum. Normal signal within portal vessels must be recognized, particularly on even-echo images or those made with software motion suppression, to avoid the misdiagnosis of dilated bile ducts in normal patients (Fig. 7-10).

At 0.6 T, T1-weighted short TR/short TE spin-echo imaging provides the greatest anatomic resolution. T2-weighted images with TE = 60 msec often fail to show bile ducts because of poor bile-fat contrast. Longer TE values have potentially greater contrast but suffer from lower SNR and therefore are often too noisy to allow

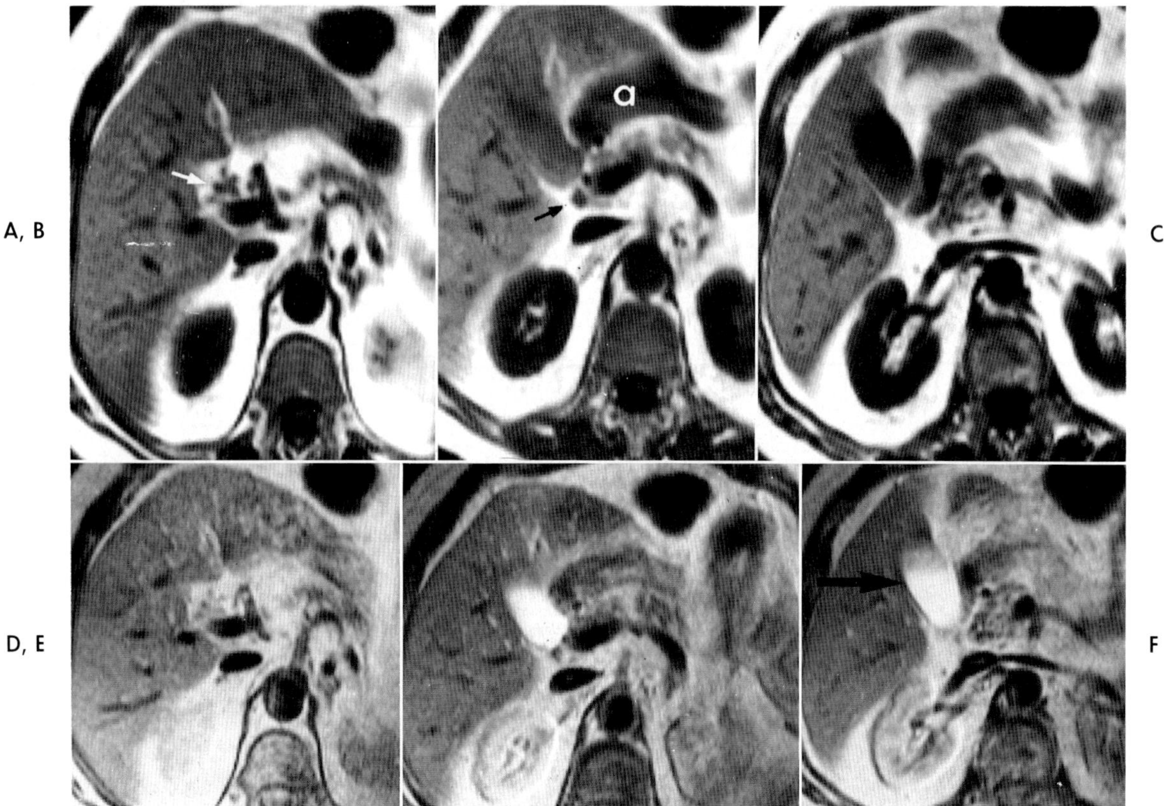

Fig. 7-8 Normal biliary anatomy at 0.6 T. Consecutive SE 260/15 images obtained at 0.6T by averaging 18 data acquisitions. **A,** Within the porta hepatis, the main portal vein is seen in cross-section. Anterior to the portal vein are multiple sections through the convoluted cystic duct *(arrow)*. The common bile duct is seen between the hepatic artery and the main portal vein. **B,** Within the pancreatic head, the distal bile duct is seen as a hypointense structure *(arrow)*. Anterolaterally, the gallbladder is partial volume averaged at this level. **C,** The fluid-filled duodenum lies between the gallbladder and pancreatic head. Branching structures within the liver are blood vessels. **D** to **F,** T2-weighted images. SE 2000 images corresponding with **A** to **C. D,** Cystic duct and common bile duct, anterior to the main portal vein, show an increase in signal intensity reflecting the long T1 and T2 relaxation times of bile. Anatomic resolution is decreased from the use of long TR, which restricts signal averaging, and long TE, which results in increased ghosting. **E,** compared with the T1-weighted image, gallbladder bile has increased signal intensity, attributable to its fluid content and long T2 relaxation time. **F,** Dilute hepatic bile is layered on top of concentrated gallbladder bile *(arrow)*. Note that bile in the cystic duct visible in **D** has the same signal intensity as unconcentrated hepatic bile supernatant in the gallbladder. Concentrated gallbladder bile is brighter due to its shorter T1 relaxation time, reflecting greater solute concentration and lower water content.

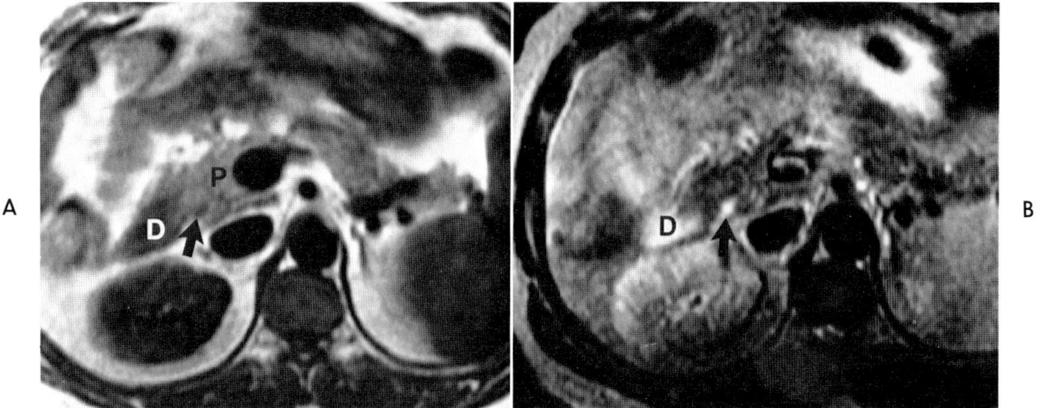

Fig. 7-9 Normal common bile duct at 1.5 T. **A,** SE 400/12 image. The common bile duct *(arrow)* is depicted as a low signal structure at the posterolateral aspect of the pancreatic head *(P)*. The pancreas has higher signal than the duodenum *(D)*. **B,** SE 2500/100 image. The common bile duct *(arrow)* and duodenal fluid *(D)* have higher signal intensity than fat.

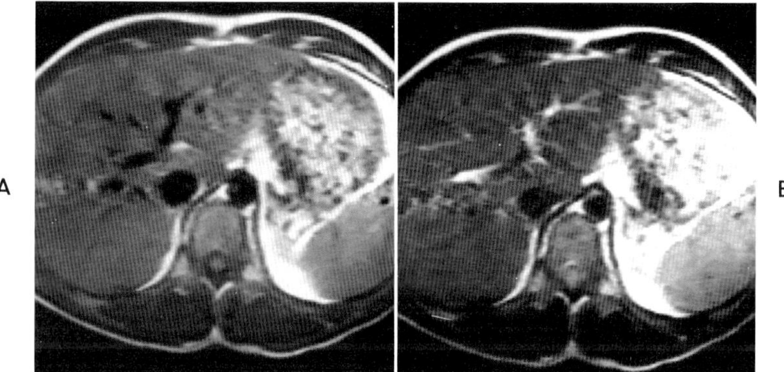

Fig. 7-10 Normal liver at 0.6 T, with even echo rephasing simulating branching bile ducts within the liver. **A,** SE 1500/32 first echo image shows the normal right and ascending left portal veins. Largest normal intrahepatic bile duct (> 6 mm) lies anterior to the right portal vein and is not resolved due to the limited spatial resolution (3.6 × 1.8 × 15 mm voxel dimensions) used in large field-of-view abdominal MRI. **B,** SE 1500/64 second echo shows increased signal intensity from portal vascular structures, known as *even-echo rephasing.* Bile (not seen) would have a much lower signal intensity with this pulse sequence. Signal from flowing blood may lie to one side of the portal vein lumen or may be offset onto adjacent liver and should not be interpreted as bile duct enlargement.

resolution of small anatomic biliary structures.

At 1.5 T, the left and right bile duct can often be identified on T2-weighted images with TE of 100 msec, adjacent to the portal veins (Fig. 7-11). At this TE, there is sufficient contrast relative to fat for bile to be depicted clearly. Conjugate spin-echo train techniques (e.g., multishot RARE, fast spin-echo) are especially effective for demonstrating bile ducts if TR ≥ 4000 msec and at least 256 phase-encoding views are acquired (see Chapter 1, T2-Weighted Images). By following anatomy on adjacent sections, the common he-

patic and common bile ducts can usually be traced toward the ampulla of Vater, although the distal-most segment is not depicted as consistently (see Figs. 1-6 to 1-9, and 7-12).

In an early study at 1.5 T without motion-artifact suppression the distal common bile duct was demonstrated in up to 70% of studies that were not considered markedly degraded by motion.[490] In our experience with flow-compensated SE images or conjugate spin-echo train techniques the distal common bile duct is identified in virtually all cases. Although the common bile

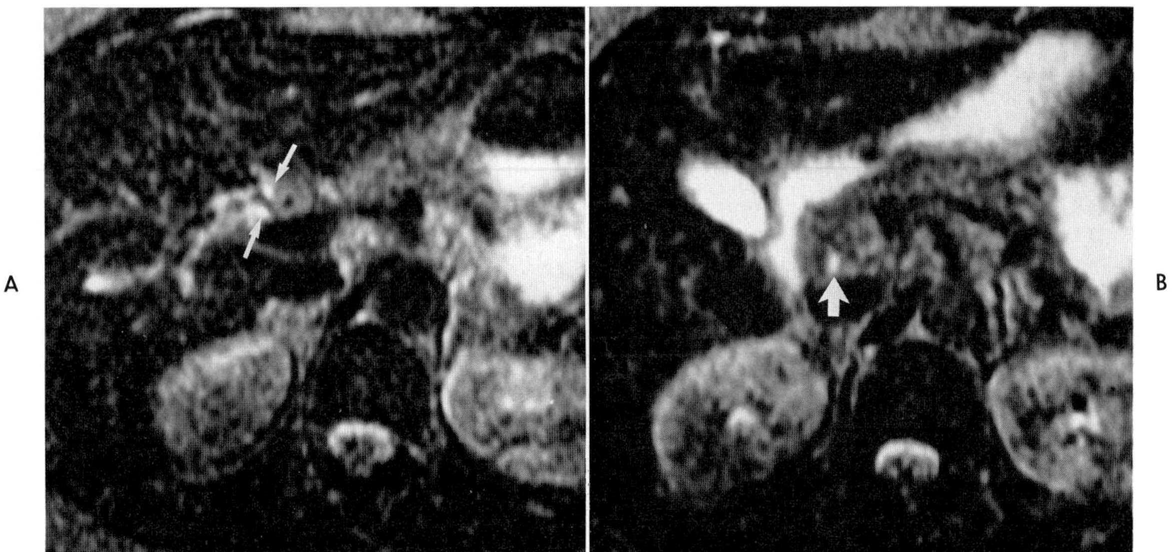

Fig. 7-11 Normal intrahepatic and extrahepatic ducts depicted on SE 2500/140 images using 5-mm–thick sections at 1.5 T. **A,** In spite of low SNR, intrahepatic ducts *(arrows)* can be seen. **B,** Inferiorly, the common bile duct *(arrow)* can be seen.

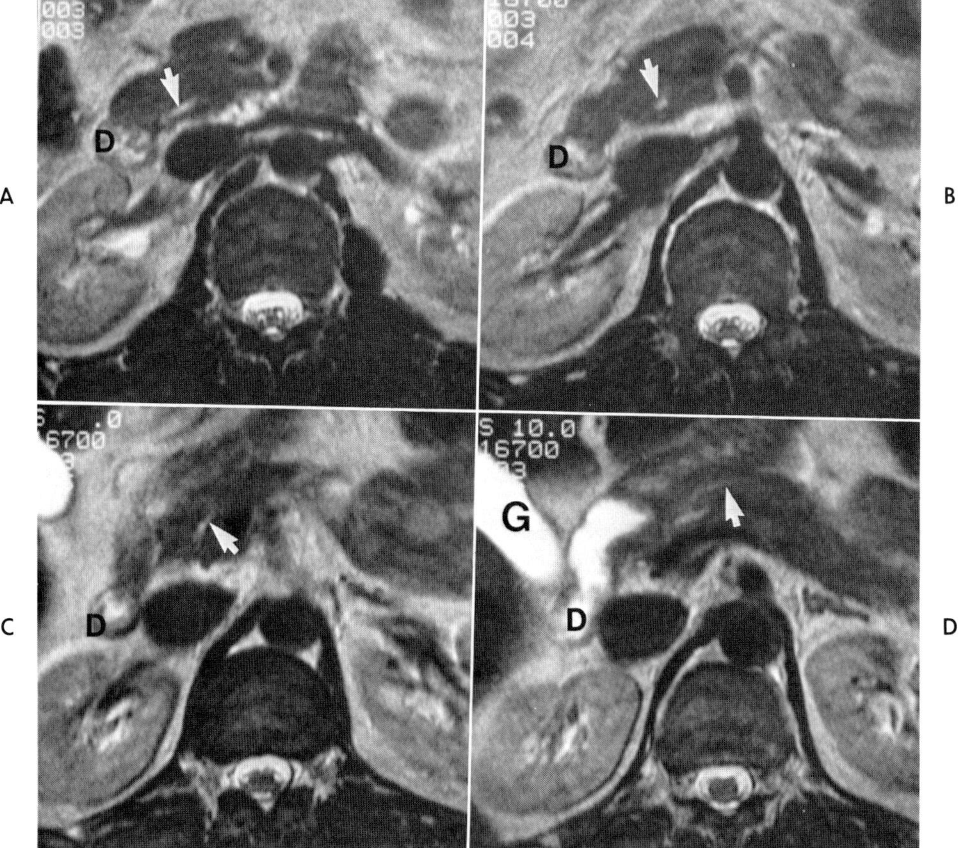

Fig. 7-12 Improved depiction of the duodenum *(D),* pancreas *(P),* and bile and pancreatic ducts *(arrows),* using conjugate (fast) spin-echo technique at 1.5 T (same patient as in Fig. 1-3). **A** to **D,** Axial images from bottom to top at the level of the pancreas (TR/TE = 5500/102). Echo train = 16 echoes per excitation, four signal averages, matrix = 512 × 256, imaging time for 17 sections = 6 minutes. Because of the long TR, intestinal fluid and bile have extremely high intensity, and depiction of small ducts is improved further by small pixel size and high SNR. G = gallbladder.

duct may be seen on T1-weighted images at 1.5 T, fat suppression improves depiction greatly.

The normal duct may measure up to 10 mm, somewhat larger than the size considered normal by CT. Motion-induced blurring, together with the larger pixel size used in MRI, probably accounts for this difference.

The normal gallbladder is readily visualized in the interlobar fissure using either T1- or T2-weighted pulse sequences (see Fig. 7-8). T2-weighted pulse sequences routinely show the gallbladder as a high signal intensity structure. With moderate to heavy T2 weighting (e.g., SE 2500/100), bile is usually brighter than cerebrospinal fluid (CSF). This is because the T1 of CSF is nearly 3 seconds, so that complete T1 relaxation does not occur.

The appearance of gallbladder bile varies on T1-weighted images, depending on gallbladder function and bile concentration. The nonaqueous fraction of normal bile is predominantly composed of bile salts and cholesterol. Unconcentrated bile, accumulated in the gallbladder after stimulation by eating or intravenous administration of cholecystokinin, has a water content of approximately 95% and shows a low signal intensity on T1-weighted images. With reabsorption of water and increased cholesterol and bile salt concentration, water content falls to approximately 84% and the T1 relaxation time decreases.[95,294] Therefore the appearance of concentrated bile on T1-weighted images is often brighter than adjacent liver. T2 relaxation times also decrease with increasing bile concentration, but the predominant effect on image signal intensity in most pulse sequences is the change in T1.

Since concentrated bile is more dense (greater specific gravity) than dilute bile, it is common to see a layering effect with dark (long T1) dilute bile on top of bright (short T1) concentrated bile. Unfortunately, a single examination showing uniform bile does not imply gallbladder disease, and layering of bile is not diagnostic of normal function. For example, layering can be seen in acute cholecystitis as inflammatory cells and debris settle within the obstructed gallbladder. It may be possible to establish gallbladder function by imaging patients in both the nonfasting and fasting states.[220] Concentration of bile in the fasting state, determined by increasing signal intensity on T1-weighted images, would indicate normal gallbladder function.

EXTRAHEPATIC VASCULAR ANATOMY

Vascular anatomy is usually defined best using "bright blood" techniques, such as single-slice gradient-echo images with short TR, short TE and gradient moment nulling (see Figs. 3-4 and 7-13) (see Chapter 3, Short TR "Angiographic" Images). "Dark blood" techniques, however, such as T1-weighted imaging with presaturation, are also useful for confirming equivocal findings.

The superior mesenteric artery arises anteriorly from the aorta at the approximate level of the renal arteries, slightly above the level of the left renal vein. The only two structures that normally cross between the aorta and the proximal superior mesenteric artery are the left renal vein and, at a slightly lower level, the horizontal portion of the duodenum.

The celiac axis arises anteriorly from the aorta slightly above the origin of the superior mesenteric artery. The length of the celiac trunk varies and splits into two large branches, the hepatic and splenic arteries, which course to the right and left, respectively. A smaller branch, the left gastric artery, ascends along the lesser curvature of the stomach.

The main hepatic artery courses towards the liver within the gastrohepatic ligament. Cephalad to the lateral border of the pancreatic head, the gastroduodenal artery descends from the main hepatic artery between the pancreas and the second portion of the duodenum. The gastroduodenal artery marks the anterolateral border of the pancreatic head, whereas the common bile duct marks the posterolateral border, separating the pancreas from the duodenum. The remainder of the main hepatic artery, now termed the *proper hepatic artery*, continues to the right where it comes to lie alongside the main portal vein.

The splenic artery undulates as it courses to the left and cephalad, toward the splenic hilum. The splenic vein is usually larger and has a straighter course along the posterosuperior border of the tail and body of the pancreas, from the splenic hilum to its confluence with

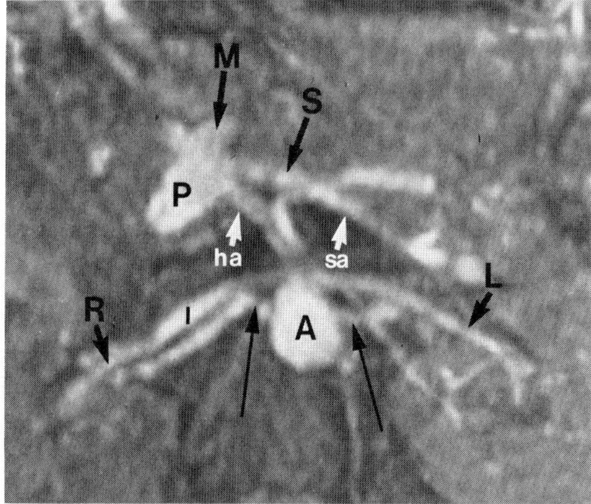

Fig. 7-13 Infrahepatic vascular anatomy depicted at 1.5 T on a 4-cm MR angiographic axial composite slab (same patient as in Fig. 7-1). The celiac axis bifurcates into the hepatic *(ha)* and splenic *(sa)* arteries. Anteriorly, the splenic *(S)* and superior mesenteric *(M)* veins join to form the portal vein *(P)*. Posteriorly, the left *(L)* and right *(R)* renal veins join the inferior vena cava *(I)*. A = aorta, *long arrows* indicate the left and right renal arteries.

the superior mesenteric vein when the main portal vein is formed.

The superior mesenteric vein, usually slightly larger than its corresponding artery, lies to the right of the artery except when displaced by a mass or in individuals with intestinal malrotation.

The pancreas is located in the retroperitoneum, oriented with its long axis transversely in the midline. The tail is usually higher than the body, so serial axial sections are usually necessary to demonstrate the entire pancreas. It the stomach is distended, or if the spleen is enlarged, the pancreas assumes a more transverse orientation. At the inferior portion of the pancreatic head, the uncinate process projects posteriorly behind the superior mesenteric vein.

The splenic vein and splenoportal junction delimit the pancreas dorsally, and behind these lie the inferior vena cava and abdominal aorta. The superior mesenteric artery and vein lie posterior to the pancreatic body, to the left of the pancreatic head, and anterior to the uncinate process. The gastric body and fundus are situated ventral to the pancreas, with the lesser peritoneal sac between the stomach and pancreas. Lateral to the pancreatic head is the descending duodenum. Jejunal bowel loops are found adjacent to the pancreatic tail, unless displaced inferiorly by a distended stomach or enlarged spleen.

PANCREAS

The pancreas remains one of the most difficult organs to image by MRI. The pancreas is surrounded by bowel, which moves during acquisition of conventional SE images, causing blurring and ghost artifact. Furthermore, the pancreas itself moves with respiration.[240] The signal intensity of unenhanced bowel lumen is unpredictable and can often mimic tumor. Vascular artifact can also degrade the pancreas. Even more than for the rest of the upper abdomen, optimum technique is essential for effective MR imaging of the pancreas. Fortunately, recent software advances now allow even the

pancreas to be imaged effectively, allowing us to make use of the significant tissue contrast available in this region.

At low- and mid-field strength, signal intensity of pancreas and liver are similar over a variety of pulse sequences and field strengths. As shown in Table 7-1 from data obtained from images at 0.35 T of 75 individuals, average T1 and T2 of normal pancreas are 448 ± 131 msec and 48 ± 6 msec, respectively. Calculations from images of eight normal individuals obtained at 0.26 T produce values of 544 ± 40 msec and 56 ± 3 msec.[240] Calculations based on spectrometer experiments indicate that T1 of liver is within 20% of pancreas at field strengths above 0.3 T, with closer agreement as field strength increases.[39] On low field images, the difference is enough so that the signal intensity of pancreas may appear slightly lower than that of the liver on T1-weighted images.[240] Liver T1 is significantly shorter than that of the pancreas at field strengths 0.1 T and below.

At 1.5 T, the normal pancreas has significantly higher signal than the liver on both T1- and T2-weighted images. It is not known why contrast relationships regarding the pancreas are different than at low field and midfield. The relative high signal of the pancreas becomes especially noticeable when motion-artifact suppression and dynamic range are optimized by fat suppression.[358] On T1-weighted images with fat suppression, the pancreas has higher signal than all tissues other than adipose, although bowel lumen may occasionally be as intense.

On T2-weighted images at 1.5 T, the pancreas often blends with fat, so fat suppression improves depiction on T2-weighted images as well. Although oral contrast helps distinguish the pancreas from bowel on T2-weighted images, the natural tissue contrast displayed on fat suppressed T1-weighted images is usually sufficient to define the pancreas even without oral contrast. Similarly, the pancreas can be delineated based on its high signal intensity even in extremely thin patients, in

Table 7-1   MRI Tissue Characteristics

Pancreas (n = 75)	Spleen (n = 42)	Liver (n = 50)	Muscle (n = 40)	Fat (n = 25)	Cancer (n = 38)
Proton density*					
0.56 ± .07	0.55 ± .16	0.67 ± .17	0.57 ± .20	1.00 ± .27	0.69 ± .18
T1 (msec)					
448 ± 131	805 ± 263	499 ± 140	663 ± 240	329 ± 117	876 ± 334
T2 (msec)					
48 ± 6	70 ± 20	48 ± 11	41 ± 11	56 ± 11	78 ± 32

Tissue parameters calculated from image intensity measurements, mean ± S.D., n = number of patients.
*Relative hydrogen density has no unit of measure.
Field strength = 0.6 T, except pancreas data (0.35 T), which is adapted from: Schmidt, H.C., et al.: J Comput Assist Tomogr 9:738, 1985; and Stark, D.D., et al.: Radiology 150:153, 1984.

whom CT often is technically inadequate. On fat-suppressed T1-weighted images with respiratory-ordered phase encoding, the common bile duct, gastroduodenal artery and pancreatic duct, as well as the margins of the entire pancreas, can be seen in most normal individuals (Fig. 7-14).

The pancreas is usually examined as part of a scan intended to evaluate the liver. When pancreas is the focus of the examination, however, certain protocol changes can be instituted for optimal imaging. Fat suppression, particularly on T1-weighted images, is especially important for imaging the pancreas. Thinner sections (0.5 or 0.75 cm) may be used to reduce partial volume artifact. Smaller field of view can improve resolution, although the entire liver should usually be included in patients with pancreatic carcinoma to exclude hepatic metastases. Thus we recommend using large field of view for conventional T1- and T2-weighted images, reducing the field of view for fat suppressed T1-weighted images and flow-sensitive gradient-echo images.

High-quality pancreatic MRI has not been available for long, and controlled studies have not yet been reported. Most of the comments on high-field pancreatic imaging included here, therefore, are based on clinical experience with approximately 100 cases, and await scientific confirmation. It is uncertain whether the superior soft-tissue contrast and vascular depiction of MRI will prove more important than the finer resolution and lower sensitivity to motion of CT.

If indeed MRI is shown to have advantages over CT, it is also uncertain whether these advantages will improve clinical management sufficiently to justify the increased cost of MRI. One must remember that most patients with pancreatic adenocarcinoma have unresectable carcinomas by the time they present for imaging. For pancreatitis, CT may remain the preferred modality for several years because of the need for unambiguous imaging of bowel. The inability of MRI to identify small calcifications also limits its ability to distinguish chronic pancreatitis from cancer. Further experience with improved oral contrast and optimized high-speed imaging may provide solutions to these problems.

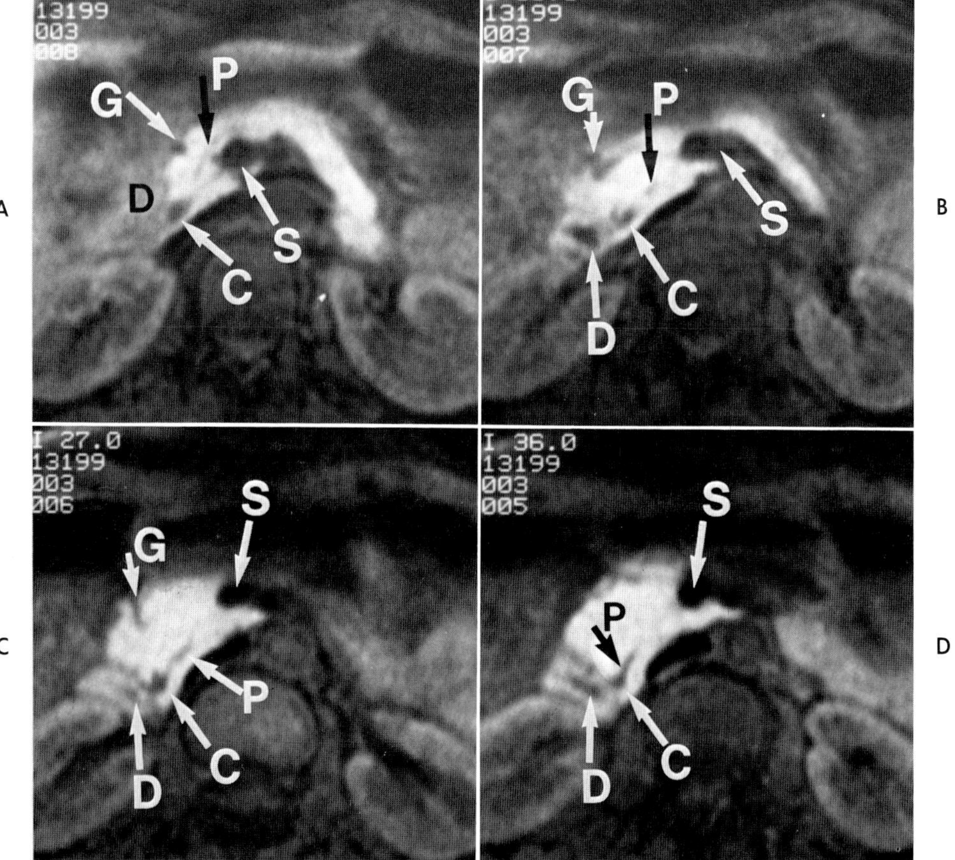

Fig. 7-14   Optimized SE imaging of the pancreas at 1.5 T via fat suppression. **A** to **D,** T1 weighted (TR/TE = 400/14) images from top down. The normal pancreas is more intense than other viscera. *C* = common bile duct, *D* = duodenum, *G* = gastroduodenal artery, *P* = pancreatic duct, *S* = superior mesenteric vein.

SPLEEN

The spleen is a smooth intraperitoneal organ that is attached to the retroperitoneum by fatty ligaments containing its vascular pedicle (Fig. 7-15). The borders of the spleen are usually convex laterally and concave medially, with occasional lobulations. The size of the spleen is quite variable and may in fact decrease after abdominal trauma and increase shortly thereafter.[172]

The spleen is a unique immunologic organ with a large fractional blood content and relatively long T1 and T2 relaxation times (see Table 7–1) (Fig. 7-16). Indeed, the magnetic characteristics of normal splenic tissue (hydrogen density, T1, T2, and chemical shift) resemble the average tissue characteristics of cancer metastatic to the liver. This allows the spleen to be used as a model of cancer metastatic to the liver for optimization of pulse sequences (see Chapter 1, Tissue Contrast).

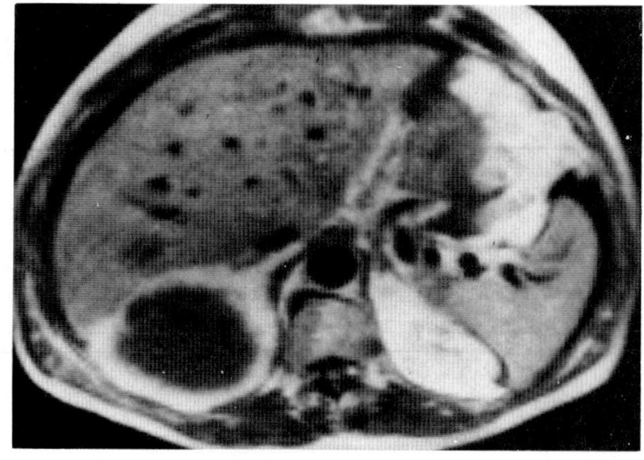

Fig. 7-15 Ascites outlines the peritoneal surfaces of the spleen and liver. The spleen is attached at its hilum to the fatty gastrolienal and lienorenal ligaments. A simple cyst is seen at the upper pole of the right kidney.

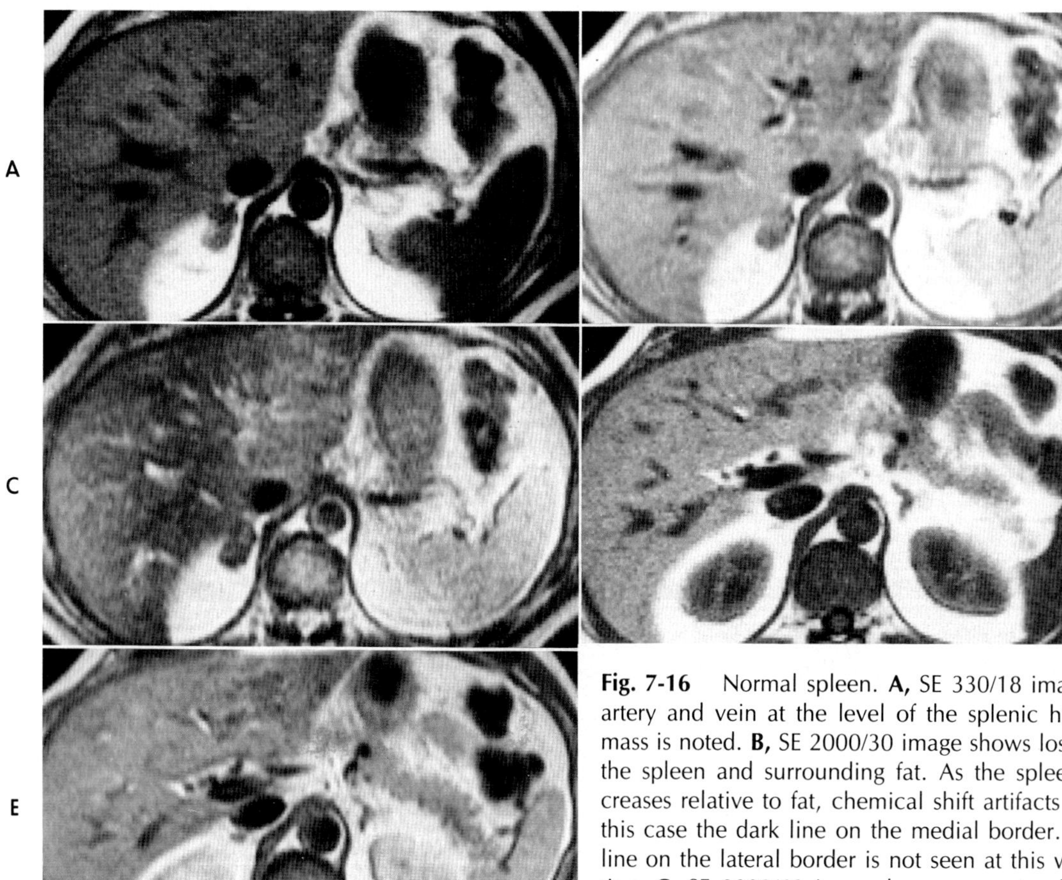

Fig. 7-16 Normal spleen. **A,** SE 330/18 image shows the splenic artery and vein at the level of the splenic hilum. A right adrenal mass is noted. **B,** SE 2000/30 image shows loss of contrast between the spleen and surrounding fat. As the spleen signal intensity increases relative to fat, chemical shift artifacts become apparent, in this case the dark line on the medial border. A comparable bright line on the lateral border is not seen at this window and level setting. **C,** SE 2000/60 image becomes grainy because of decreased SNR. Further loss of spleen-fat contrast is seen. The right adrenal mass remains the same signal intensity as liver, consistent with its clinical diagnosis: benign adenoma. **D,** Two centimeters caudal to **A.** The pancreatic tail is seen to enter the splenic hilum. The spleen tends to take the impression of structures in contact with it; at this level its inferior margin is concave, accommodating the left kidney. **E,** SE 2000/30 image.

The splenic vein is imaged on SE images as a signal void dorsal to the pancreatic body and tail. The splenic artery sometimes can be traced from the celiac axis and is typically more tortuous than its corresponding vein. Vessels arborizing within the spleen cannot be traced beyond the hilus (central third).

Pulse sequences used to survey the spleen are usually the same as those used for the liver. Indeed, the spleen is a familiar organ because it is included in every MR examination of the liver. Thus routine imaging of the liver provides a baseline for understanding the variations in the normal MR appearance of the spleen. Images with T1 and T2 contrast dependencies are acquired so that variations in overall splenic T1 and T2 can be estimated and so that focal abnormalities can be detected. Although axial images corresponding to the CT examination are used most commonly to evaluate the spleen, coronal images can be used to assess splenic size and to demonstrate the relationship of the spleen to the stomach, kidney, splenic colonic flexure, and to the diaphragm.

Images of the spleen can be degraded by motion artifacts. Transmitted cardiac pulsation, bowel peristalsis, and respiratory excursion all contribute to the noise. Pseudogating of respiratory motion to the step time can produce a particularly difficult artifact. Usually appearing on the medial aspect of the spleen, this artifact often resembles a focal lesion but only on one pulse sequence. Unfortunately, many true lesions may be visible on only one pulse sequence as well, so that great care is necessary in the interpretation of unexpected focal lesions in the spleen. If necessary, reversing the gradients or changing the echo time can eliminate the defect.

Motion of the spleen itself during data acquisition can lead to phase displacement of signal arising from the spleen, artifactually reducing the spleen signal intensity. Motion-artifact–suppression techniques, such as gradient moment nulling, can correct for this signal loss (Fig. 7-17, see Chapter 2, Gradient Moment Nulling).[353]

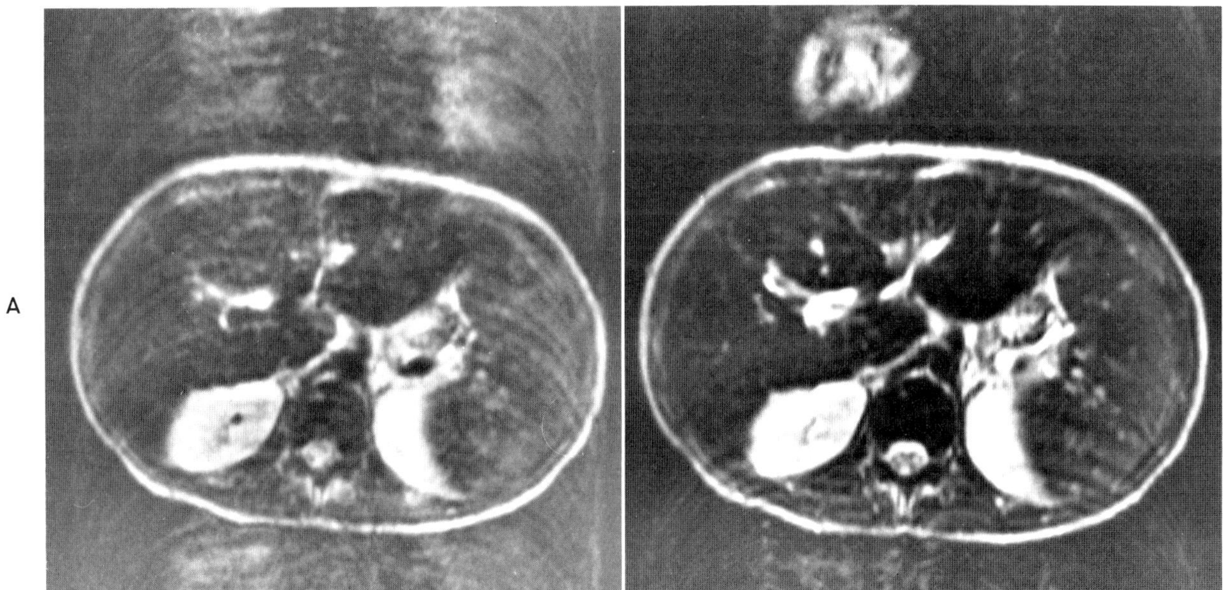

Fig. 7-17 Effect of motion suppression for imaging the spleen. Both images are symmetric second-echo SE 2500/80 images obtained at 1.5 T in a patient with chronic lymphocytic leukemia and fungal septicemia. **A** was obtained with respiratory-encoded (ordered) phase encoding. Uncompensated motion along imaging gradients produces phase changes that lead to ghost artifacts along the phase-encoded (anteroposterior) axis. **B** was obtained with gradient moment nulling. Artifacts are significantly reduced, permitting demonstration of multiple focal splenic lesions thought to represent fungal abscesses. (From Mitchell, D.G., Vinitski, S., Burk, D.L., et al.: Radiology 169:155-160, 1988.)

Comparison with Computed Tomography

LIMITATIONS OF COMPUTED TOMOGRAPHY

Computed tomography (CT) is currently the standard modality for preoperative detection of focal liver lesions.* In one study, liver function tests were normal in 33% of patients in whom metastases were depicted by CT.[398]

In spite of its wide acceptance, recent data suggest that the sensitivity of contrast-enhanced CT for detecting individual hepatic lesions is only 34% to 37%, and the sensitivity for identifying patients with one or more

---

*5, 30, 133, 139, 146, 337

lesions is only 74%.[146,200,430,513] Indeed, the false-negative rate for CT accounts for most cancer deaths in patients who have previously undergone curative excision of primary cancers.[37,58,304]

Most centers administer iodinated contrast material to improve the accuracy of lesion detection by CT, despite the inconvenience, cost, and associated risks. Unfortunately, contrast administration may obscure metastases from hypervascular,[43] breast,[107] or other primary malignancies (see Figs. 5-9 and 8-1 to 8-4). Therefore both noncontrast and contrast-enhanced scans should be performed if possible. Most centers infuse 40 to 60 g io-

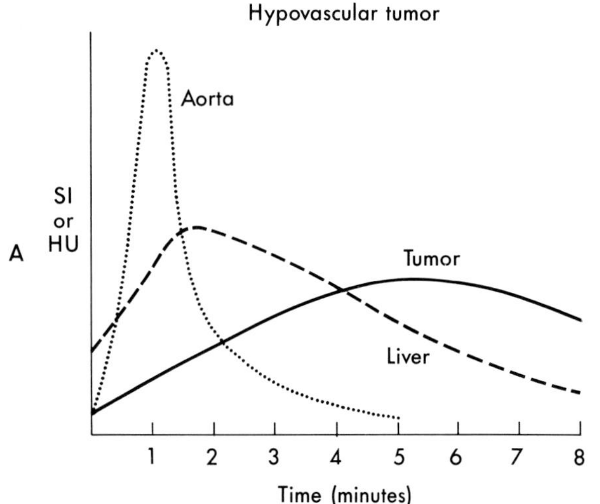

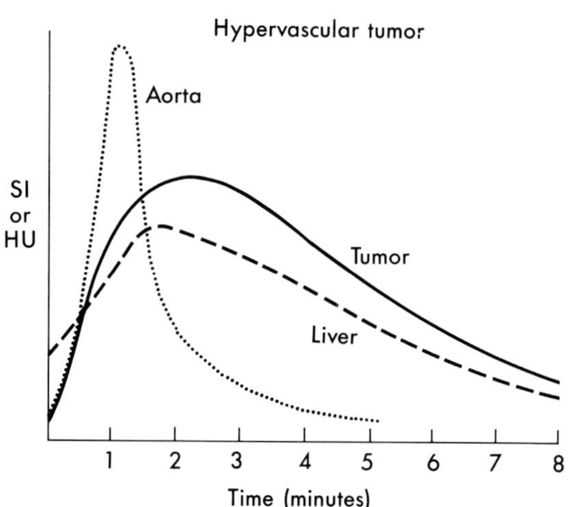

Fig. 8-1 Contrast-enhanced imaging of liver cancer. Intravenous administration of radiographic contrast media (or alternatively gadopentatate dimeglumine) by bolus abruptly increases intravascular (aortic) concentration followed by rapid distribution into the extravascular extracellular space. Clearance from the liver lags behind clearance from the intravascular space. **A,** Hypovascular tumors show delayed enhancement with maximal lesion-liver contrast at 1 to 3 minutes. Since tumor tissue has "leaky" capillaries and a large extracellular space, delayed enhancement may exceed that of liver tissue. **B,** Hypervascular tumors may show greater enhancement than the liver. Depending on vascularity and size of the extracellular compartment, tumor-liver contrast may be increased, decreased, or unchanged at various time points.

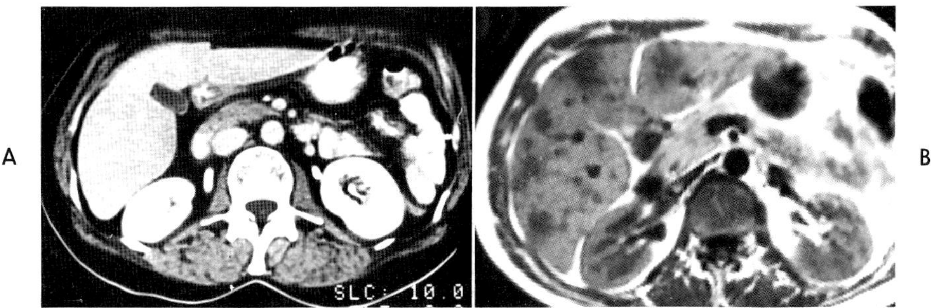

Fig. 8-2   Metastatic breast cancer. **A,** CT scan performed with dynamic bolus contrast administration was interpreted as normal. **B,** SE 300/14 image at 0.6T, obtained the same day, showing numerous metastases.

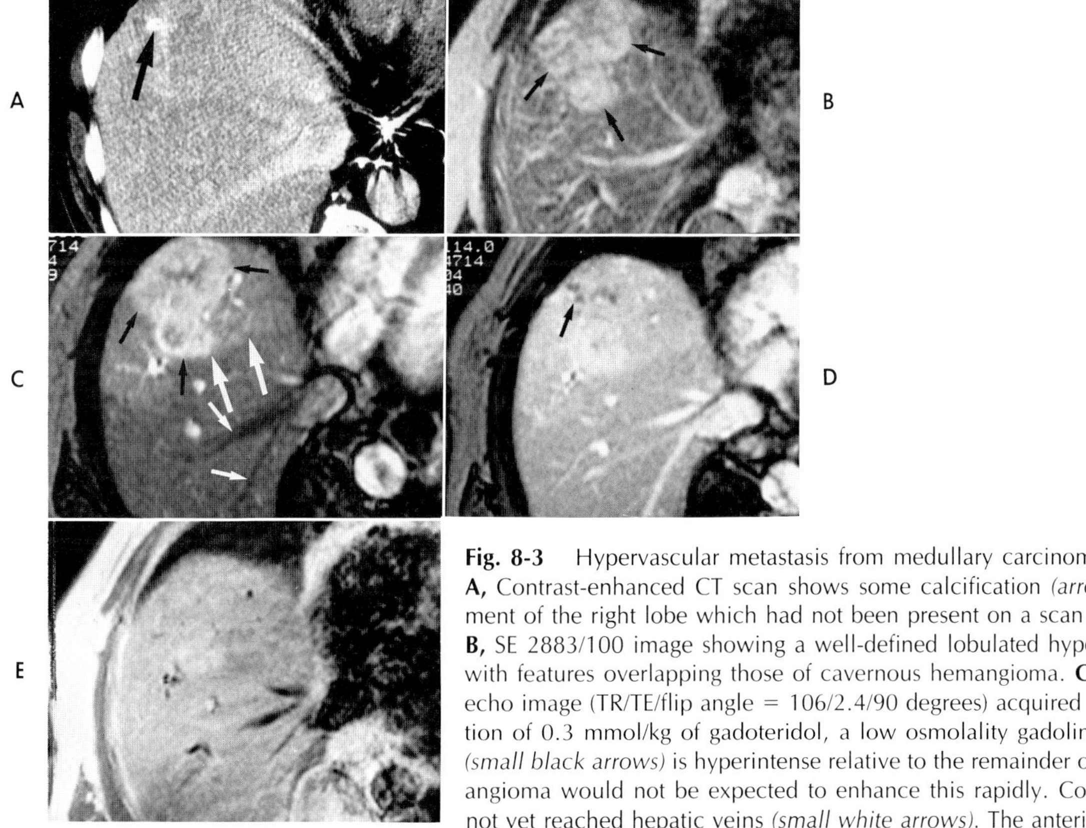

Fig. 8-3   Hypervascular metastasis from medullary carcinoma of the thyroid gland. **A,** Contrast-enhanced CT scan shows some calcification *(arrow)* in the anterior segment of the right lobe which had not been present on a scan performed 2 years ago. **B,** SE 2883/100 image showing a well-defined lobulated hyperintense mass *(arrows)*, with features overlapping those of cavernous hemangioma. **C,** T1-weighted gradient-echo image (TR/TE/flip angle = 106/2.4/90 degrees) acquired immediately after injection of 0.3 mmol/kg of gadoteridol, a low osmolality gadolineum chelate. The mass *(small black arrows)* is hyperintense relative to the remainder of the liver. A large hemangioma would not be expected to enhance this rapidly. Contrast enhancement has not yet reached hepatic veins *(small white arrows)*. The anterior portion of the liver is enhanced more than the posterior aspect, with a straight margin *(large white arrows)* suggesting vascular cause. This probably indicates increased arterial perfusion. **D,** With same imaging and photographic technique, 20 seconds later, the remainder of the liver has increased signal intensity and the hepatic veins have filled. The mass remains slightly more intensity than liver. *Arrow* indicates probable location of clacification. **E,** SE 500/11 image 15 minutes after contrast administration. The mass is only minimally hyperintense to liver.

ogeneous enhancement shortly after bolus injection, potentially mimicking lesions.[366] Regenerative nodules are isointense or hypointense on T2-weighted images,[262] in contrast to malignancies which are virtually always hyperintense. Heterogeneous fatty infiltration is also unlikely to cause hyperintensity on T2-weighted images, and can be characterized with confidence by using chemical shift imaging. These issues are explored in greater detail in later chapters.

COMPARATIVE STUDIES

In most comparisons, MRI has had greater* or similar[21,378,430,608] accuracy compared with contrast-enhanced CT (Figs. 8-2 to 8-4). These studies must be read critically, however, since it is nearly impossible to eliminate all sources of potential bias from comparative imaging studies; no study comparing MRI with CT performed thus far is immune from criticism.

In this section, we review the experience of four investigative centers who have attempted to compare the accuracy of MRI and CT for the detection of focal liver lesions. These centers are the Massachusetts General Hospital (MGH), the National Institutes of Health (NIH), Emory University, and the Mallinckrodt Institute of Radiology.

---

*36, 74, 148, 432, 454, 500, 564, 626

Massachusetts General Hospital

In the first comparative hepatic imaging study using optimized MRI techniques, a 0.6 T system was used at MGH to image 135 subjects, including 57 with metastases. MRI identified 64% of proven metastases, compared with 51% for CT (p<.001).[500] The sensitivity for identifying patients with metastases was similar, however (MRI 82%, CT 80%). In this study, spin-echo and inversion recovery T1-weighted images were most successful, with sensitivities of 64% and 65%, respectively, compared with 43% for T2-weighted sequences.

For a screening technique, sensitivity and specificity are both important. Since most patients do not have liver metastases, a high false-positive rate (low specificity) may lead to inappropriate treatment or additional tests. The specificity of MR in this series was 99% versus 94% for CT (p<.05).[500] Receiver operating characteristic (ROC) analysis of this data showed that MR was a better test than CT for screening patients at risk to develop hepatic metastases (Fig. 8-8).

The major limitation of this study was the lack of standardization of CT examinations, resulting in a significant bias in favor of MRI. CT examinations were included from multiple institutions and were thus considered representative of the "state of the community." MRI examinations, on the other hand, had rigorously optimized technique, arrived at based on careful consid-

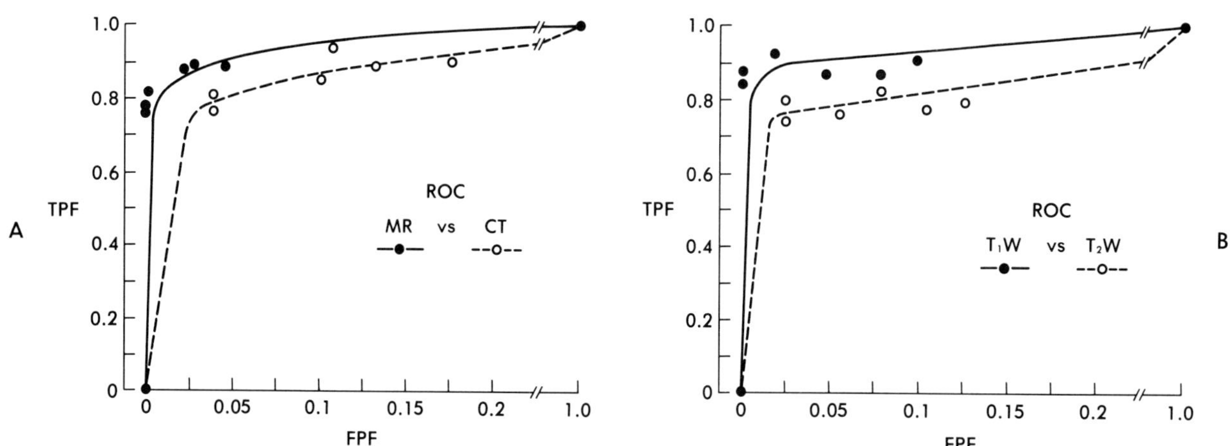

Fig. 8-8 Receiver operating characteristics (ROC) curves for the diagnosis of metastatic liver cancer at 0.6 T. The true-positive fraction is on the abscissa. **A,** ROC curves for a 1-hour, four-pulse sequence MR examination and contrast-enhanced CT. The area under the MR curve is greater than the area under the CT curve; therefore MR was superior for this test group of 90 patients. **B,** ROC curves for T1-weighted IR 1500/450/18 and T2-weighted SE 2000/120 pulse sequences. The T1-weighted technique outperformed the T2-weighted technique at every confidence level. Note that the T1-weighted pulse sequence alone outperformed CT **(A).** ROC curves are the accepted format for comparative analyses of the performance of diagnostic tests. (From Stark, D.D., Wittenberg, J., Butch, R.J., et al.: Radiology 165:399-406, 1987.)

erations of tissue contrast and motion-artifact suppression. TR was optimized to achieve optimum T1 contrast at 0.6 T, and TE was reduced beyond the manufacturer's capability by increasing gradient strength and sampling faster (see Chapter 1, Tissue Contrast). Motion artifact was reduced by obtaining the average of more than 10 signals, a practice that has never been implemented at many centers, although the resulting examination time is not longer than that of most T2-weighted images. It must also be noted that only the T1-weighted SE sequences were optimized, using appropriately minimized TR and TE and multiple averages to reduce motion-induced artifact. In contrast, the T2-weighted sequences did not include any artifact suppression or bandwidth optimization. The potential of optimized T2-weighted images to detect liver lesions, as well as techniques at other field strengths, was not evaluated.

In spite of these deficiencies, this study was important in that it showed that the accuracy of the community standard, CT, could be exceeded by optimized midfield MRI. Subsequently, other centers were given added impetus to investigate abdominal MRI and to compare it with higher quality CT examinations.

National Institutes of Health

At the NIH, earlier investigations had established the utility of using a soluble intravenous liposoluble contrast agent, EOE-13, to label the reticuloendothelial system for hepatic CT. In one study from this institution, 77% of lesions were detected by CT with EOE-13, compared with only 34% by CT enhanced by conventional water-soluble contrast. Although this agent has not been available at most other centers because of undesirable side effects, its availability at the NIH has provided these investigators with an effective "gold standard" for the detection of hepatic metastases.

Like the early work at the MGH, investigators at the NIH found midfield (0.5 T) T2-weighted images suboptimal, detecting only 53% of lesions in a study of 25 patients with a total of 162 lesions.[430] This disappointing sensitivity was similar to the performance of noncontrast CT (50%). As at MGH, however, bandwidth was not optimized and motion artifact was not suppressed. T1-weighted images had significantly higher sensitivities of 96% and 90% for SE 300/26 and STIR (TR/TI/TE = 1500/100/30), respectively. In fact, the sensitivity of these MRI techniques was at least as good as the 88% sensitivity of EOE-13 enhanced CT.

In a later prospective study at this institution, including 20 patients with surgically proven lesions, the authors compared midfield MRI with three different CT techniques, each of which has been shown to be more sensitive than bolus-enhanced CT. These included EOE-13 enhanced CT, CT with arterial portography (CTAP), and CT 4 to 6 hours after a large dose of water-soluble iodinated contrast (delayed CT).[574] There was no significant difference between the sensitivities of SE 300/20 MRI (84%), EOE-CT (83%), CTAP (78%), and delayed CT (82%). The sensitivity of SE 2000/80 MRI (64%) was significantly lower, even though gradient moment nulling and four averages were used to suppress motion-induced artifact. False-positive rates were lowest for SE 300/20 MRI (3%), and highest for CTAP (31%). It is not certain why the results of CTAP are inferior to those reported by other institutions.[200,324,378] Reporting on many of the same patients, these investigators also noted comparable sensitivity (90%) at 1.5 T, using an IR technique with TR/TI/TE = 2000/600/20.[430]

The major deficiency of these studies is that MRI was not compared with the current community standard, bolus-enhanced CT. It is notable, however, that MRI performed similar to other CT techniques that compare favorably with bolus enhancement.[336]

Emory

Investigators at Emory have had considerable experience with hepatic imaging at both 0.5 T and 1.5 T. To investigate 0.5 T MRI, these investigators collaborated with investigators at New York University.[74] Bolus-enhanced and delayed CT were compared with SE 250-300/20 and IR 1200-1400/400/20-30 techniques. Unfortunately, no motion-artifact suppression was used.

Of 59 patients in the study, 27 patients had a total of 93 lesions, although not all were surgically proven. Sensitivities were bolus CT (90%), delayed CT (83%), combined CT (96%), IR MRI (90%), SE MRI (81%), and combined MRI (91%).

In this study, MRI and CT were comparable for detection of hepatic metastases. Four of the 32 patients without metastases had extrahepatic disease detected by CT but missed by MRI. Thus the results of this study supported the continued use of CT for screening patients with suspected metastases, although the MRI techniques that were used were suboptimal in that motion artifact was not suppressed.

Subsequently, hepatic imaging at 1.5 T was evaluated in collaboration with investigators from the Medical College of Wisconsin.[564] Here again, unfortunately, MRI technique was not standardized. Of 69 patients, only 32% had T2-weighted images with gradient moment nulling, whereas 35 patients had T2-weighted images with no motion-artifact suppression. In spite of this limitation, the sensitivity of T2-weighted images for confident detection of hepatic lesions (78%) was comparable with that of bolus-enhanced CT (70%) and delayed CT (71%). For lesions smaller than 1 cm, however, the sensitivity of T2-weighted MRI (76%) was significantly greater than that of bolus-enhanced CT (56%) and delayed CT (31%) (p<.006). The shortest TE available at that time for T1-weighted images was 20 msec. Thus these images were inferior to CT and

T2-weighted MRI. In five patients, lymph nodes were seen only by CT, although three patients had adrenal masses seen only by MRI.

In a small series involving 43 patient studies comparing CTAP and delayed CT with MRI performed at either 0.5 or 1.5 T, CTAP was the most sensitive modality (85%).[378] The combined sensitivity of CTAP and delayed CT (85%) was not significantly better. Importantly, the highest sensitivity (96%) resulted when the results of CTAP and MRI were combined, indicating that CTAP and MRI may be complimentary for appropriate patients.

Mallinckrodt

Early Mallinckrodt studies, performed at 0.35 T, were compromised by machine restrictions that required TEs of 30 msec or longer. MRI and CT were comparable.[199] In a more recent study, these investigators restricted their analysis to 37 lesions in eight patients verified pathologically after partial hepatic resection.[200] This is considerably more sensitive than simple surgical inspection, which misses approximately 6% of lesions noted at autopsy.[336] CTAP was most sensitive (81%), followed by MRI (57%), and delayed CT (52%). Importantly, the sensitivity of bolus-enhanced CT, the current standard of practice, was only 38%. Of 18 lesions smaller than 1 cm, CTAP detected 61% and MRI 17%, whereas delayed and bolus-enhanced CT detected none.

ABDOMINAL LYMPH NODES

Although the consensus appears to be building that MRI is more accurate than CT for detecting, characterizing, and excluding liver lesions, CT remains the current clinical standard at most centers. One reason for this is the current superiority of CT at most centers for detecting extrahepatic abdominal pathology.[21,74,564] Since extrahepatic lesions detectable by CT occur in 10% of patients at risk for hepatic metastases, the choice between CT and MR is complex.[5,200] The need to detect extrahepatic lesions must be balanced against the risk and cost of CT contrast material, the relative availability and cost of MRI and CT, and the superiority

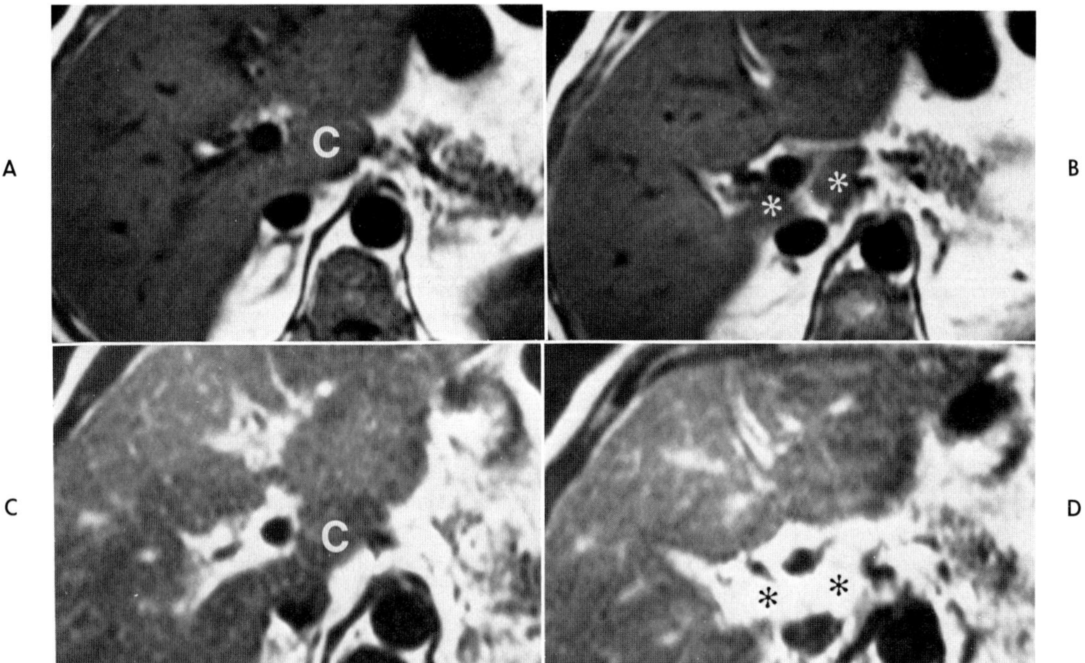

Fig. 8-9 Surgically proven periportal lymph nodes missed by CT, detected definitively by comparison of T1-weighted and T2-weighted MR images at 1.5 T. **A,** SE 400/12 image shows a slightly prominent caudate lobe (C). **B,** Inferior to **A,** two soft tissue structures are identified (asterisks) that are consistent with either the inferior portion of caudate lobe or large lymph nodes. The CT scan was interpreted similarly. **C,** SE 2500/100 image corresponding to **A,** depicting the enlarged caudate lobe (C). **D,** SE 2500/100 image corresponding to **B.** The lymph nodes (asterisks) are more intense than fat, excluding the possibility of partial volume effect from caudate lobe. At surgery, large lymph nodes were found, but they were due to inflammation.

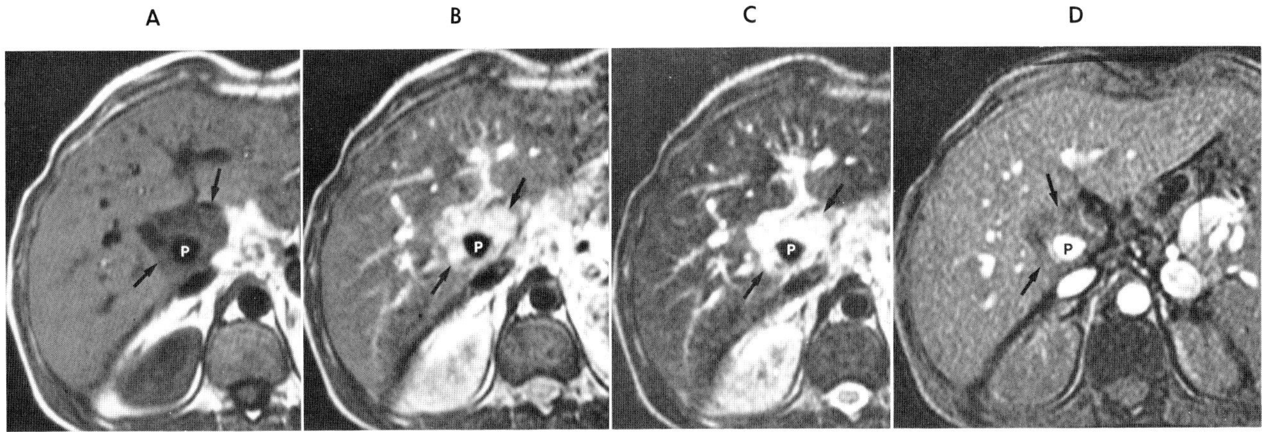

Fig. 8-10   Benign periportal lymph nodes *(arrows)* in a patient with viral hepatitis, depicted at 1.5 T. *P* = portal vein. **A,** SE 400/12. **B,** SE 2500/50. **C,** SE 2500/100. **D,** Gradient-echo image (27/7.4/20 degrees). The nodes are confluent but do not compress the portal vein. This is typical of benign lyphadenopathy.

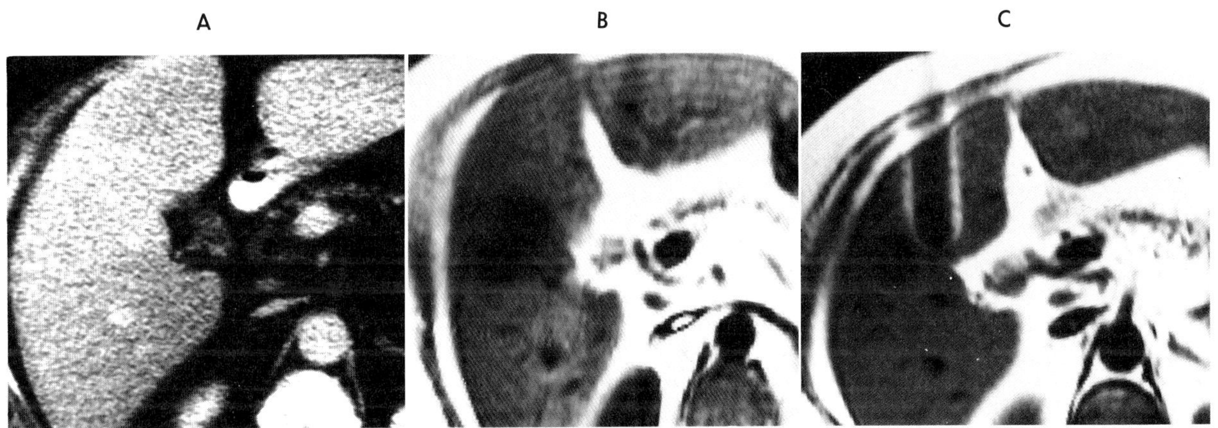

Fig. 8-11   MR detection and guided biopsy at 0.6 T in a patient having an elevated carcinoid embryonic antigen (CEA) titer. No previous evidence of recurrence or metastatic disease. **A,** Dynamic bolus contrast-enhanced CT scan is normal. **B,** SE 260/15 MR image showed a pair of 2-cm metastases in the right hepatic lobe. **C,** Histologic proof was required to justify chemotherapy or excisional surgery. MR was used to guide percutaneous fine-needle biopsy. The needle tip is positioned within the more anterior lesion. A ferromagnetic artifact consisting of a dark central region and two parallel bright lines outlines the needle shaft.

of MRI for imaging the liver itself.

Effective suppression of motion-induced artifact and the use of thinner sections improves depiction of abdominal lymph nodes. Careful comparison of T1-weighted and T2-weighted images is necessary for detection of lymph nodes, since nodes may be nearly isointense with liver on T1-weighted images and nearly isointense with fat on T2-weighted images (see Figs. 1-3, 8-9 and 8-10). The ability to distinguish confidently between liver and lymph node on T2-weighted images is a significant advantage of MRI over CT, provided motion artifact is controlled sufficiently.

Ultrafast MRI techniques are likely to improve the efficacy and decrease the cost of MRI. Routine use of faster pulse sequences and oral contrast medium is also likely to improve detection of extrahepatic disease. The accuracy and speed of MRI will also be improved by the use of appropriate contrast enhancement. The wider availability of MR guided liver biopsies (Fig. 8-11) will expand the clinical utility of MRI even further.[367] It is our opinion that MRI will replace CT as the primary modality for imaging the liver and upper abdomen.

PART

II

FOCAL HEPATIC DISEASE

At most centers, suspected focal pathology is the major indication for hepatic imaging. Success at this endeavor depends on high spatial resolution, high contrast between lesion and hepatic parenchyma, and the ability to distinguish between significant and insignificant pathology. Although the spatial resolution of CT remains superior, MRI has higher contrast resolution and is more capable of characterizing focal lesions. In this section, we examine the MRI features of various focal lesions and how they differ from each other.

On T1-weighted images, the liver and pancreas have higher signal intensity than most other nonfatty tissues in the abdomen. The short T1 relaxation times of liver and pancreas are probably due to the large surface area of endoplasmic reticulum in organs such as these that are active in protein synthesis.[57,153,346] Thus, even though the signal intensity on T1-weighted images of malignant lesions may resemble that of other solid organs, there is usually abundant contrast between liver and lesion.

Although the increased sensitivity of MRI compared with other modalities is important, its ability to characterize pathology is an even greater advantage (Table II-1). T2-weighted sequences show significant differences in the internal structure

Table II-1   MRI Features of Focal Hepatic Lesions

| | Signal Intensity Relative to Liver | | | | | |
	T1	T2	Margins	Central Features	Ring, Halo, or Target	Capsule
Benign						
Cavernous hemongioma	−	+ +	smooth lobulated	homogeneous, or sparse, low signal defects	−	−
Cyst	− −	+ +	smooth	homogeneous	−	−
Metastases	−	+	indistinct	homogeneous or heterogenous	+	−
Hepatocellular						
Hepatocellular carcinoma	−,0,+	−,0,+	variable	heterogeneous or nodular	rare	+
Hyperplastic nodule	0,+	−,0	smooth	homogeneous	−	−
Focal nodular hyperplasia	−,0	0,+	smooth	scar	−	−
Hepatocellular adenoma	−,0,+	0,+	smooth	homogeneous or scar	−	rare

of various hepatic tumors.[451] Furthermore, tissue signal-intensity relationships or ratios on T1-weighted images, assessed visually or by measurement, can usually distinguish hemangiomas and cysts from malignant tumors. However, less common benign lesions that are composed of solid tissue may have features similar to those of malignant lesions. T1-weighted images are valuable for diagnosing and characterizing well-differentiated hepatocellular tumors. T1 and T2 calculations derived from a series of images confirm differences among hepatic lesions but are unreliable in individual cases, require strict attention to consistent methodology, and are seldom used for clinical diagnosis.

Most reports on MRI features of focal lesions have emphasized the distinction between metastases and common benign lesions, such as cavernous hemangiomas and cysts. It is important to recognize hepatocellular tumors as a third category, however, since benign and malignant hepatocellular tumors share certain histologic and imaging features that often complicate diagnosis. We also consider other focal lesions, such as abscess and hemorrhage.

Hepatic Metastases

The liver is the most common site in which remote metastases occur. Accurate diagnosis of hepatic metastases is critical for management of patients with gastrointestinal, pancreatic, breast, lung, and other malignancies. It is estimated that more than 3 million patients annually undergo screening examinations by CT, sonography, scintigraphy, or MRI, primarily to detect hepatic metastases. Among hospitalized patients, metastases are the most common liver tumor. In the general population, however, cavernous hemangiomas are more common and can mimic the appearance of metastases when imaged by CT, sonography, or scintigraphy.

We recommend MRI as the initial screening test for patients at risk for hepatic metastases. In selected patients, such as potential candidates for surgical resection of hepatic metastases, CT with arterial portography (CTAP) is a valuable second test to exclude additional lesions. CTAP is too expensive and invasive, however, for initial screening.

Metastases often have homogeneous internal morphology and well-defined margins,[49] but 25% have a central increase in signal intensity on T2-weighted images, indicating increased water content, necrosis, and/or hemorrhage.[187,451,607] This morphology is depicted as a target configuration (Figs. 9-1 to 9-6). T1-weighted images may show this finding as a central decrease in signal intensity (see Figs. 9-1 and 9-4). This appearance is not seen in hemangiomas or cysts. Discrepant signal features between the central and peripheral portions of a mass are a strong indicator of malignancy, since benign lesions should not have central necrosis or reactive changes in adjacent hepatic parenchyma. Confusion can occur, however, because of central scars that may be present in benign or malignant hepatocellular masses.

Approximately 20% of metastases on T2-weighted images have a bright halo surrounding a less intense nodule (Figs. 9-7 and 9-8). This finding is not seen on T1-weighted images. Peripheral halos can also be seen with hepatocellular carcinoma but have not been reported with benign noninflammatory lesions.[187,453,607] When histologic findings were correlated with high-resolution MRI findings of resected colorectal metastases to liver, the peripheral high signal represented viable tumor surrounding low-signal necrosis, rather than peritumoral edema (see Fig. 9-7) (see also Color Plate IV).[399] True peritumoral edema may occur, however, if the tumor causes vascular and/or biliary obstruction (see Figs. 9-1 and 9-2). Rarely, low-signal capsules may surround hepatic metastases (Fig. 9-9), although this finding is far more common with hepatocellular carcinoma.

With heavily T2-weighted sequences, tumors other than hemangiomas and cysts show a loss of intensity and margin sharpness (Figs. 9-8, 9-10 and 9-11).[49,451,607] Tumors with central liquefaction necrosis or increased vascularity often have long T2 relaxation times and may have relatively increased signal intensity on late-echo images. However, necrotic tumors nearly always have irregular internal morphology, mural nodules, a solid tissue rim, or an indistinct interface with adjacent liver, distinguishing them from hemangiomas or cysts (see Figs. 9-2, 9-3, 9-12, and 9-13).[187,450,607] Furthermore, MR often detects multiple additional solid metastases without necrosis. However, inproper photography compressing the dynamic range for depiction of high-signal tissues can interfere with differential diagnosis (Fig. 9-13). Images should be photographed so high-signal masses are bright but not absolute white. Rarely, hypervascular metastases can mimic hemangiomas on unenhanced images (Fig. 9-14). Dynamic imaging may help in these cases, showing early enhancement.

Metastases from malignant melanoma may be hyperintense on T1-weighted images and hypointense on T2-weighted images (Fig. 9-15). Studies with melanoma metastatic to brain indicate that the paramagnetic effects of melanin are an important cause of this unusual signal pattern.[12] Hemorrhagic tumors may also have foci of high signal on T1-weighted images (see Figs. 9-4 and 9-5).

Administration of extracellular contrast agents such as gadopentatate dimeglumine provides an additional parameter for characaterizing focal hepatic masses. Even hypervascular tumors, which are supplied almost entirely by hepatic arteries, usually have less blood pool than the liver, which receives approximately two thirds of its perfusion from the portal vein. Contrast between liver and malignant lesions is therefore increased in

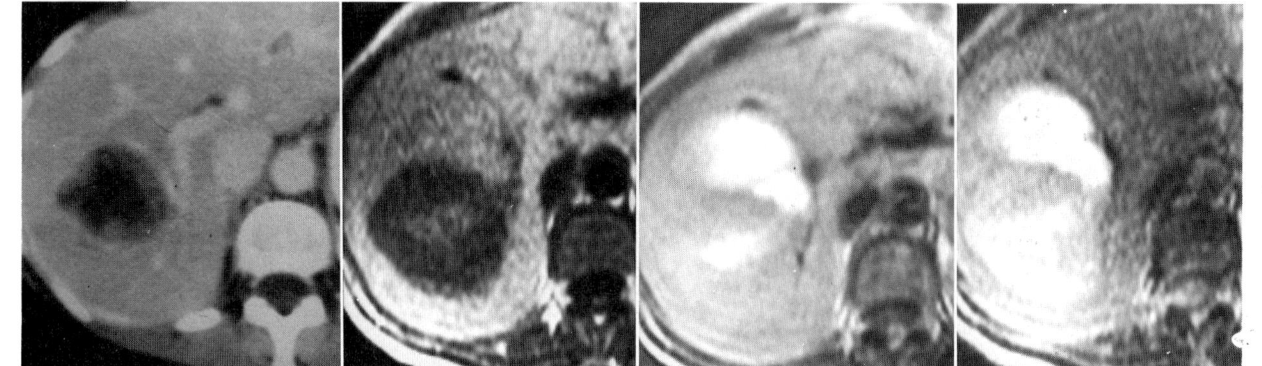

Fig. 9-3   Central necrosis within colloid carcinoma metastatic from the colon. **A,** SE 2500/80 image depicts central necrosis *(N)* with peripheral intermediate intensity. **B,** Histologic section from the center of the tumor showing mucin and debris, accounting for high intensity. (From Outwater, E., Tomaszewski, J.E., Daly, J.M., et al.: Radiology 180:327-332, 1991.)

Fig. 9-4   Hemorrhage into a necrotic breast metastasis. **A,** CT scan shows rim enhancement. **B,** SE 260/18 image at 0.6 T shows a right hepatic lobe lesion with a bull's-eye on the T1-weighted images. Note elevation of the right portal vein. **C,** SE 2000/60 T2-weighted image shows central hypointensity, corresponding to the center of the bull's-eye on the T1-weighted images. This central collection is seen extending to the margin of the lesion, where a second high-intensity collection is elevating the right portal vein. On the T1-weighted image **(B)** the fluid is higher in signal intensity than tumor (and isointense to liver), since it contains paramagnetic hemoglobin degradation products. **D,** SE 2000/120 image.

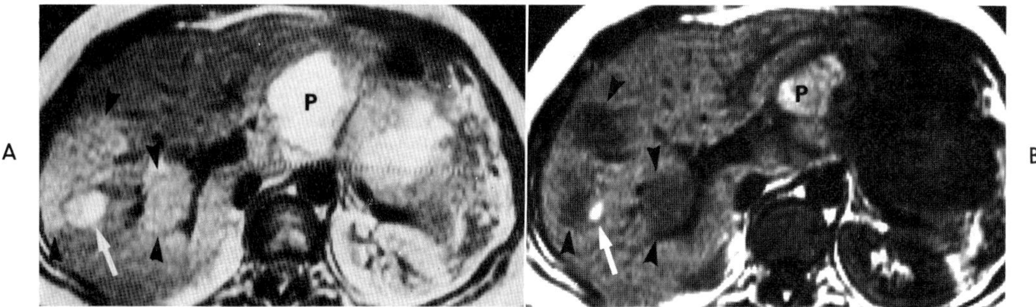

Fig. 9-5   Hemorrhage into metastatic pancreatic islet cell cancer. **A,** SE 2000/60. Areas of tumor tissue are heterogeneous, irregular, and poorly defined *(arrowheads)*. Hemorrhage into primary pancreatic tumor *(P)* is also seen. **B,** IR 1500/450/30. Areas of tumor tissue are of low intensity *(arrowheads)*. Hemorrhage *(arrow)* has high signal intensity and can thereby be distinguished from normal blood-filled cavernous hemangiomas.

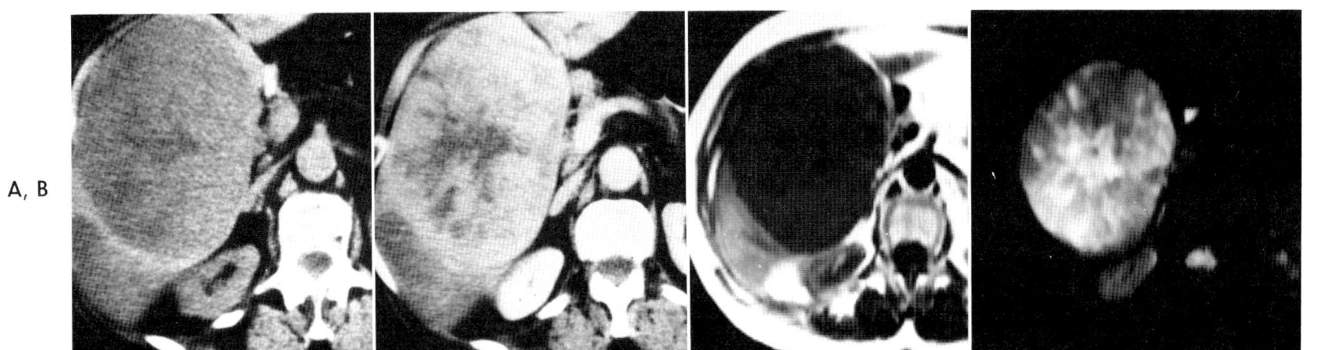

Fig. 9-6   Asymptomatic 80-year-old woman with a mass palpated during a routine physical examination. Liver function tests were normal. Biopsy was obtained after MR findings contradicted other imaging studies. **A,** Noncontrast CT scan. A giant cavernous hemangioma was suspected. **B,** Bolus contrast, hemangioma protocol shows peripheral rim enhancement and hyperintensity relative to surrounding liver. Cavernous hemangiomas of this size rarely fill in completely. **C,** SE 300/14 image at 0.6 T shows a sharply circumscribed lesion with some barely perceptible internal inhomogeneity. **D,** SE 2400/180 image demonstrates grape-like low-intensity nodules separated by high-intensity central fluid. Biopsy confirmed the MR diagnosis of necrotic neoplasm (anaplastic sarcoma).

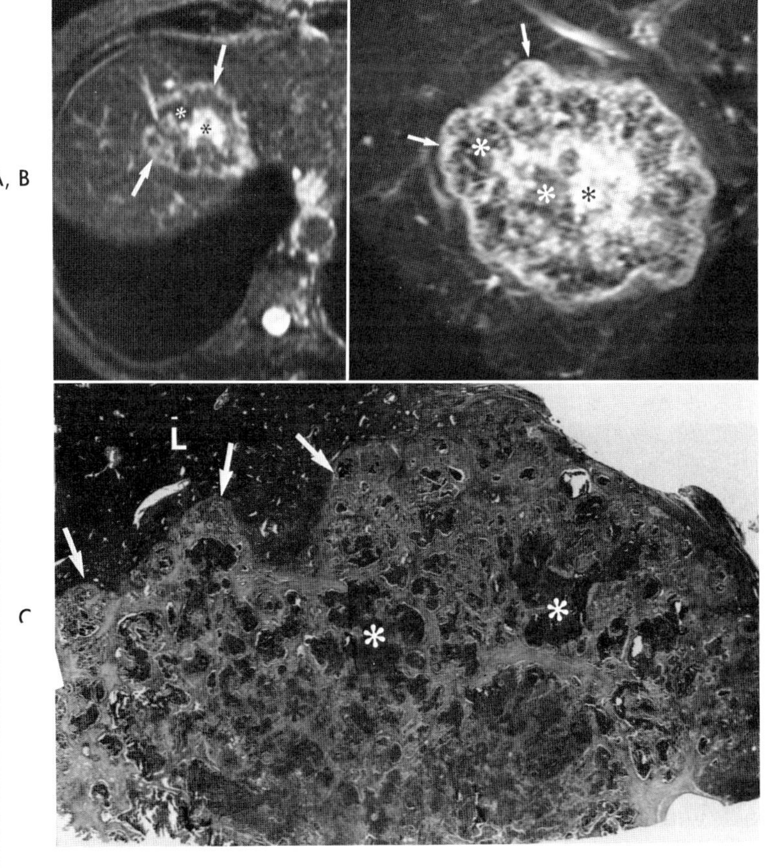

Fig. 9-7   Peripheral halo secondary to proven viable tumor with central low signal secondary to coagulative necrosis. **A,** SE 2500/80 image at 1.5 T shows a heterogeneous tumor that has low signal *(white asterisk)* except for the center *(black asterisk)* and a peripheral rim *(arrows)*. **B,** SE 2500/80 image obtained with a surface coil of left lobectomy specimen shows the same signal characteristics. **C,** Histologic section of right half of tumor (trichrome stain) shows advancing cellular tumor rim *(arrows)*. Areas of low signal on MR images correspond to coagulative necrosis *(white asterisks)*, which are stained dark red, and fibrosis, which are stained blue. High intensity foci in **A** and **B** represent accumulations of cell debris *(black asterisks)* in the center of the tumor. *L* = liver. (See Color Plate IV.) (From Outwater, E., Tomaszewski, J.E., Daly, J.M., and Kressel, H.Y.: Radiology 180:327-332, 1991.)

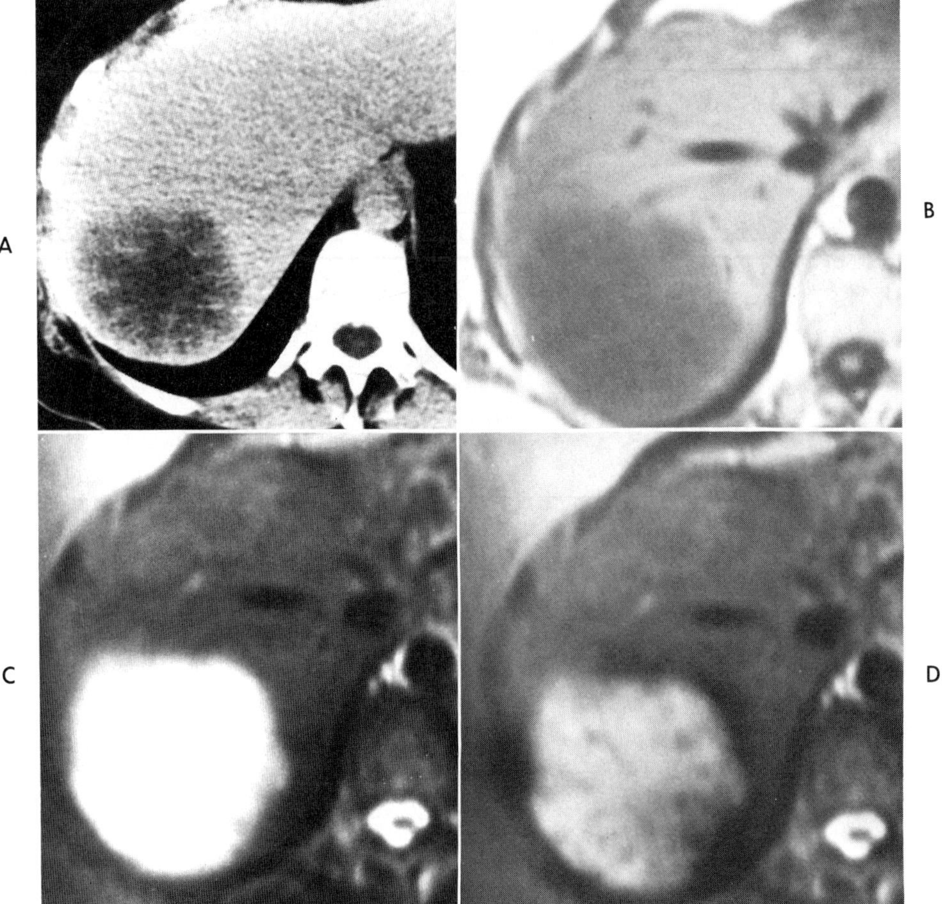

Fig. 9-13 Necrotic metastasis from colorectal carcinoma. **A,** Contrast-enhanced CT image shows a low-attenuation lesion with decreased attenuation centrally. **B,** Axial SE 600/20 image at 1.5 T shows the lesion to be larger than indicated by the CT scan. **C,** Axial T2-weighted (SE 2500/80) image shows marked hyperintensity, consistent with necrosis. Distinction from hemangioma is difficult from this image due to improper photography. **D,** With proper photography, the lesions is less intense than cerebrospinal fluid and has complex internal morphology and indistinct margins.

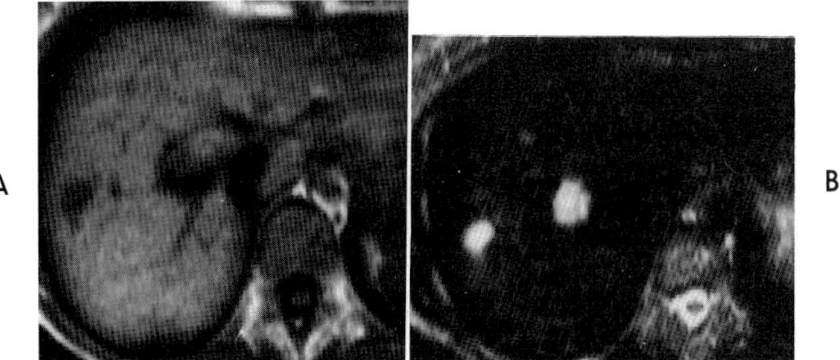

Fig. 9-14 Islet cell cancer metastatic to the liver. **A,** IR 1500/450/20 image at 0.6 T shows two focal hepatic lesions, 1.5 and 2.0 cm in size. **B** SE 2000/180 image shows the lesions to have an extremely high signal intensity, indistinguishable from cavernous hemangioma. The lesions are too small for evaluation of internal morphology.

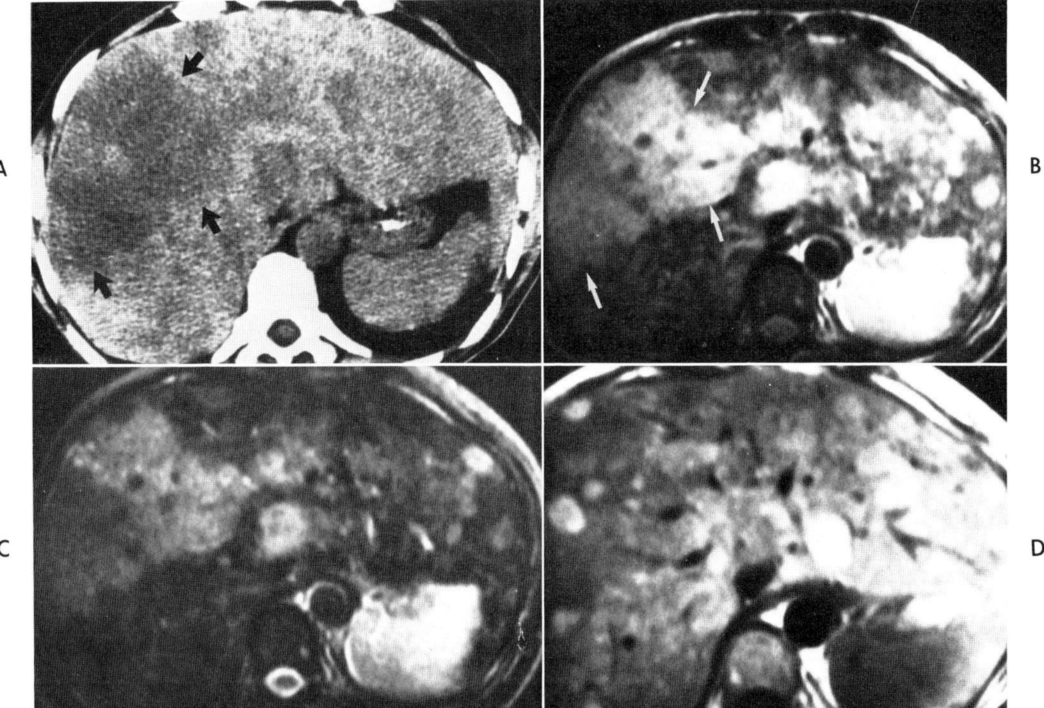

Fig. 9-15 Anomalous signal characteristics in metastases from malignant melanoma. **A,** CT scan without contrast reveals a heterogeneous liver, most consistent with widespread metastases. There are no foci of high signal to suggest hemorrhage. Note the wedge-shaped region of low attenuation in the anterior segment of the right lobe *(arrows),* suggestive of segmental vascular obstruction. **B,** Corresponding T2-weighted image (SE 2500/50) reveals a wedge-shaped hyperintense zone *(arrows),* corresponding to the low attenuation zone seen in **A. C,** SE 2500/100 image. **D,** Axial T1-weighted image (SE400/12) at 1.5 T reveals numerous high-signal masses throughout the liver. Corresponding image with fat suppresion demonstrated high signal of the masses, proving that the high signal was not due to fat. Most of the lesions that were hyperintense in **B** and **C** are isointense with liver. Several hyperintense lesions can be seen, however, which were not seen on the T2-weighted images.

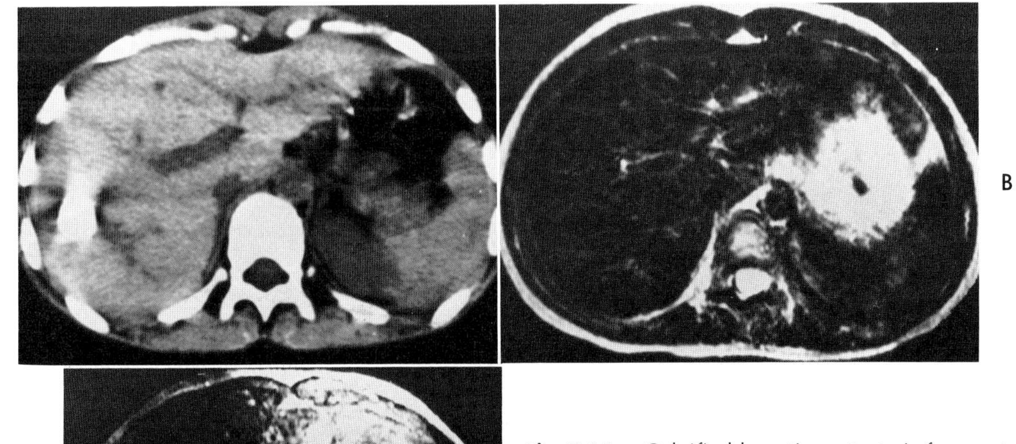

Fig. 9-16 Calcified hepatic metastasis from osteogenic sarcoma. **A,** Unenhanced CT scan reveals a densely calcified mass in the right lobe. **B,** SE 2000/100 image. The mass *(arrow)* has low signal. **C,** Gradient-echo image (50/18, flip angle 30 degrees). The rim of the tumor is more obvious on the gradient-echo image. The liver and spleen have decreased intensity because of transfusional siderosis. (Courtesy L. te Strake.)

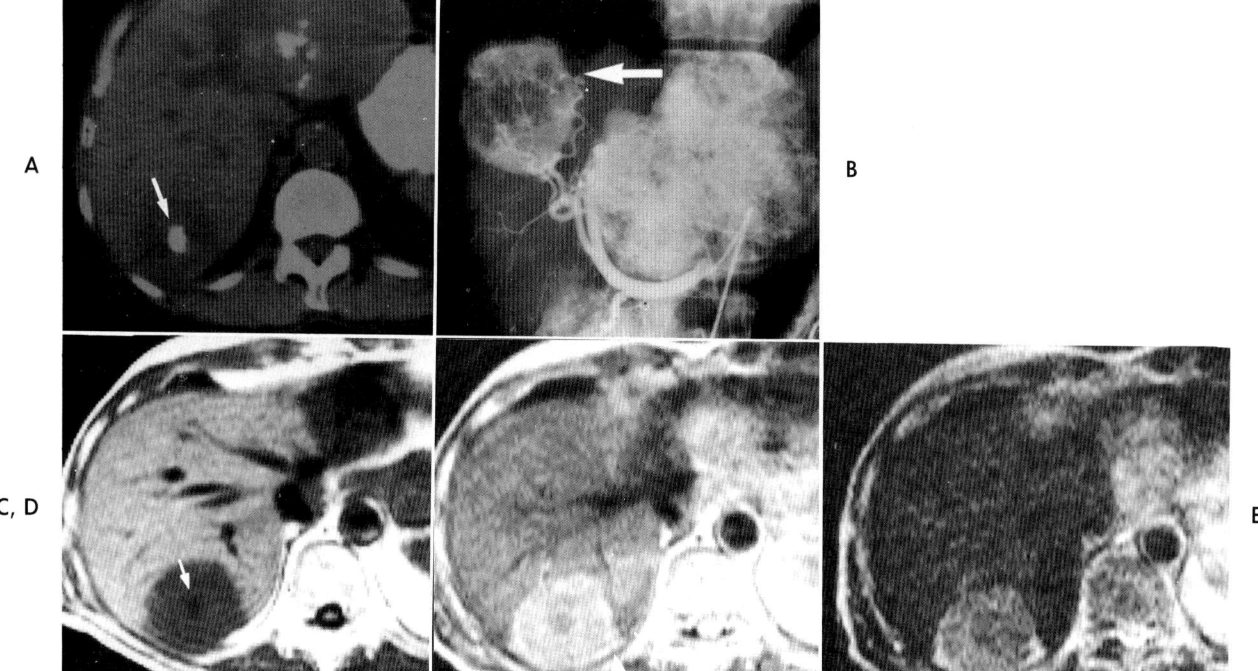

Fig. 9-17 Metastatic pancreatic islet cell cancer. Hypervascular gastrinoma metastases show MR features that suggest a specific diagnosis of metastatic cancer. **A,** CT scan shows calcified hepatic metastases. **B,** Angiogram demonstrates hypervascularity of the metastasis in the right hepatic lobe *(arrow)*. **C,** SE 260/18 image at 0.6 T. The central calcification *(arrow)* is shown as a focal region of low signal intensity. **D,** SE 2000/60 image shows a peripheral high-intensity rim *(arrow)*. **E,** SE 2000/120 image better shows the rim, and loss of lesion-liver CNR clearly distinguishes this tumor from cavernous hemangioma.

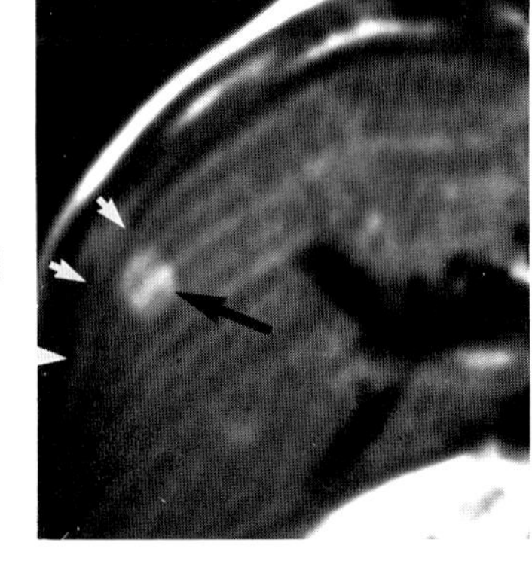

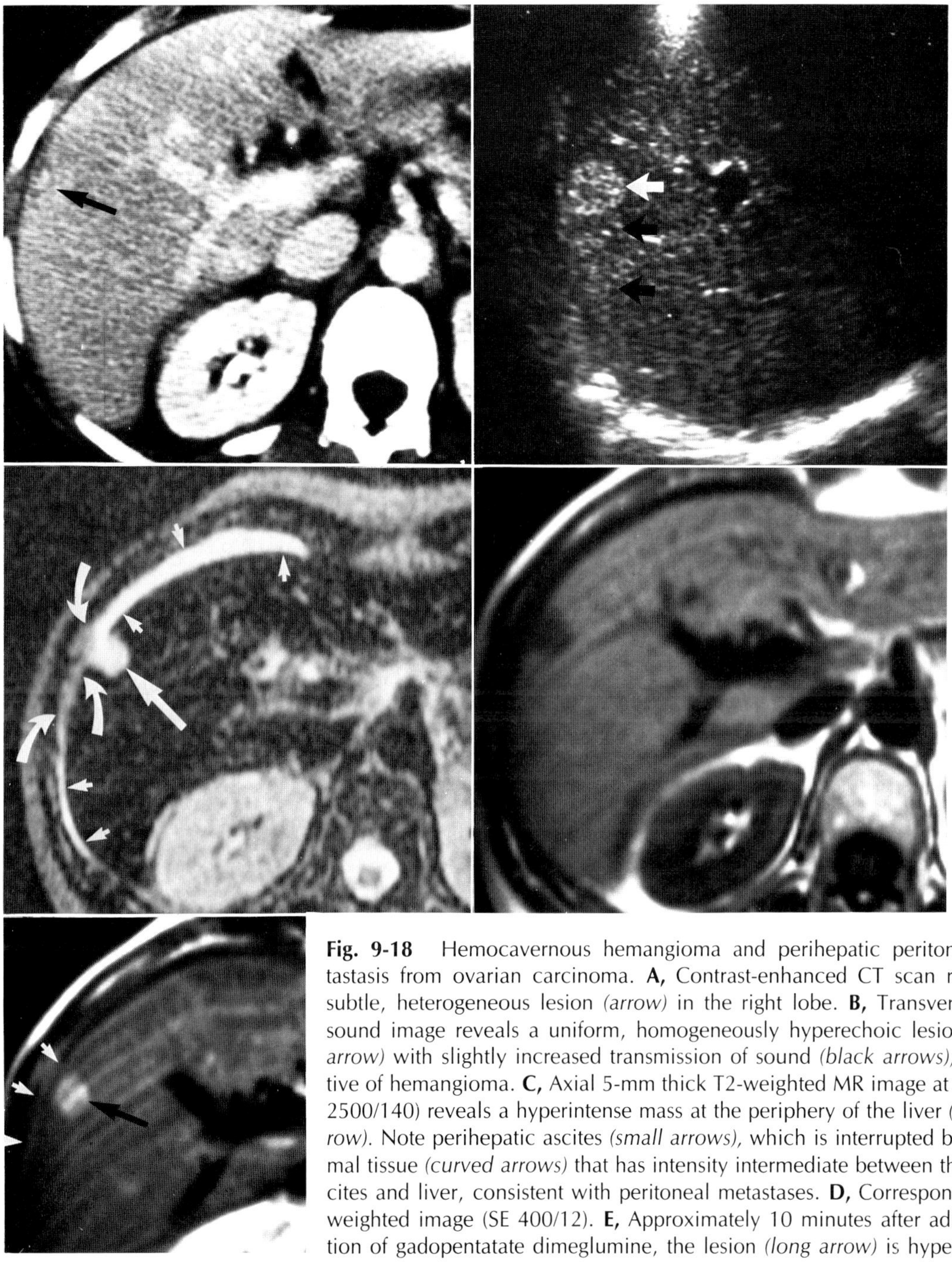

Fig. 9-18 Hemocavernous hemangioma and perihepatic peritoneal metastasis from ovarian carcinoma. **A,** Contrast-enhanced CT scan reveals a subtle, heterogeneous lesion *(arrow)* in the right lobe. **B,** Transverse ultrasound image reveals a uniform, homogeneously hyperechoic lesion *(white arrow)* with slightly increased transmission of sound *(black arrows),* suggestive of hemangioma. **C,** Axial 5-mm thick T2-weighted MR image at 1.5T (SE 2500/140) reveals a hyperintense mass at the periphery of the liver *(large arrow).* Note perihepatic ascites *(small arrows),* which is interrupted by abnormal tissue *(curved arrows)* that has intensity intermediate between that of ascites and liver, consistent with peritoneal metastases. **D,** Corresponding T1-weighted image (SE 400/12). **E,** Approximately 10 minutes after administration of gadopentatate dimeglumine, the lesion *(long arrow)* is hyperintense, consistent with cavernous hemangioma. Note, however, that the adjacent peritoneal metastases *(small arrows)* have enhanced slightly and are now more intense than the perihepatic ascites (compare with **D**).

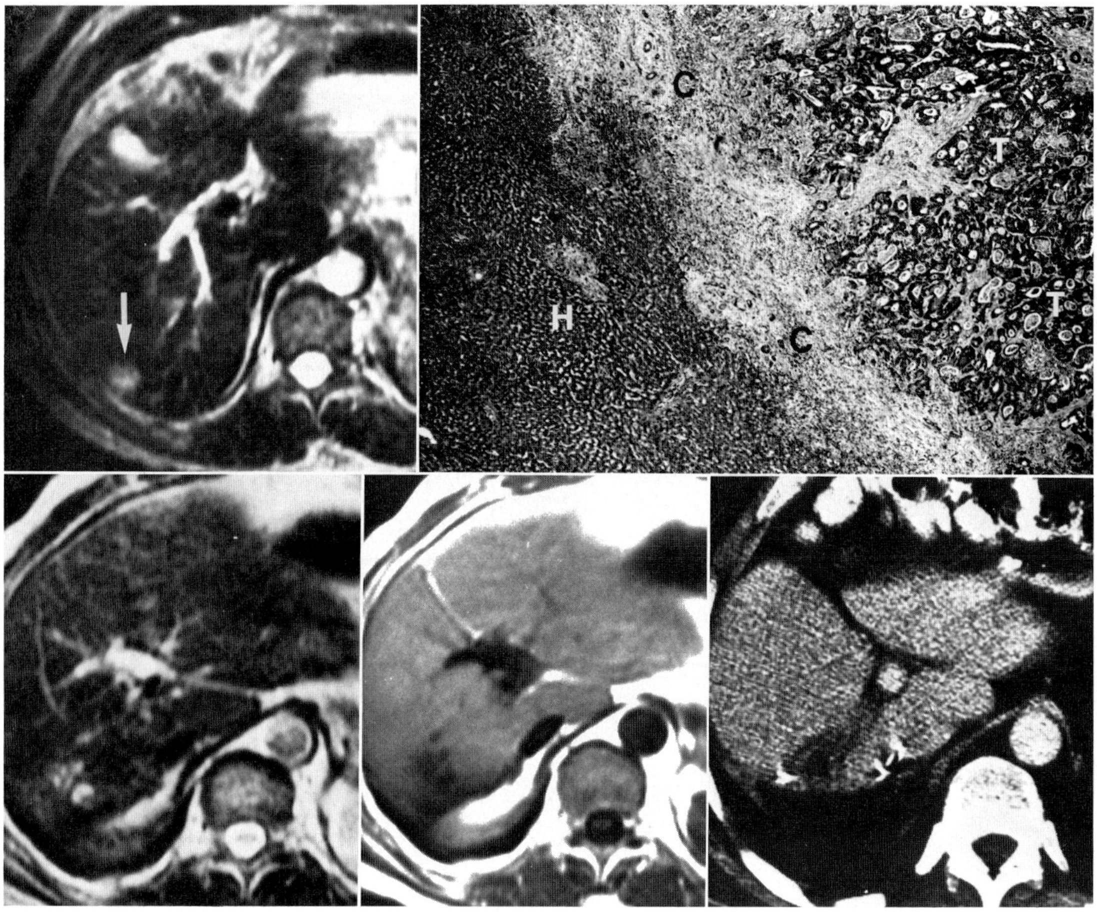

Fig. 9-19 Solitary metastasis from colonic carcinoma treated by segmental resection. **A,** Preoperative T2-weighted image at 1.5 T (SE 3000/80) reveals a solitary heterogeneous lesion *(arrow)* in the posterior segment of the right lobe. The margins are not distinct, and it is much less intense than the cerebrospinal fluid. **B,** Histologic section at the margin between tumor *(T)* and hepatic parenchyma *(H),* demonstrating a reactive pseudocapsule *(C),* accounting for the indistinct margin. **C,** After surgery (SE 2500/100), some high signal is noted at the site of resection, but there is no tumor mass. **D,** Corresponding T1-weighted (SE 400/12) image. **E,** Corresponding CT image. Follow-up scan 1 year later (not shown) was unchanged.

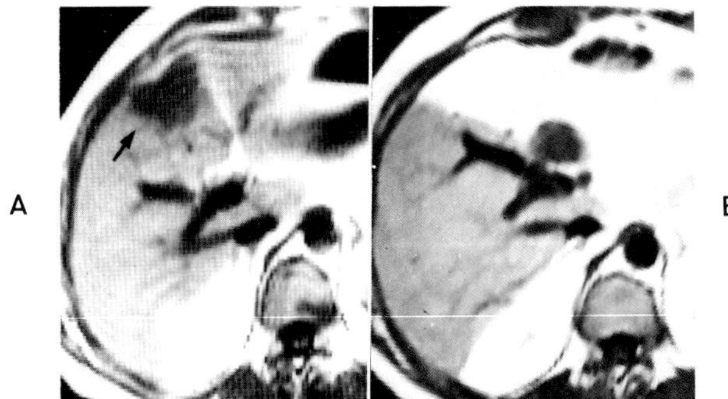

Fig. 9-20 Resection of metastatic colon cancer by extended left hepatectomy. **A,** SE 260/15 image at 0.6T. A solitary metastasis is seen in the medial segment of the left hepatic lobe. **B,** Postoperative SE 260/14 image show no evidence of recurrence. The left lobe was removed by dissection anterior to the right portal vein.

Common Benign Hepatic Lesions

Cavernous hemangiomas and cysts are far more common than other benign hepatic lesions. They may be difficult to distinguish from each other on unenhanced MR images, but this distinction is not important since neither of these lesions requires treatment. Fortunately, hemangiomas and cysts can be distinguished from malignant tumors by MRI in the vast majority of patients.

CAVERNOUS HEMANGIOMA

Cavernous hemangioma is the most common benign hepatic neoplasm. Experience with imaging techniques, such as sonography, MR, and angiography, suggests that its worldwide incidence is approximately 15%.[165,231,493]

Cavernous hemangiomas are composed primarily of large vascular lakes and channels (Fig. 10-1). Many of these channels undergo thrombosis and fibrous organization. Capillary hemangiomas, consisting of normal caliber capillaries, are rare in adults. Complications are rare, and ensue only when large lesions rupture. Most lesions change little if at all over time, however, rapid growth can occur.[519]

Other Imaging Modalities

The major hazard of cavernous hemangiomas is their incidental discovery on abdominal sonograms, CT scans, or scintigrams obtained for other reasons, complicating these patients' management (Figs. 10-1 to 10-4). The angiographic appearance of cavernous hemangioma is usually characteristic, with delayed but persistent accumulation of contrast. Extremely slow flow, however, may cause even large hemangiomas to appear avascular by angiography.[91]

In most instances, hemangiomas have a distinctive appearance on sonography, with the unusual combination of increases in both echogenicity and transmission of sound (see Fig. 10-1). Sonography is not specific, however, since 15% to 20% of cavernous hemangiomas are hypoechoic (see Fig. 10-4).[42,161,228,522] In fact, the echogenicity of cavernous hemangiomas can vary with increasing transducer pressure.[79] Furthermore, cancer can be uniformly hyperechoic and therefore mimic cavernous hemangiomas.

In the past, CT scanning has been advocated for non-

invasive differential diagnosis of cavernous hemangioma. Unfortunately, the single-slice methodology for diagnosing cavernous hemangiomas by CT is incompatible with the bolus-contrast sequential table incrementation technique used routinely in screening CT examinations. To evaluate lesions detected by routine CT, the patient must return for a second examination.

Smaller lesions are difficult to characterize by dynamic CT because of slice misregistration on sequential scans. Additionally, the following strict criteria are required to make a specific diagnosis of cavernous hemangioma by CT: (1) diminished attenuation on the precontrast scan, (2) peripheral enhancement during dynamic scanning, and (3) complete isodense fill in on delayed scans more than 15 minutes after contrast administration. These criteria are seen in only 52% of hemangiomas (see Figs. 10-2 and 10-3).[42,138,145] With less strict criteria, erroneous diagnoses occur.

Scintigraphy with technetium-labeled erythrocytes (blood-pool study) allows a specific diagnosis of cavernous hemangioma (see Fig. 10-4).[47,50,360,419] Unfortunately, the blood-pool study is a secondary test that adds time and cost to the initial screening examination, and provides no additional information if cavernous hemangioma is not diagnosed. Although single photon computerized emission tomography (SPECT) has improved the scintigraphic evaluation of small lesions, cavernous hemangiomas as large as 2 cm may be missed.* Additionally, blood-pool scintigraphy cannot differentiate between metastases and cysts. Occasionally, false-negative results may be obtained for large hemangiomas.[222]

We recommend blood-pool scintigraphy only for cases that satisfy all of the following criteria: (1) solitary or multiple lesions, each of which are at least 2 cm in diameter, (2) features on other imaging modalities that suggest cavernous hemangiomas, and (3) no other indication for comprehensive hepatic imaging, such as a known primary neoplasm or abnormal liver function tests. Conversely, we recommend MRI for (1) small lesions, (2) lesions with findings suggestive of malignancy, such as ill-defined borders, or (3) patients who

---

*33, 47, 222, 265, 552

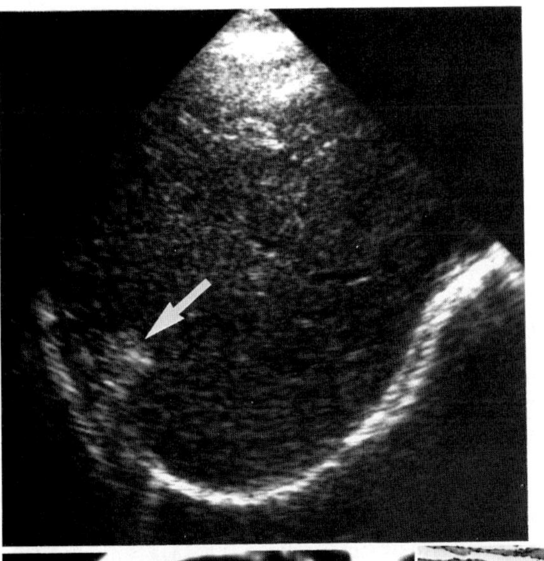

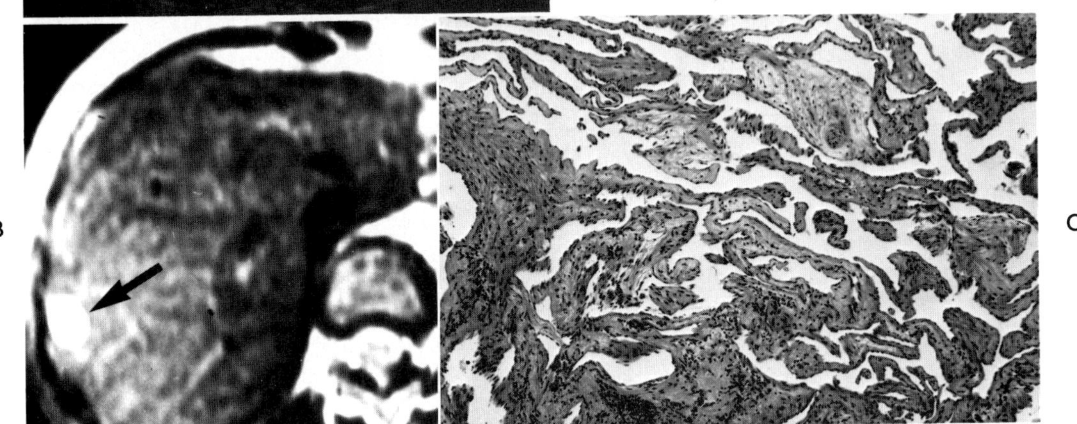

Fig. 10-1 Cavernous hemangioma: typical sonographic, magnetic resonance and histologic appearance. **A,** Transverse ultrasound image reveals a hyperechoic peripheral right hepatic lesion *(arrow)*. **B,** Corresponding T2-weighted MR image at 1.5 T (2500/80) reveals bright homogeneous signal intensity with distinct borders and no adjacent hepatic reaction *(arrow)*. **C,** Histologic section depicting abundant vascular spaces.

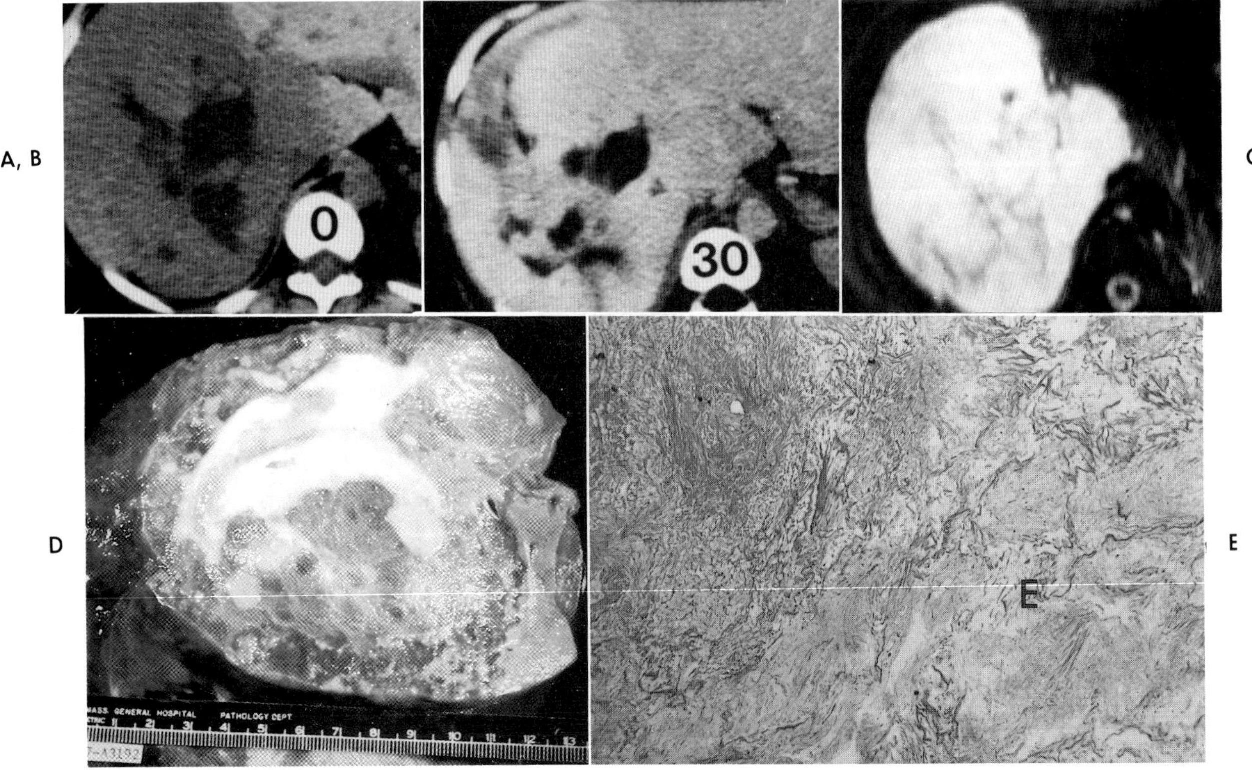

Fig. 10-2 For legend, see opposite page.

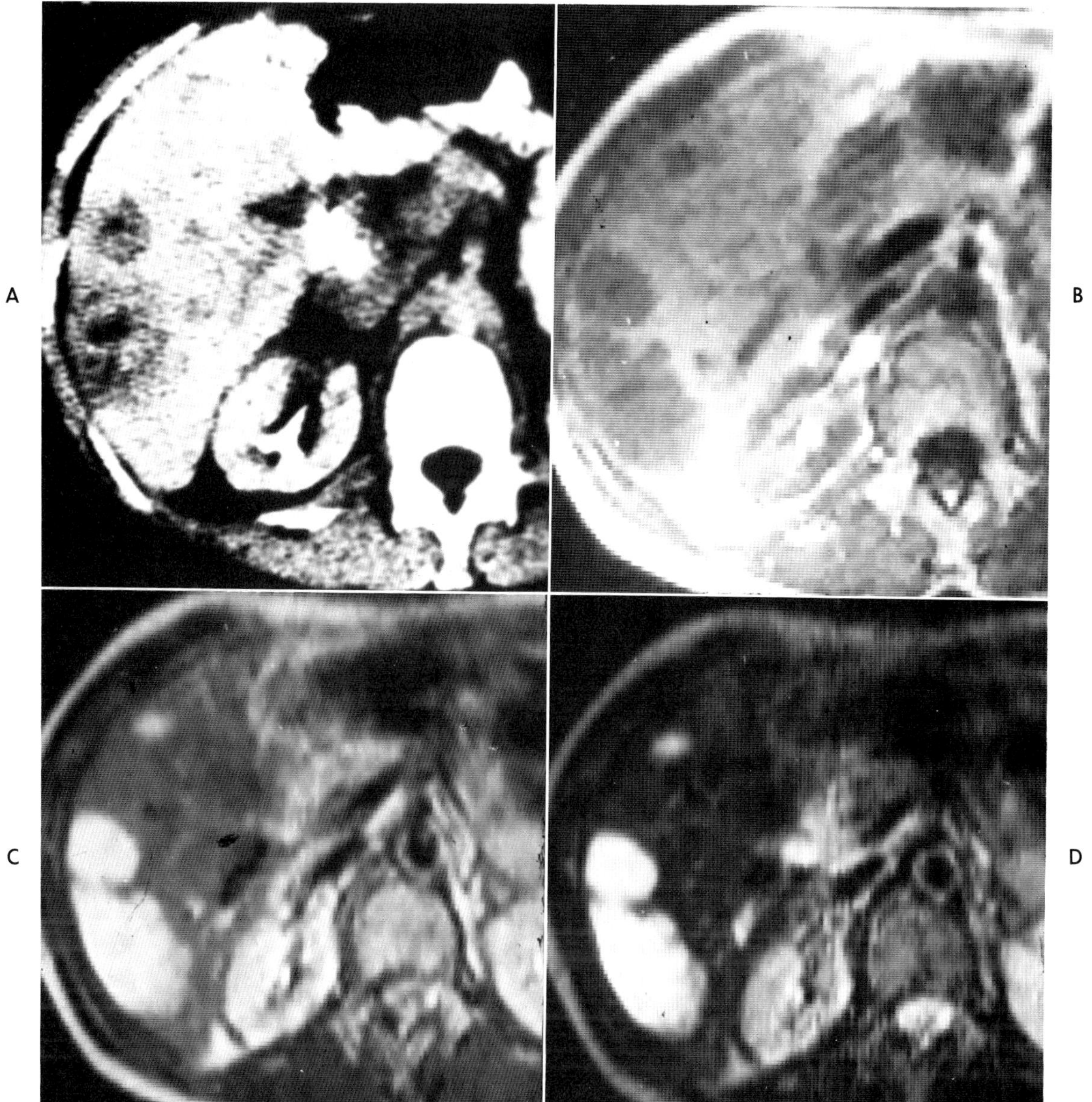

Fig. 10-3 Cavernous hemangiomas in a breast cancer patient with abdominal pain. **A,** Contrast-enhanced CT scan shows typical findings for multiple hepatic metastases. **B,** SE 300/14 MR image at 0.6 T is nonspecific for differential diagnosis. **C,** SE 2400/60 image shows additional lesions. **D,** SE 2400/120. Homogeneity and intensity of all three lesions match that of the cerebrospinal fluid. The MR diagnosis of cavernous hemangioma was proved by a 1-year follow-up examination

Fig. 10-2 Giant cavernous hemangioma with internal scar shown at 0.6 T. **A,** Precontrast CT scan shows a complex mass. **B,** Dynamic bolus technique with 30-minute delayed scan fails to fulfill criteria for the diagnosis of a cavernous hemangioma. **C,** SE 2400/180 image shows the entire mass to have a high signal intensity, confirming the long T2 relaxation time characteristic of cavernous hemangioma. **D,** Pathologic specimen confirms the diagnosis of cavernous hemangioma with a central scar. **E,** Histologic specimen reveals loose edematous tissue *(E)* within the tumor scar (H & E staining; original magnification, ×31). Although this tissue did not enhance on CT scans, its long T2 relaxation time causes it to behave like the remainder of the cavernous hemangioma, and it does not usually interfere with the correct diagnosis by MR criteria. (From Rummeny, E., Weissleder, R., Sironi, S., et al: Radiology 171:323-326, 1989.)

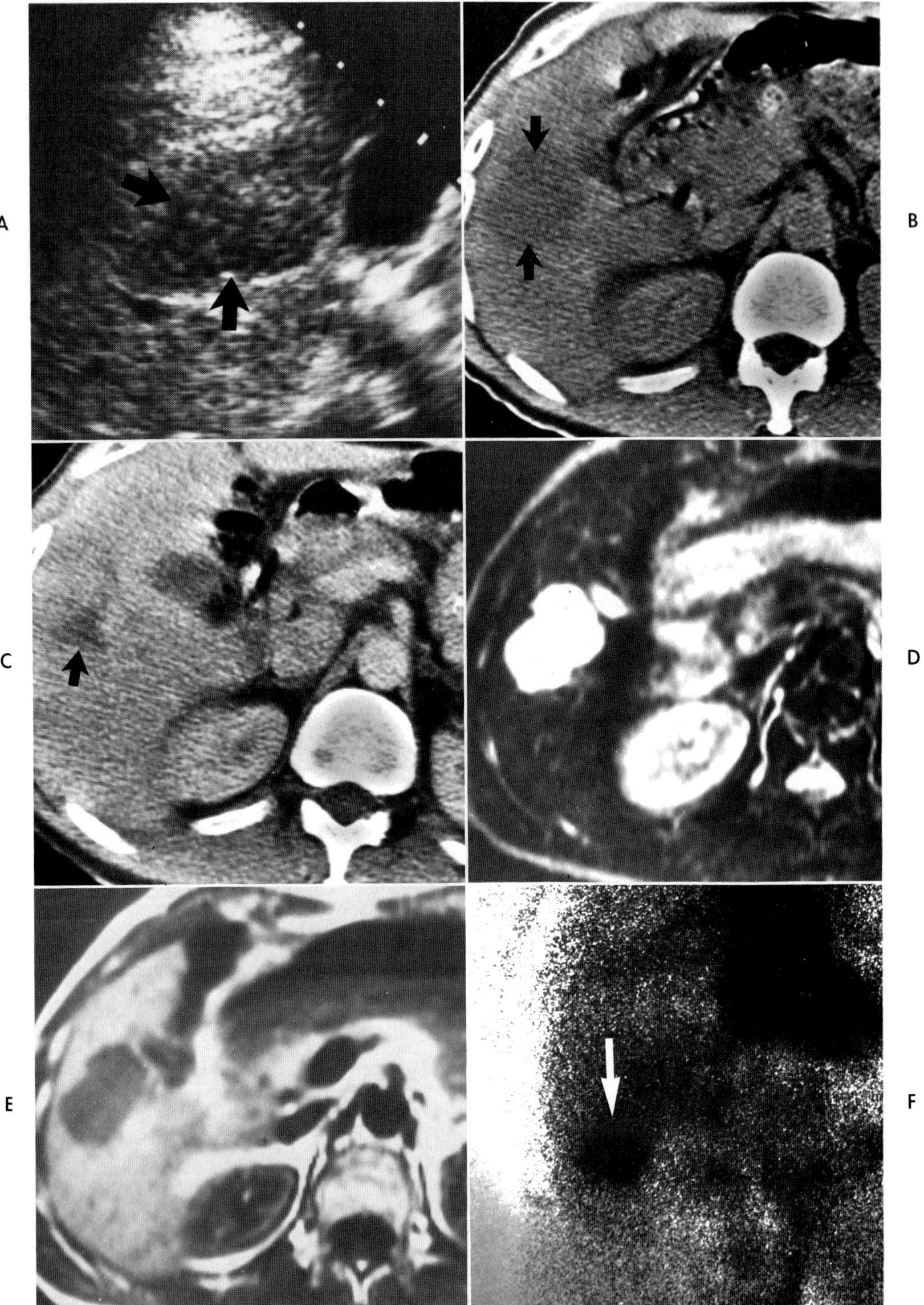

Fig. 10-4 Cavernous hemangioma: nonspecific sonographic and CT appearance, typical magnetic-resonance and blood-pool appearance. **A,** Right transverse ultrasound image reveals a hypoechoic mass *(arrows)* in the right lobe with minimally increased transmission of sound. **B,** CT scan without contrast depicts a low-attenuation mass *(arrows)*. **C,** After administration of contrast material, a central region of nonenhancement is noted *(arrow)*. **D,** The corresponding T2-weighted MR image at 1.5 T (SE 2500/100) is diagnostic of a benign lesion. **E,** SE 400/12 image. **F,** Blood-pool phase of tagged red blood cell study reveals a mass with an increased blood pool *(arrow)*, diagnostic of cavernous hemangioma.

would benefit from hepatic MRI of the remainder of the liver, even if the lesion in question proves to be a hemangioma. For instance, a patient with a recently diagnosed malignancy and a 2-cm hemangioma detected incidentally by sonography or CT may have small metastases visible only by MRI.

MRI Features

MRI is more sensitive than other imaging methods, and is at least as specific, for diagnosing cavernous hemangiomas.[33,231,493,568] Cavernous hemangiomas differ from all other hepatic masses in that they are essentially a lake of slowly flowing blood. The high intensity of cavernous hemangiomas is probably due to the extremely long T2 relaxation time of the abundant free fluid in blood. At 0.6 T, the T2 relaxation times of cavernous hemangiomas (150 $\pm$ 45 msec) are significantly longer than primary or metastatic liver cancer (78 $\pm$ 32 msec).[493] At 1.5 T, where T2 relaxation times may be shorter, calculated T2 greater than 88 msec is useful for diagnosing hemangioma.[295,393] In clinical practice, however, T2 values as reported in the literature should not play a primary role for differential diagnosis because of their inaccuracy and dependence on numerous technical factors.

Signal-intensity ratios, using normal liver tissue as a reference, have been useful in distinguishing cavernous hemangioma from metastases (Fig. 10-5). Using liver tissue as a reference may lead to errors, however, since intensity and T2 of liver may vary, depending on its content of fat, iron or edema.[341] On T2-weighted images, nearly all hepatic lesions are more intense than liver, but the degree of hyperintensity and morphologic characteristics differ in consistent ways. Isointensity with cerebrospinal fluid (CSF) is a more reliable and practical criterion for diagnosis of cavernous hemangiomas (see Figs. 10-1 to 10-4); metastases are rarely as bright as CSF on heavily T2-weighted images, except for central necrosis.

Bile or gastric fluid are less reliable references than CSF, since their T1 relaxation times are often less than that of CSF and hemangioma. Since the T1 of CSF is approximately 2000 msec,[83] recovery of longitudinal relaxation is incomplete even with "long" TR. Hemangiomas may not be as intense as bile or gastric fluid, but they should be as bright as CSF.

Extremely T2-weighted pulse sequences are most reliable in distinguishing cancer from hemangioma.[117,493] TE values of 60 msec are not reliable for distinguishing cancerous lesions from hemangiomas. Late echoes with TE of at least 100 msec are most useful in distinguishing cavernous hemangioma from solid neoplasms. At low field and mid field, echo times as long as 150 msec are preferred.

Cavernous hemangiomas, cysts, and malignancies have significantly different T1 relaxation times.[49,404]

Conventional T1-weighted images are not helpful for characterizing most hepatic lesions, however. This is probably because all nonhepatocellular lesions have low SNR, and small differences between lesions are lost in background noise. T1 differences have been used to separate cavernous hemangiomas, cysts, and metastases on inversion recovery images, however, since these images have a larger and more flexible dynamic range for depiction of T1 contrast. Lesions can be characterized on inverions recovery images by finding the TI that causes the lesions to become isointense with background noise.[404]

Morphologic criteria must be examined to supplement evaluation of relative intensity.[49,607] Cavernous hemangiomas are well circumscribed and tend to be homogeneous, whereas cancers are heterogeneous and have ill-defined margins or rings. Cavernous hemangiomas are commonly lobulated (see Figs. 10-3 and 10-4), but their borders should never be irregular, spiculated, or indistinct. Hemangiomas do not have low-signal capsules or

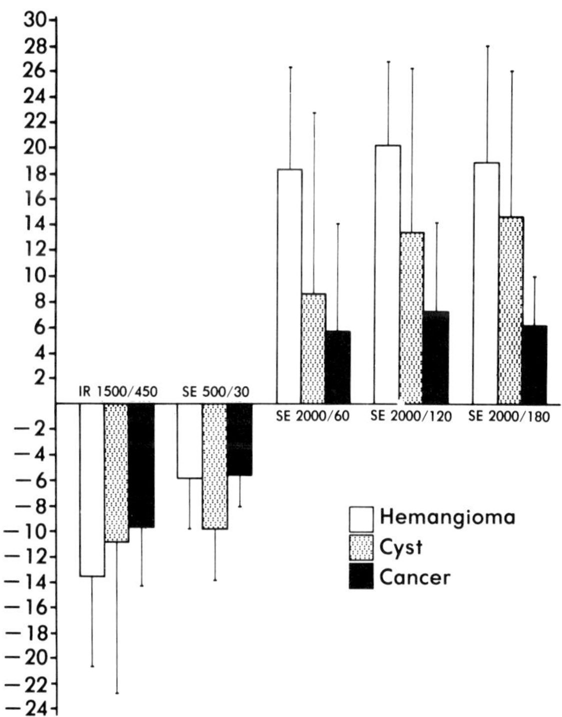

Fig. 10-5 Bar diagram displaying contrast-to-noise ratios (CNR) for focal hepatic lesions imaged using different MRI pulse sequences. Positive lesion-liver CNR values correspond to hyperintense lesions (T2-weighted pulse sequences) and negative CNR values correspond to hypointense lesions (T1-weighted pulse sequences). The T1-weighted images show little tissue specificity; however, cysts are generally darker than cancer or hemangioma on SE 500/30 images. Cancer is most reliably distinguished from hemangioma or cysts on SE 2000/180 images.

intermediate-intensity zones of edema, which are often present at the periphery of malignant lesions.

Cavernous hemangiomas frequently show complex internal architecture by sonography, CT, blood-pool scintigraphy or MRI.[77,440,522] Cavernous hemangiomas frequently degenerate, forming internal cysts or fibrotic scars that occasionally calcify (Figs. 10-5 and 10-6). All of these features confound differential diagnosis by conventional imaging techniques, including angiography. Whereas fibrous components commonly cause discreet low-signal areas within cavernous hemangiomas, especially large ones,[77] virtually all cavernous hemangiomas are primarily hyperintense on heavily T2-weighted images, and the borders should always be distinct. Rarely, heavily fibrotic hemangiomas overlap the appearance of cystic metastases, causing ambiguous MR features in only 5% of cases.[493]

Occasionally, hemangiomas less than 2 cm may not be characterized adequately by MRI.[236] This is a difficult clinical problem, since other modalities are even less successful at characterizing these lesions. One approach is to obtain an additional sequence with thin (5-mm) sections to reduce the influence of partial volume effects (Fig. 10-7).

Dynamic MR imaging after administration of contrast material may help confirm the diagnosis of hemangioma if T2-weighted images are equivocal (see Figs. 6-3, 10-6, 10-8).* Cavernous hemangiomas show peripheral enhancement immediately after a bolus of gadopentetate dimeglumine, but the remainder of the lesion usually requires more time to fill in.[307,392] The fill in is often clumplike, due to the large intercommunicating vascular lakes (Fig. 10-8). Most hemangiomas fill in completely within 5 to 30 minutes, analogous to the enhancement pattern reported for dynamic CT.[145] Persistent hyperintensity 15 minutes after administration of gadopentatate dimeglumine is strong support for the diagnosis of hemangioma.

The diagnosis of small hemangiomas may benefit from gadopentetate-dimeglumine–enhanced multislice MRI. These lesions are difficult to characterize using the single-slice, dynamic-bolus CT technique[139,145] because of slice misregistration from inconsistent position of the diaphragm during suspended respirations.

It must be remembered that gadopentatate dimeglumine is a nonspecific extracellular agent, analogous to iodinated vascular contrast, rather than a blood-pool agent. Delayed images after administration of gadopentatate dimeglumine depict the combination of blood-pool and interstitial enhancement and are therefore less specific than RBC-scintigraphy. For this reason, tumors with large interstital spaces (e.g., edematous tumors and hypervascular tumors) can mimic the enhancement pattern of hemangiomas. Additionally, large hemangiomas with scar tissue may not fill in completely.

The specificity of contrast-enhanced MRI is likely to improve when blood-pool agents are developed for MRI. Meanwhile, enhancement techniques should supplement, rather than replace, conventional T2-weighted SE techniques for characterizing liver lesions. Contrast-enhanced MR images provide valuable physiologic information not available from unenhanced images; final MRI diagnosis should incorporate all infomation available, rather than rely on a signal parameter or pulse sequence.

CYSTS

Cysts of the liver are less common than cavernous hemangiomas and are seldom if ever symptomatic. Cysts are usually discovered incidentally during sonographic or CT examinations. Although sonographic features are highly diagnostic, cysts can be confused with malignant lesions by CT.[22,45]

Simple cysts have even longer T1 and T2 relaxation times than hemangiomas (T2 = 243 ± 163 msec), since they contain more than 95% water. Heavily T2-weighted images show cysts and cavernous hemangiomas to have a similarly high-signal intensity (Fig. 10-9). Since the T2 relaxation times of these lesions are so long, TEs in common clinical use are not long enough to depict reliably the T2 differences between hemangiomas and cysts.

The T1 differences between hemangiomas and cysts can be depicted on T1-weighted or intermediate images. Cysts are often less intense than hemangiomas on these images, although these differences are more apparent on images with intermediate-to-long TR (e.g., 2000 msec), because of higher SNR of the lesions (see Fig. 10-9).[49,493] Longer TR (e.g., greater than 5000 msec), as may be used with multiecho conjugate (fast) spin echo or echo planar images, is less likely to distinguish hemangiomas and cysts. These two benign lesions can be differentiated unambiguously by administering contrast material, although this is not important clinically.

The intensity of cysts on T1-weighted or intermediate images can vary, however, if protein and/or hemorrhage is present within cyst fluid. These materials can shorten T1 and therefore cause hyperintensity (Figs. 10-10 and 10-11).

Multiple cysts of variable intensity, presumably caused by multiple episodes of intracystic hemorrhage, have been described in patients with polycystic liver disease (see Fig. 10-11).[90] This MRI appearance is similar to that of renal cysts present with autosomal dominant polycystic kidney disease.[211] In some patients, all cysts may have low intensity (Fig. 10-12).

---

*113, 191, 308, 471, 560

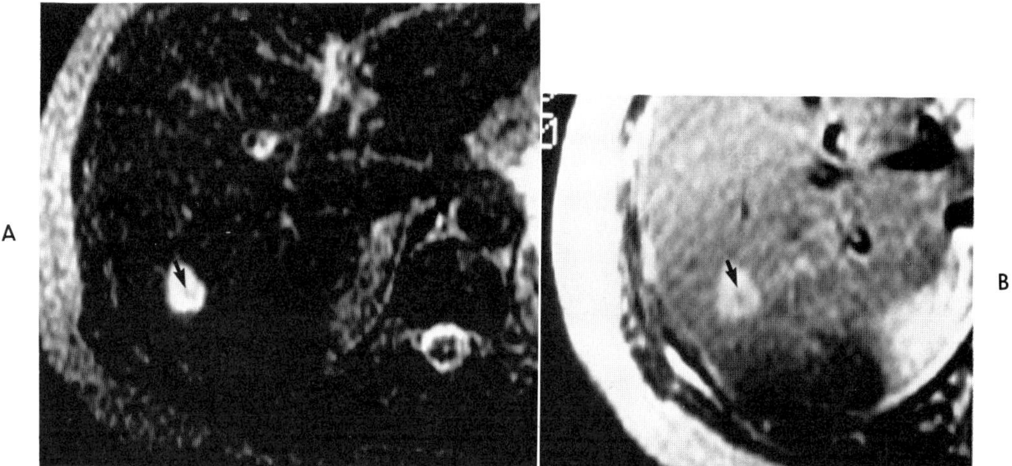

Fig. 10-6 Cavernous hemangioma with central scar depicted with T2-weighted and blood-pool enhanced T1-weighted images at 1.5 T. **A,** SE 2500/140 image with 5-mm thickness depicts a central defect *(arrow)* within an otherwise well-defined hyperintense lesion. **B,** SE 400/12 image approximately 15 minutes after administration of gadopentatate dimeglumine has a similar appearance.

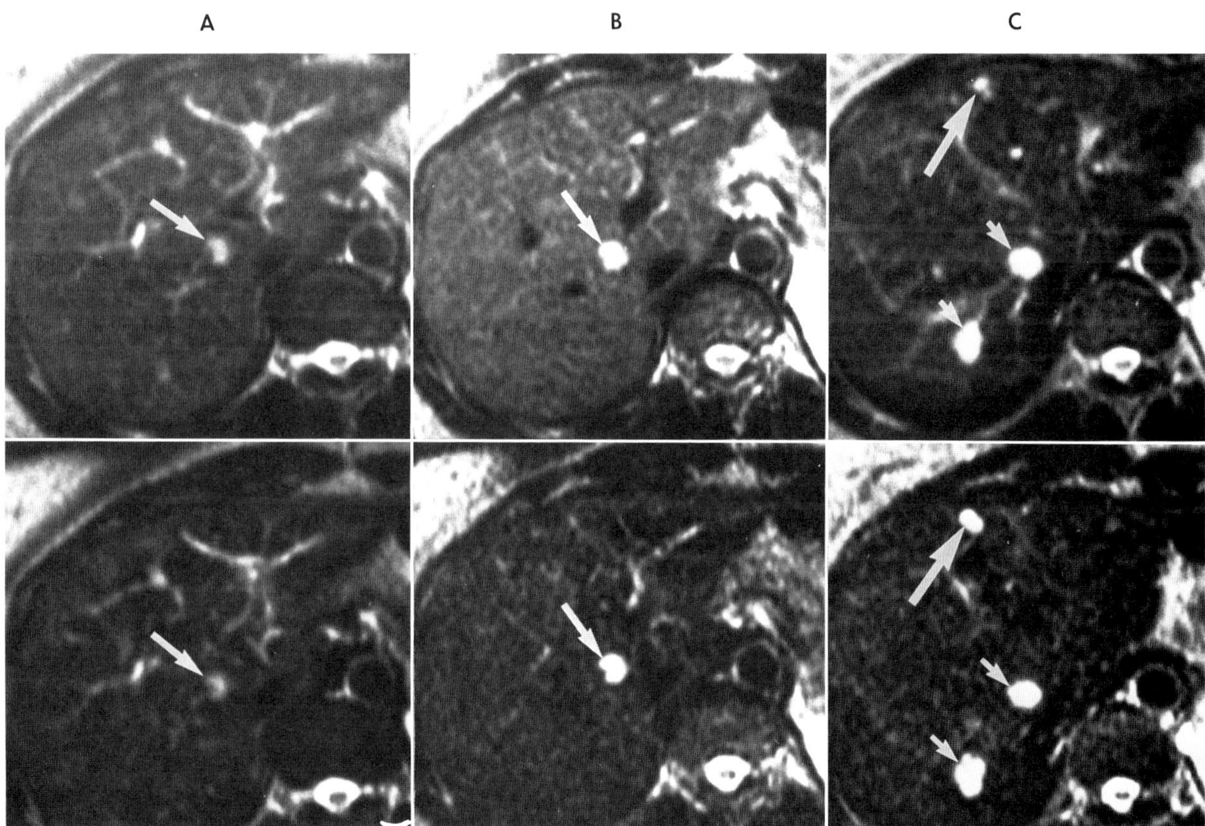

Fig. 10-7 Value of thin sections and long TE for diagnosing small hemangiomas at 1.5 T. **A,** With 10-mm thick sections, the small mass *(arrow)* lateral to the inferior vena cava is less intense than cerebrospinal fluid, with SE 2500/100 *(top)* and SE 2500/120 *(bottom)*. **B,** With 5-mm thick sections, the mass has sharp borders and is isointense with cerebrospinal fluid on both. SE 2500/70 *(top)* and SE 2500/140 *(bottom)*, diagnostic of hemangioma or cyst. **C,** At a higher level, three additional lesions are noted. Two masses in the right lobe *(short arrows)* are diagnostic of hemangioma or cyst with both techniques, but the smaller lesion in the left lobe *(long arrow)* is nonspecific with 10-mm thick section *(top; SE 2500/120)*, but diagnostic with 5-mm thick section *(bottom; SE 2500/140)*. Although longer TE may improve specificity, the use of thinner sections may be more important for small lesions.

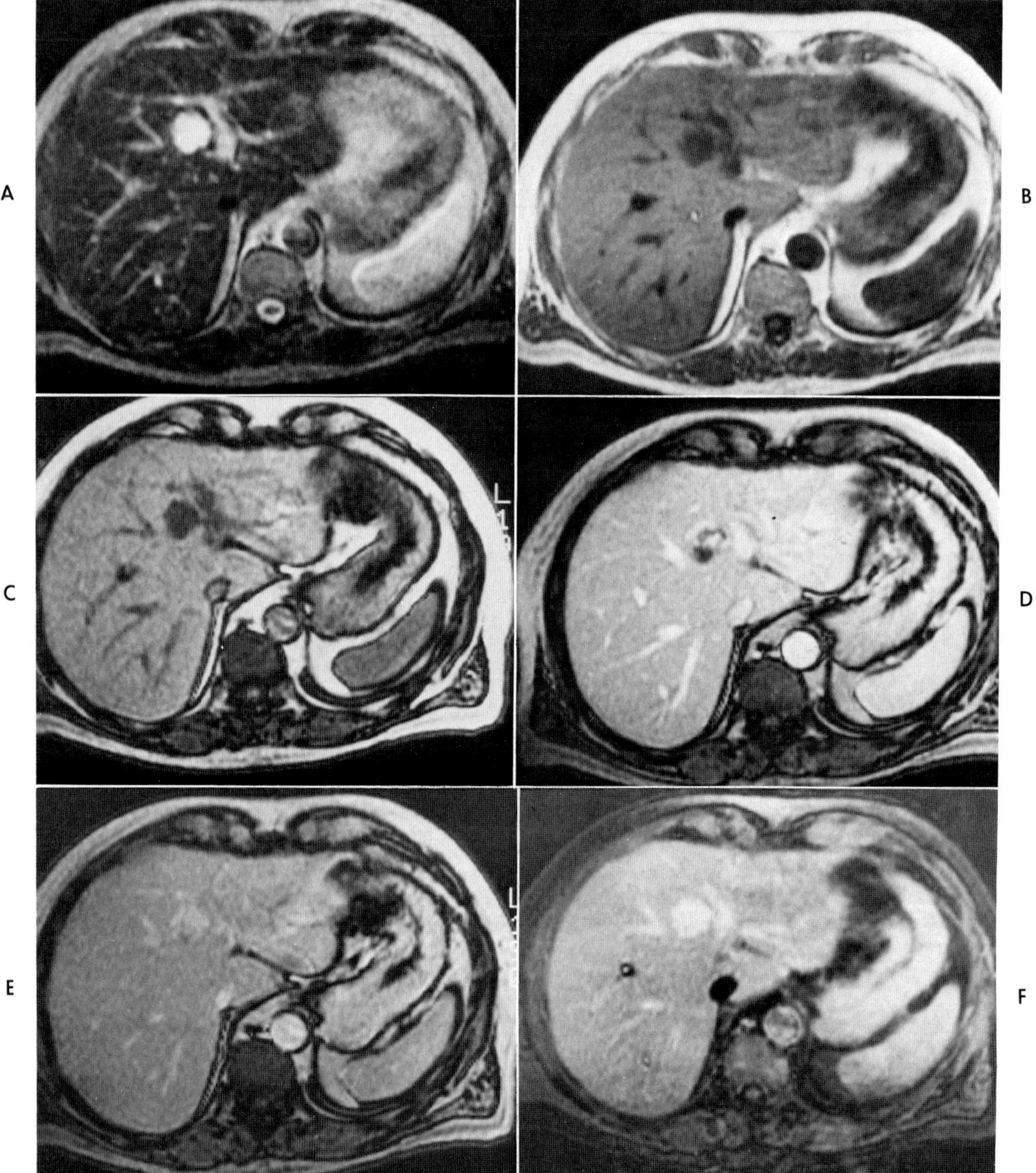

Fig. 10-8 Cavernous hemangioma with typical spin-echo and enhancement characteristics at 1.5 T. **A,** SE 2500/100 image depicts the hemangioma as a well-defined lesion isointense with cerebrospinal fluid. **B,** SE 400/12 image shows a well-defined lesion. **C,** T1-weighted gradient-echo image (TR/TE/flip angle = 102/2.3/90 degrees). **D,** As in **C,** within 30 seconds after administration of gadopentatate dimeglumine. Clumplike hyperintensity has developed resulting from filling of large vascular spaces with contrast. **E,** As in **D,** approximately 2 minutes later. The lesion has filled in and is now nearly isointense with hepatic vessels. **F,** SE 500/14 image with fat suppression, approximately 15 minutes after administration of gadopentatate dimeglumine. The lesion is homogeneously hyperintense.

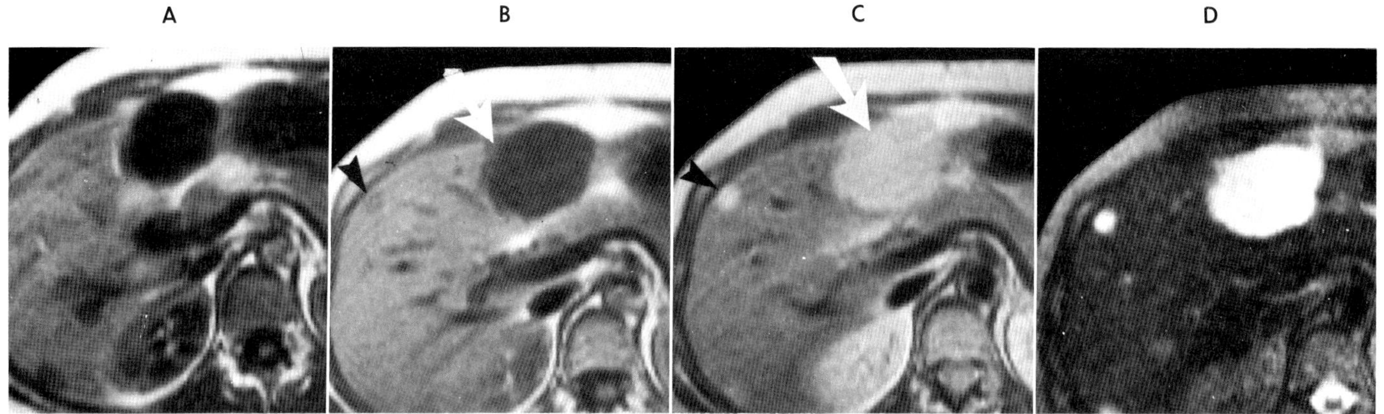

Fig. 10-9   Cysts versus hemangioma: differential diagnosis by MRI at 0.6 T. **A** to **D,** A 7-centimeter cyst *(arrow)* and multiple 1-cm hemangiomas *(arrowhead).* **A,** IR 1500/450/30. **B,** SE 500/30. **C,** SE 2000/60. **D,** SE 2000/180. The most useful images for distinguishing cyst from hemangioma have substantial but competing contrast from both T1 and T2 differences (e.g., SE 500/30, SE 2000/60). On these images, cysts have a lower signal intensity than cavernous hemangioma, since cysts have a longer T1 relaxation time and are less completely remagnetized between pulses. At TE = 30 to 60 msec, T2 differences contribute little to image signal intensity differences between cysts and hemangiomas.

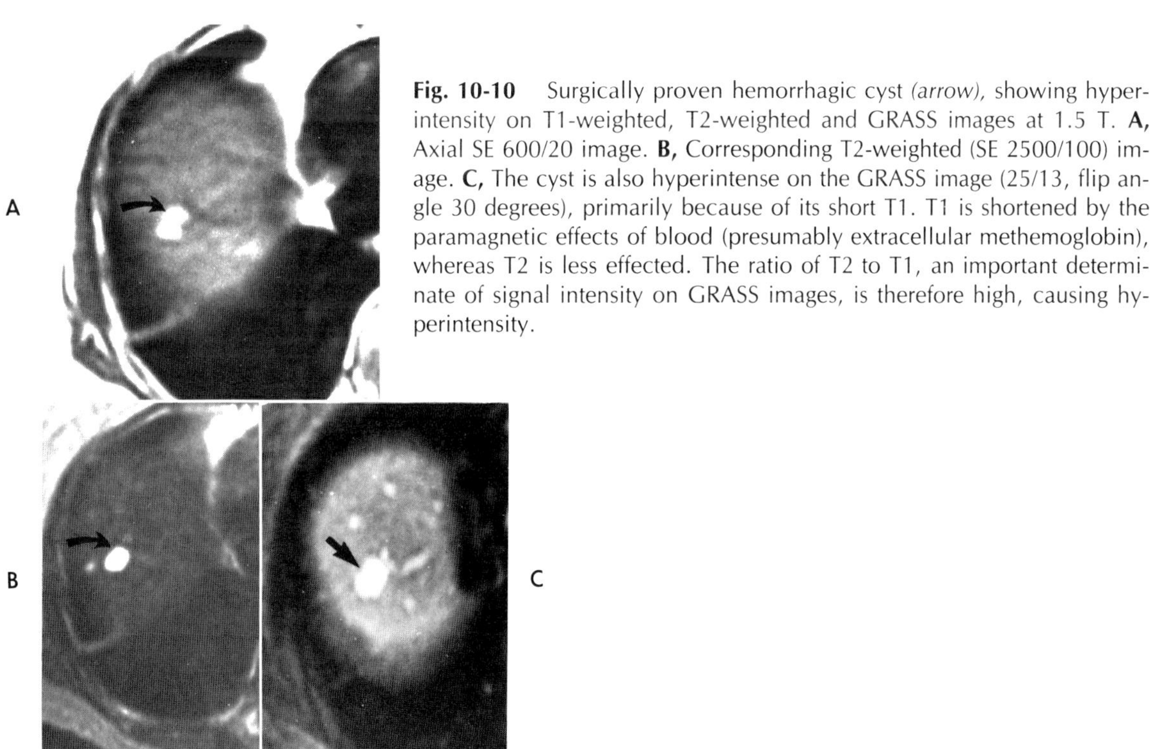

Fig. 10-10   Surgically proven hemorrhagic cyst *(arrow),* showing hyperintensity on T1-weighted, T2-weighted and GRASS images at 1.5 T. **A,** Axial SE 600/20 image. **B,** Corresponding T2-weighted (SE 2500/100) image. **C,** The cyst is also hyperintense on the GRASS image (25/13, flip angle 30 degrees), primarily because of its short T1. T1 is shortened by the paramagnetic effects of blood (presumably extracellular methemoglobin), whereas T2 is less effected. The ratio of T2 to T1, an important determinate of signal intensity on GRASS images, is therefore high, causing hyperintensity.

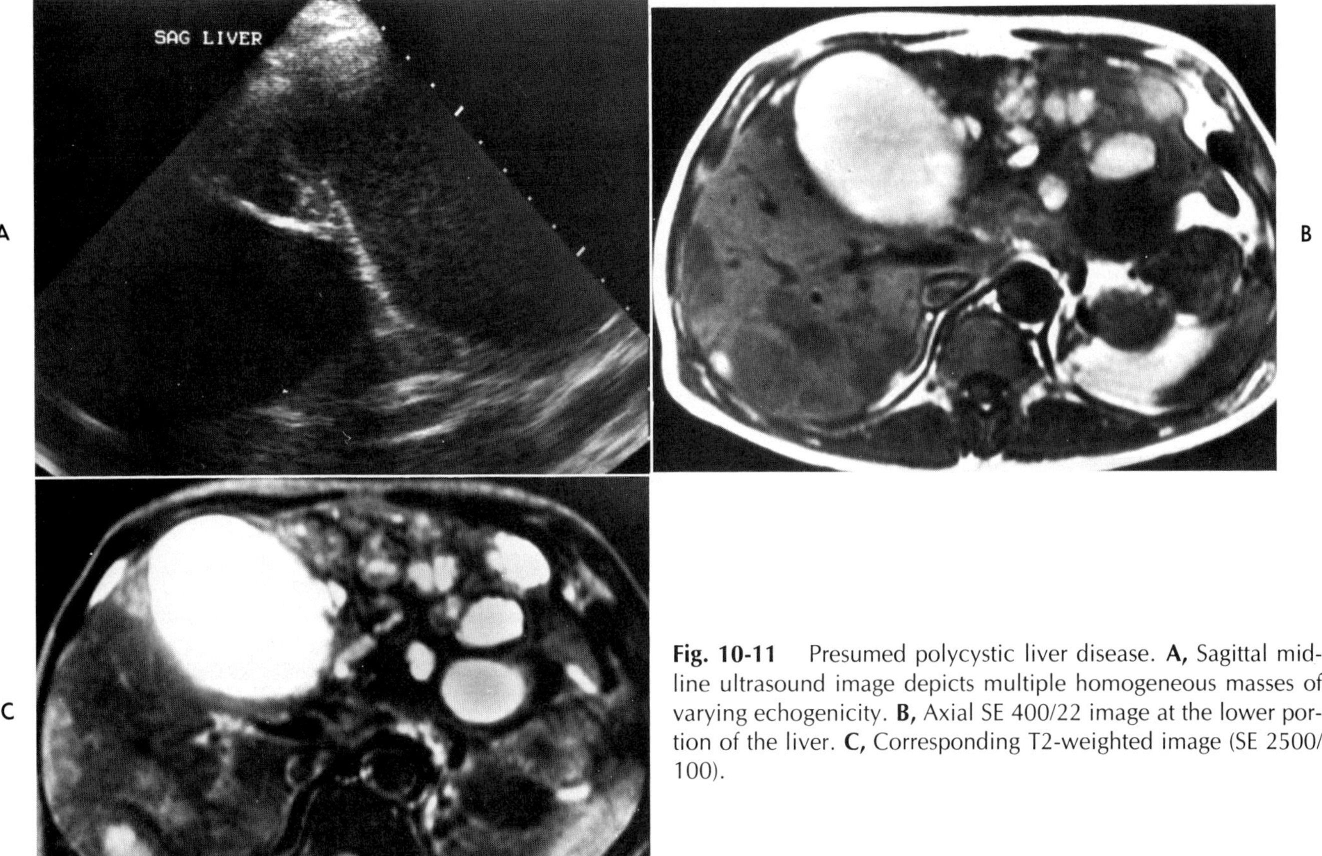

Fig. 10-11 Presumed polycystic liver disease. **A,** Sagittal midline ultrasound image depicts multiple homogeneous masses of varying echogenicity. **B,** Axial SE 400/22 image at the lower portion of the liver. **C,** Corresponding T2-weighted image (SE 2500/100).

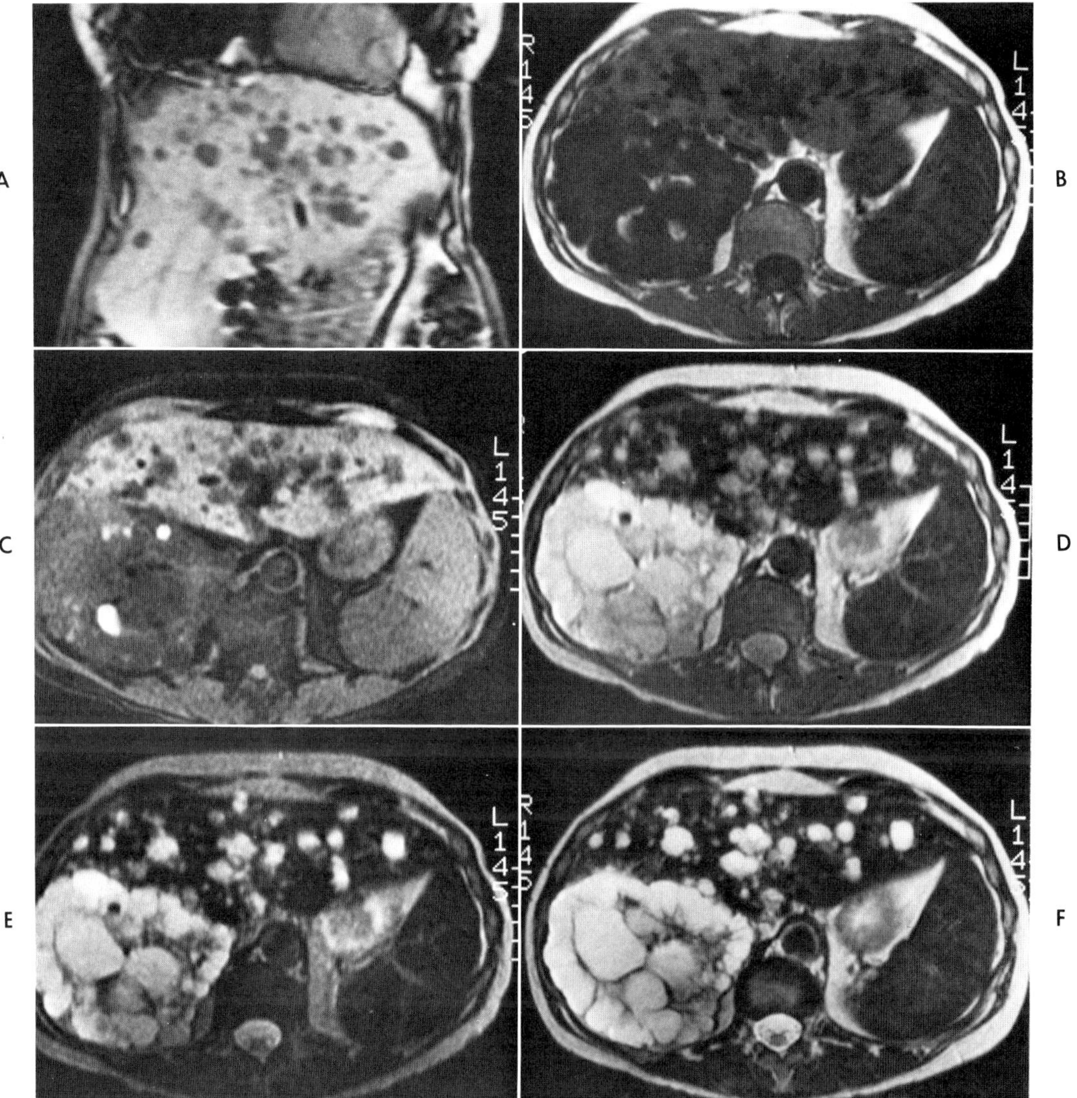

Fig. 10-12   Polycystic kidney and liver disease in a patient with transfusional siderosis, at 1.5 T. **A,** Coronal T1-weighted gradient-echo image (57.2/2.4/90 degrees) reveals multiple cysts in the liver. **B,** SE 467/12 image reveals numerous cysts within the kidney *(large arrows),* some of which have high signal indicative of hemorrhage *(curved arrows).* Several cysts are also present in the liver *(small arrows).* **C,** Corresponding SE 500/13 image with fat suppression. **D,** SE 2500/50 image. The liver and spleen have low signal resulting from transfusional siderosis (see Chapter 16). **E,** SE 2500/100 image. **F,** Multiecho conjugate (fast spin echo) image (TR/TE = 5000/85). Echo train = 16, matrix = 256 × 256, four signals averaged, acquisition time = 5:20, compared with 12:59 for **D** and **E.**

Hepatocellular Carcinoma

Hepatocellular carcinoma (HCC) is the most common hepatic malignancy in Asia because of the prevalence of hepatitis B.[110,235] HCC is usually associated with chronic liver disease, such as alcoholic cirrhosis, chronic active hepatitis, or hemochromatosis. In one prospective series of Asian patients with cirrhosis, HCC developed within 6 years in more than 50% of patients with viral hepatitis and in 22% of patients without viral hepatitis who drank excessively.[395]

Small HCC lesions are usually well differentiated, with vascularity similar to that of the adjacent liver.[255,260,373] These small lesions are often missed by angiography (Fig. 11-1).* For similar reasons, arterial signals may not be obtained by Doppler ultrasound.[387] Small lesions may also be missed by ultrasound or CT (Fig. 11-2).[386,624] Arterial portography and intraarterial injection of iodized oil improve the sensitivity of CT (94% and 82%, respectively, in one series), but even these techniques are relatively insensitive for small daughter lesions (38% and 50%).[386] Serum α-fetoprotein levels are usually normal with small HCC lesions.[395]

Slow-growing HCC is frequently surrounded by a fibrous capsule (Figs. 11-3 and 11-4).[109,235,441,618] Large HCC lesions are usually hypervascular, often with prominent arteriovenous shunting (Fig. 11-5). Advanced tumors commonly have necrosis and hemorrhage (Figs. 11-3 and 11-6) and/or invasion of portal and hepatic veins (Figs. 11-7 to 11-9).

Solitary HCC (50% of cases) can be treated by surgical resection if the patient's hepatic functional reserve is sufficient. If it is not, or if the tumor is multinodular or diffuse (Figs. 11-11 and 11-12), alternative treatments include embolization, percutaneous injection of ethanol, chemotherapy, radiation therapy, or hepatic transplantation.[386,481,525,624] Hepatic transplantation should only be considered for small solitary tumors in patients with end-stage hepatic disease.

Diagnosis of HCC is complicated by focal manifestations of cirrhosis. In one series, 15 of 100 patients with cirrhosis who were screened by CT had focal abnormalities. Only one patient had HCC, whereas the other 14

had focal fatty infiltration or regenerative nodule.[201]

The reported sensitivity for imaging-guided percutaneous biopsy of HCC ranges from 69%[51] to 90%.[44] In one report, 12 of 62 focal lesions detected by ultrasound were diagnosed as regenerative nodules based on negative guided biopsy. On follow-up examination, however, 10 of these 12 lesions were found to be HCC lesions.[424] Some of these cases may represent HCC developing within regenerative nodules, whereas others may have been false-negative biopsy results from the similarity between well-differentiated HCC and normal hepatic tissue.[260,373]

SIGNAL INTENSITY

Advanced HCC is usually hypointense on T1-weighted images and hyperintense on T2-weighted images, similar to metastases.[78,230,391,565] The signal intensity of HCC is more variable than that of other tumors, however. Well-differentiated HCC is often isointense on T1-weighted images (see Figs. 11-8, 11-9, 11-11, and 11-12) and may even be hyperintense in up to 30% of cases (Figs. 11-3, 11-4, 11-10, and 11-12 to 11-14).[109,110,258,371,444] In this respect, HCC is similar to other tumors of hepatocellular origin.[349]

Hyperintense HCC lesions sometimes contain abundant intracellular triglyceride.[109,453,619] Fat is more common in small well-differentiated HCCs than in large undifferentiated tumors, probably resulting from the defective release of fat produced within partially functioning malignant hepatocytes. Chemical shift imaging can provide confirmatory evidence of intratumoral fat by demonstrating a decrease in tumor signal intensity on an opposed-phase or fat-suppressed image compared with an in-phase image acquired using similar TR and TE (see Fig. 11-10). Fat is extremely rare within metastases or other malignancies but is an occasional finding in hepatocellular masses, such as hepatic adenoma, focal nodular hyperplasia, and regenerative nodules (see Chapter 12).

In many instances, hyperintensity of HCC on T1-weighted images is not due to fat (see Figs. 11-3, 11-4, and 11-12 to 11-14),[349] although the reason for this is unknown. Intratumoral copper is commonly increased in hyperintense HCC,[110,258] although it may not necessarily be the direct cause of high signal.

*197, 489, 514, 521, 524, 621

Text continues on p. 108.

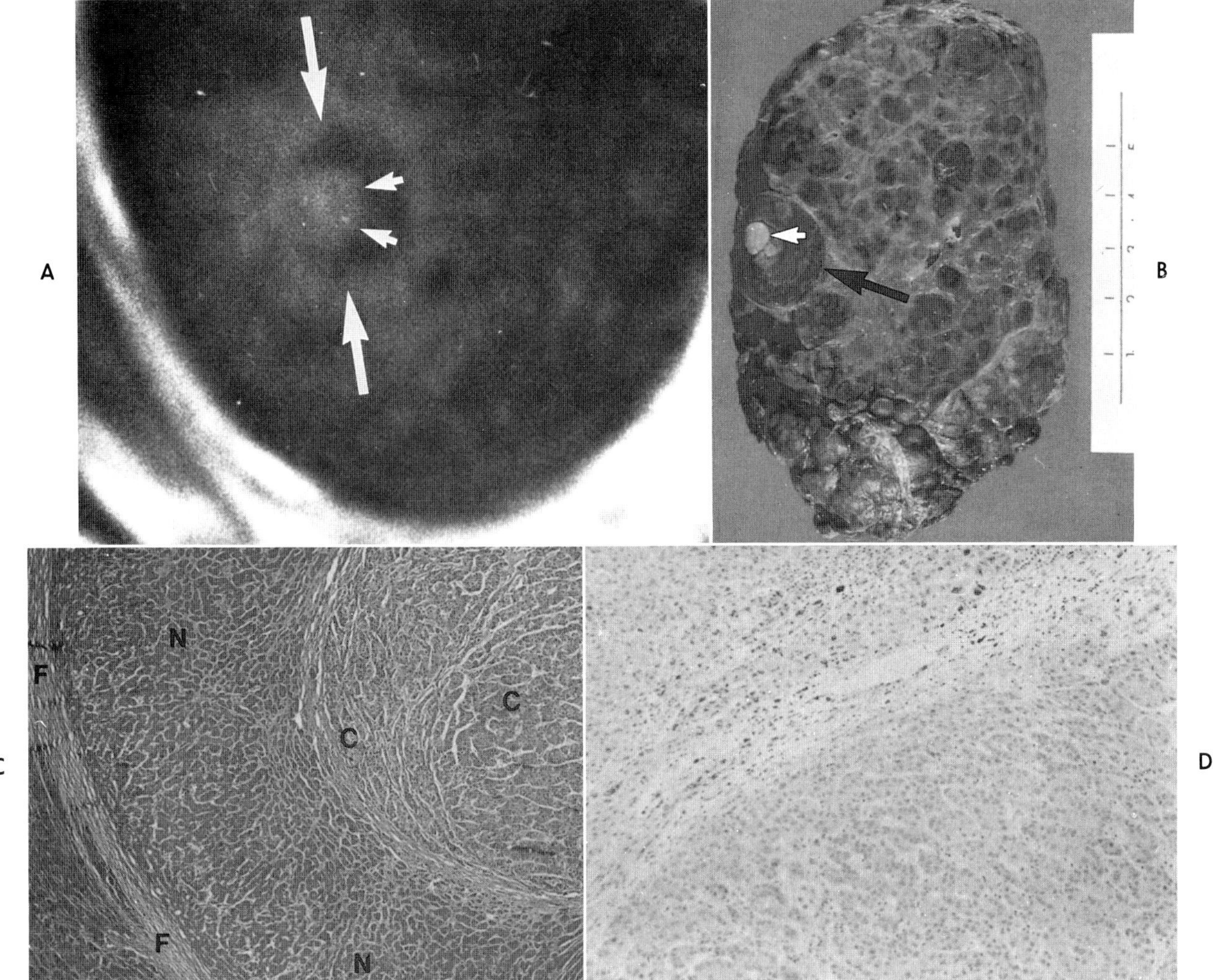

Fig. 11-1   Small hepatocellular carcinoma within a large siderotic regenerative nodule (nodule-within-nodule), resected at surgery. Serum α-fetoprotein was normal. **A,** Axial MR image at 1.5 T (SE 400/12) at the dome of the liver reveals a 2-cm low-signal mass *(large arrows)* with an isointense focus *(small arrows)* within it. Preoperative hepatic arteriogram revealed changes of cirrhosis but no evidence of malignancy. **B,** Cut section of the liver, removed at surgery for transplantation. A 5-mm hepatocellular carcinoma *(small white arrow)* is noted within a siderotic nodule *(large black arrow)*. Numerous smaller siderotic nodules are noted throughout the liver. **C,** Histologic section (H & E) reveals a well-differentiated carcinoma *(C)* within a regenerative nodule *(N)*, surrounded by a fibrous septation *(F)*. **D,** Iron stain reveals dense staining for iron within the regenerative nodule but no staining within the tumor. Iron was markedly increased throughout the liver, consistent with hemochromatosis. (From Mitchell, D.G., Rubin, R., Siegelman, E., et al.: Radiology 178:101-103, 1991.)

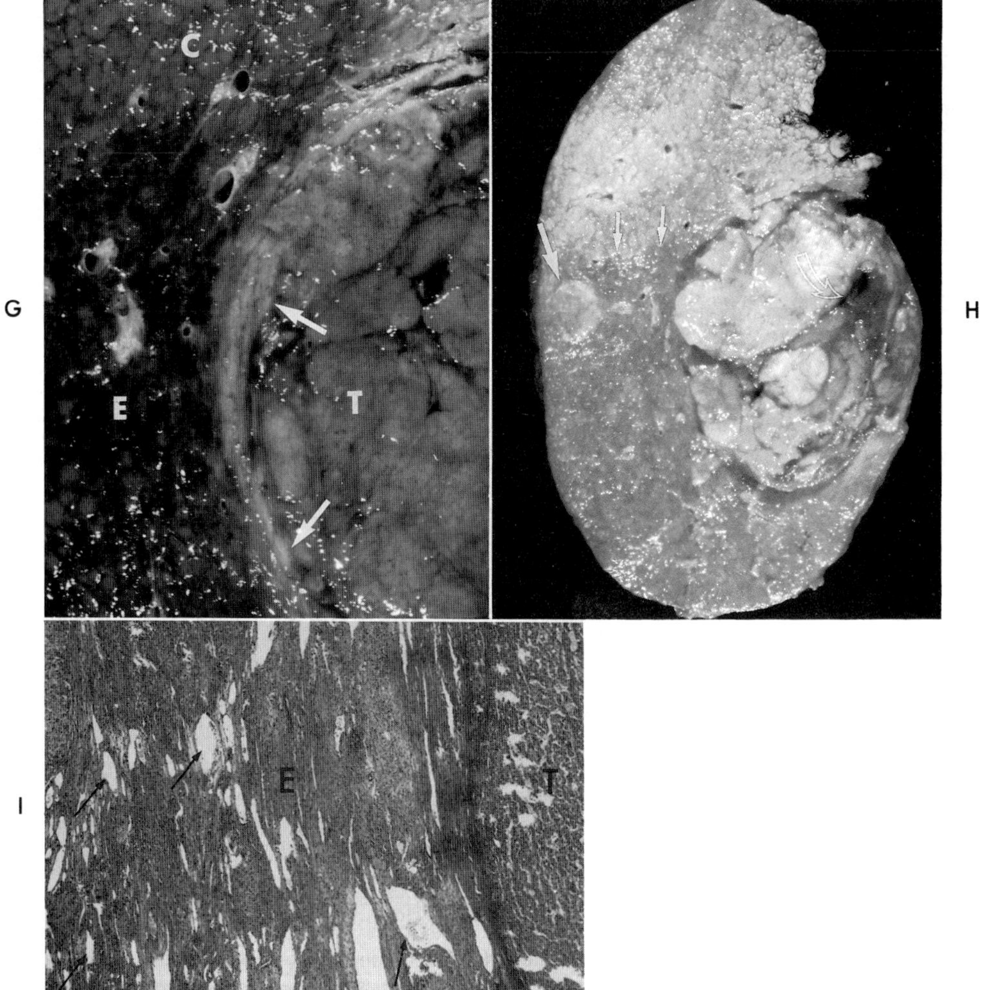

Fig. 11-3, cont'd.   Encapsulated hepatocellular carcinoma with necrosis and peritumoral edema. **G,** Surgical specimen sectioned in transverse plane corresponds to **A** and **B.** Tumor *(T),* fibrous capsule *(arrows),* and edematous parenchyma *(E)* are demonstrated. **H,** Surgical specimen corresponding to **D** and **E,** demonstrating necrosis *(curved arrow),* edematous parenchyma (small arrows), and accessory nodule *(large arrow).* **I,** Histologic specimen (magnification ×31) of edematous hepatic parenchyma *(E),* of right lobe with dilated lymphatic and venous channels *(arrows);* adjacent tumor tissue *(T).* No gross fat is visible within the tumor. (From Rummeny, E., Weissleder, R., Stark D.D., et al.: AJR 152:63-72, 1989.)

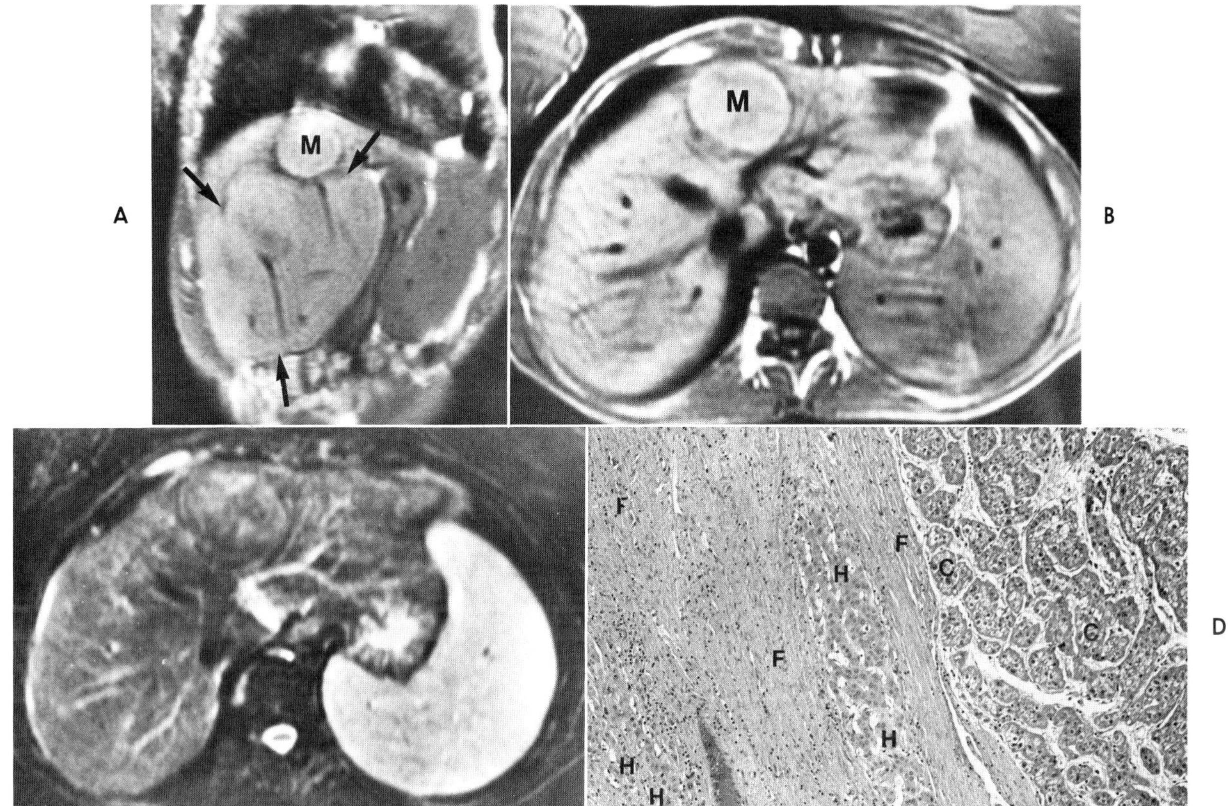

Fig. 11-4 Encapsulated solitary hepatocellular carcinoma with subtle signal characteristics, in a patient with massive regeneration of the right lobe. **A,** Coronal SE 500/20 image at 1.5 T through the anterior portion of the liver reveals a slightly hyperintense mass *(M)* superiorly in the medial segment of the left lobe, and a regenerative mass *(arrows)* inferiorly. **B,** Axial SE 400/20 image at the superior portion of the liver reveals a hyperintense encapsulated mass *(M)* between the medial and left hepatic veins. **C,** Corresponding SE 3000/100 image. The mass is only minimally hyperintense. **D,** Histologic section at the border between cancer and parenchyma (H & E). The hepatocellular carcinoma *(C)* is well differentiated, and there is no evidence of fat. The capsule is composed of hepatocytes *(H)* and abundant fibrous tissue *(F)*. (From Mitchell, D.G., Palazzo, J., Hann, H-W.Y.L., et al.: J. Comput. Assist. Tomogr. 15:762-769, 1991.)

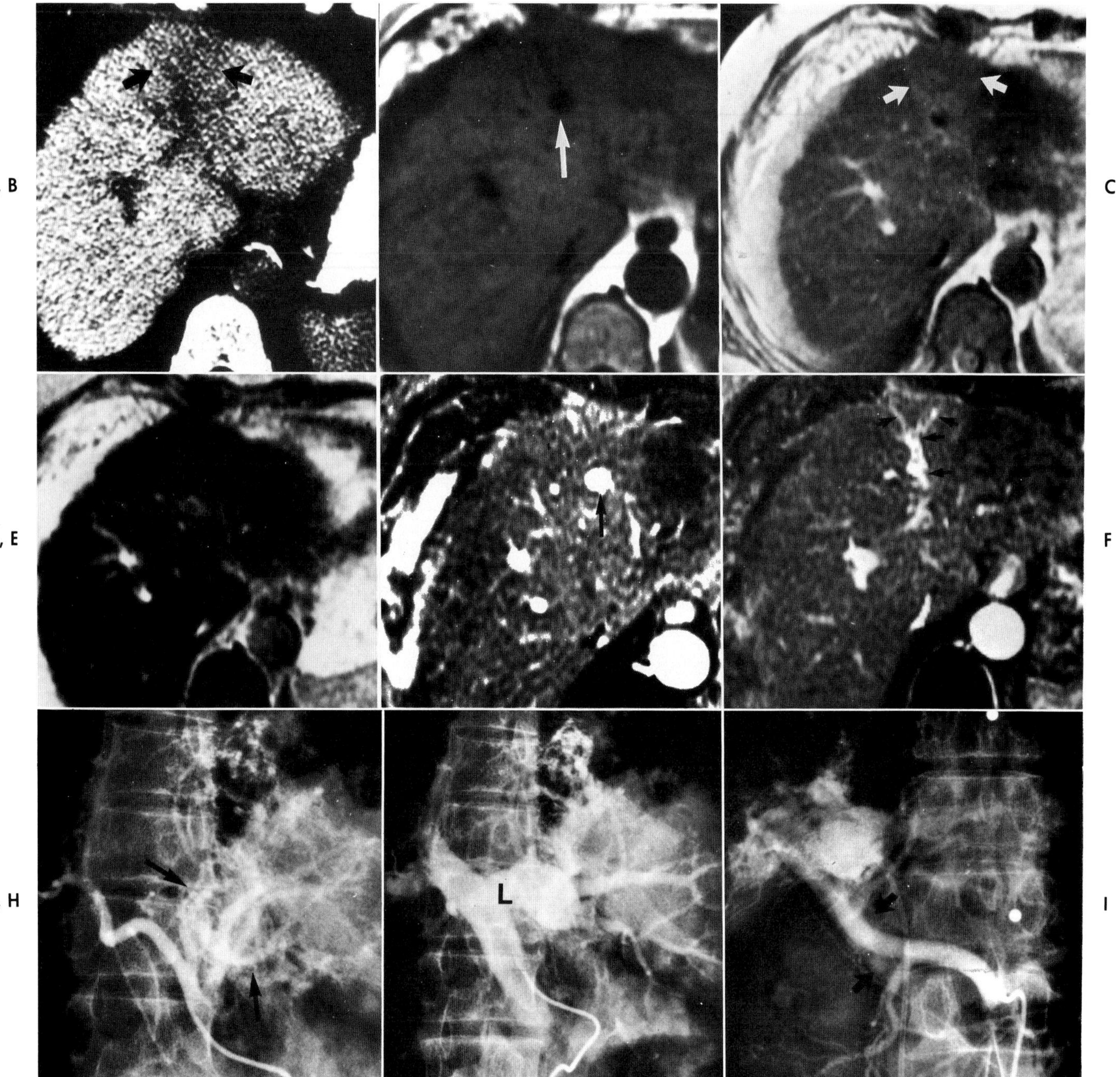

Fig. 11-5   Arteriovenous shunting within a solitary hepatocellular carcinoma with subtle signal characteristics at 1.5 T. **A,** Nonenhanced CT scan reveals a low attenuation mass *(arrows)* in the medial segment of the left lobe. **B,** Corresponding SE 400/22 MR image does not depict the lesion, but an abnormal vessel *(arrow)* is seen in that region. **C,** On the mildly T2-weighted image (SE 2500/50), the lesion *(arrows)* is slightly hyperintense. **D,** On the more heavily T2-weighted (SE 2500/100) image, the lesion is nearly isointense. **E,** The corresponding GRASS image (25/13, flip angle 20 degrees) depicts the abnormal vessel *(arrow)* but not the borders of the lesion. The low signal in the lateral segment is artifact from the aorta. **F,** 1-cm cephalad, more abnormal vessels *(arrows)* are seen within the lesion. **G,** The arterial phase of an hepatic arteriogram, left posterior oblique projection, reveals an anterior hypervascular mass *(arrows)*. **H,** At a later phase, prominent vessels are seen draining into the left portal vein *(L)*. **I,** Late arterial phase, posteroanterior projection. Note early filling of the main portal vein *(arrows)*. Hepatocellular carcinoma was confirmed at surgery, but the patient's severe cirrhosis precluded resection.

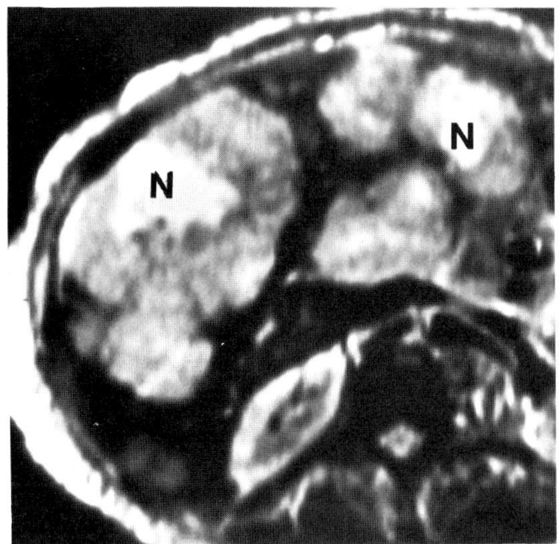

Fig. 11-6 Multifocal hepatocellular carcinoma with necrosis. Axial T2-weighted MR image at 1.5 T (SE 2500/80) reveals numerous masses, some with central hyperintensity indicating necrosis *(N)*.

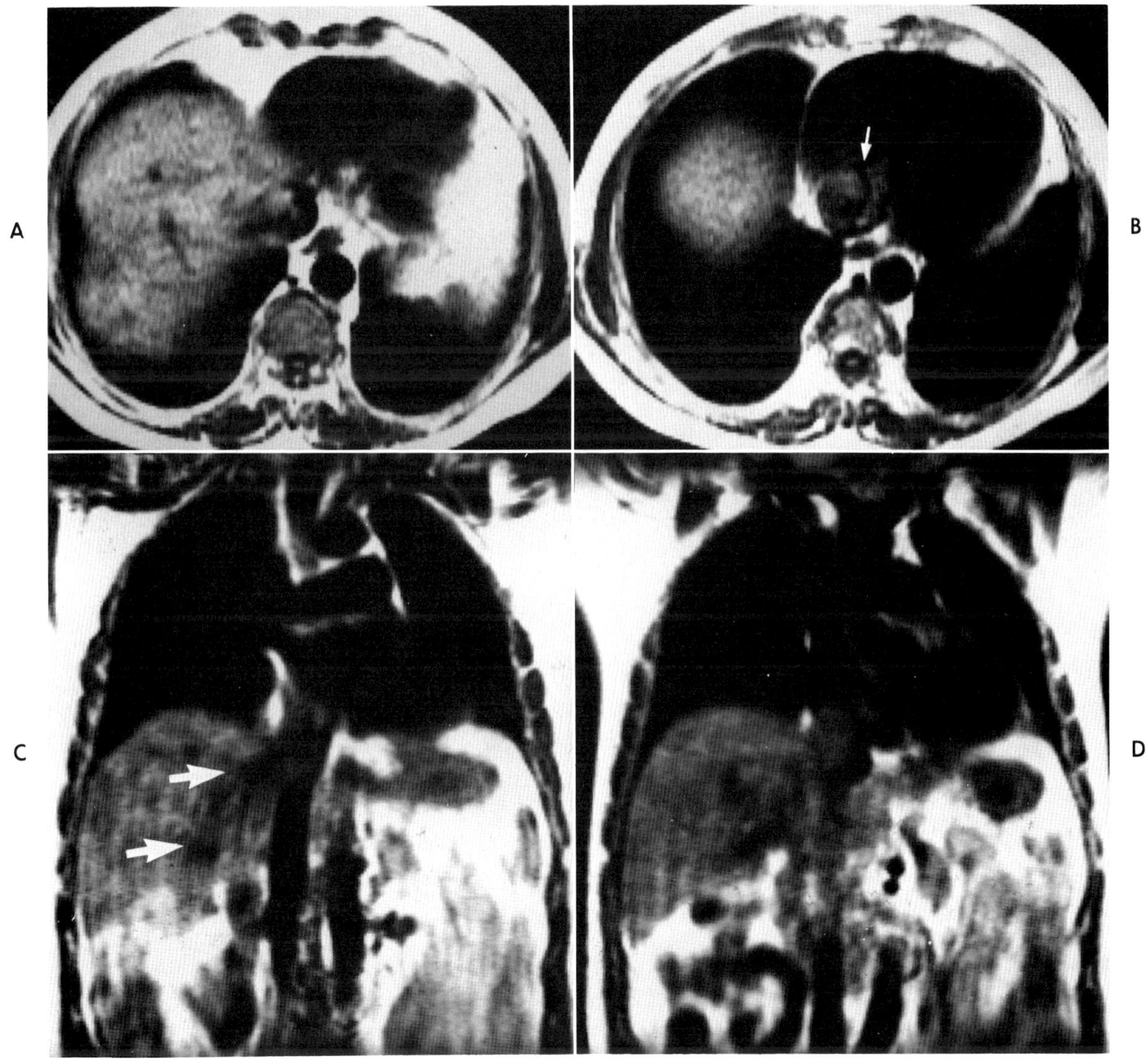

Fig. 11-7 Hepatocellular carcinoma extending through right hepatic vein and inferior vena cava into the heart. **A** and **B,** SE 260/18 images at 0.6 T. Patency of the inferior vena cava is best seen by the MR signal void. A serpiginous vessel is seen within the intracardiac portion of the tumor *(arrow)*. **C,** Coronal image shows the tumor extending through the right hepatic vein *(arrows),* into the inferior vena cava. **D,** Image 1.5 cm anterior to **C.** Tumor is seen floating in the right atrium.

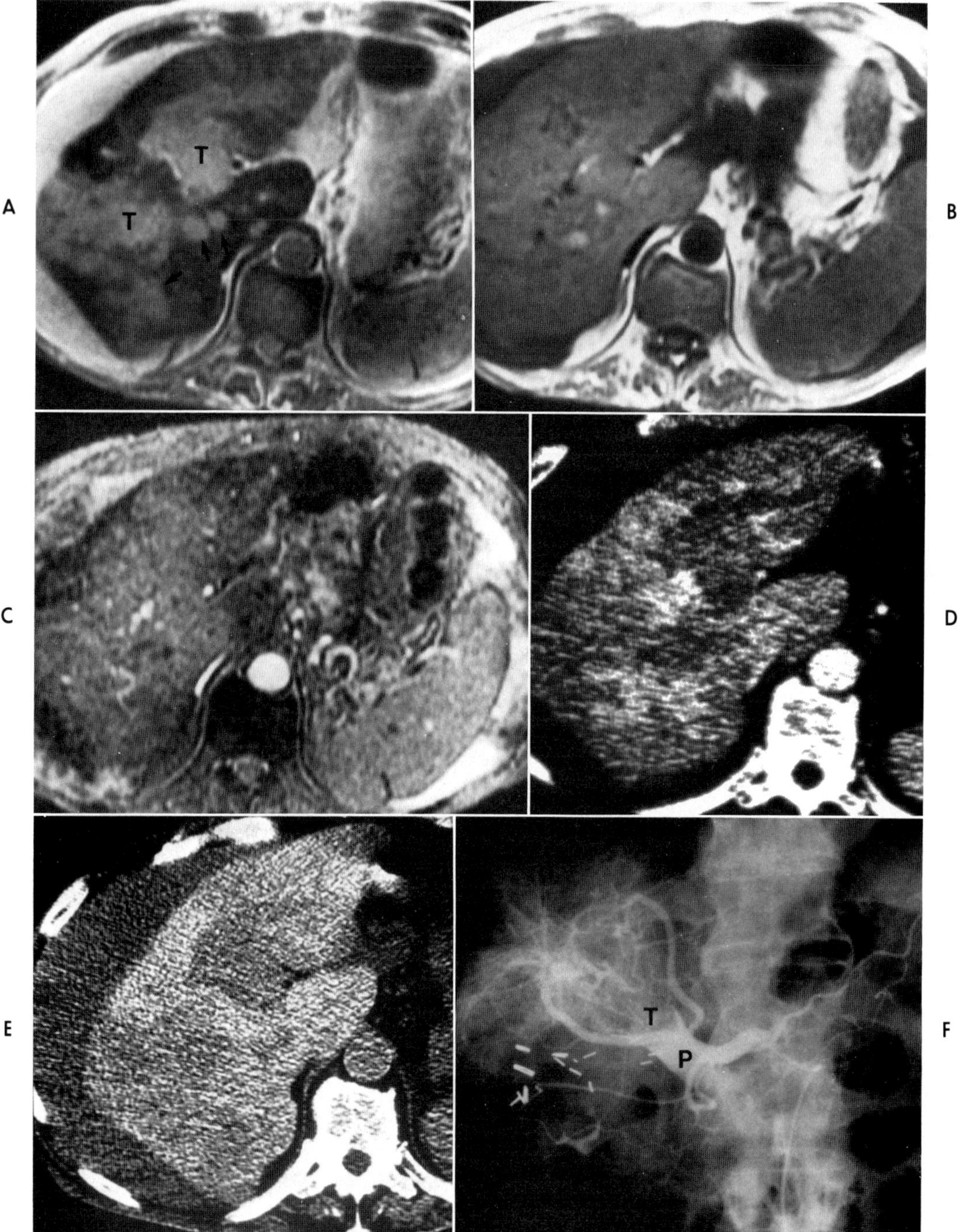

Fig. 11-8 Multifocal hepatocellular carcinoma with portal vein invasion (same patient as Fig 2-1). **A,** SE 2500/50 image at 1.5 T. High-signal tumor *(T)* fills and expands the left and right branches of the portal vein. Several other high-signal masses can be seen *(arrows)*. **B,** Corresponding SE 400/12 image. The tumor is minimally more intense than liver. **C,** Corresponding GRASS (25/13, flip angle 20 degrees) image, confirming portal vein thrombus. **D,** Corresponding CT portogram. Portal vein invasion is confirmed, but the lesions are less well defined than in **A. E,** Corresponding CT scan 4 hours after **D. F,** Hepatic arteriography, arterial phase. Note rapid shunting into the portal vein *(P)*, the distal portion of which is filled with thrombus *(T)*.

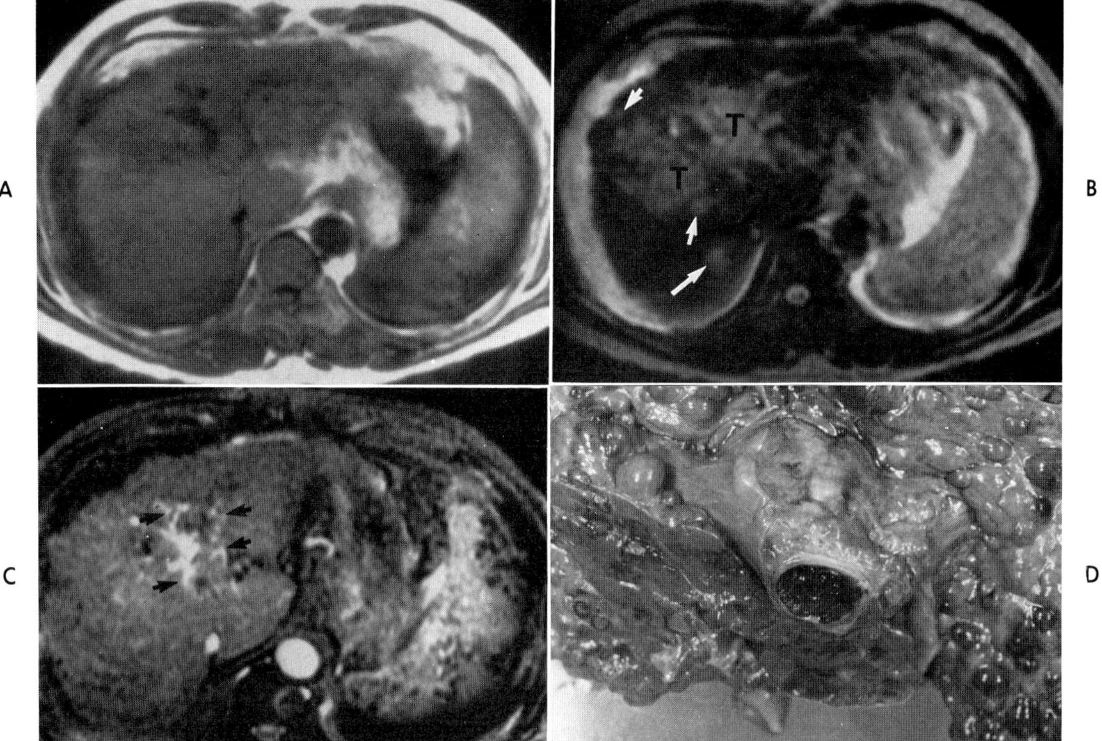

Fig. 11-9 Multifocal hepatocellular carcinoma with portal vein invasion. **A,** Axial SE 600/20 image at 1.5 T at the level of the porta hepatus depicts liver nodularity consistent with cirrhosis. There is no distinct mass, but the portal bifurcation is obliterated. **B,** Corresponding T2-weighted (SE 2500/100) image reveals high-signal tumor *(T)* in the expected position of the portal bifurcation, with several additional masses peripherally *(arrows)*. **C,** Corresponding gradient-echo image (GRASS 25/13, flip angle 20 degrees) fails to detect the mass, but collateral portal vessels *(arrows)* are depicted. Low-signal nodules in the spleen are consistent with siderotic (Gamma-Gandy) nodules, a consequence of portal hypertension **D,** Gross specimen. Tumor thrombus is noted within the portal vein. Note the nodular surface of the liver, indicating cirrhosis.

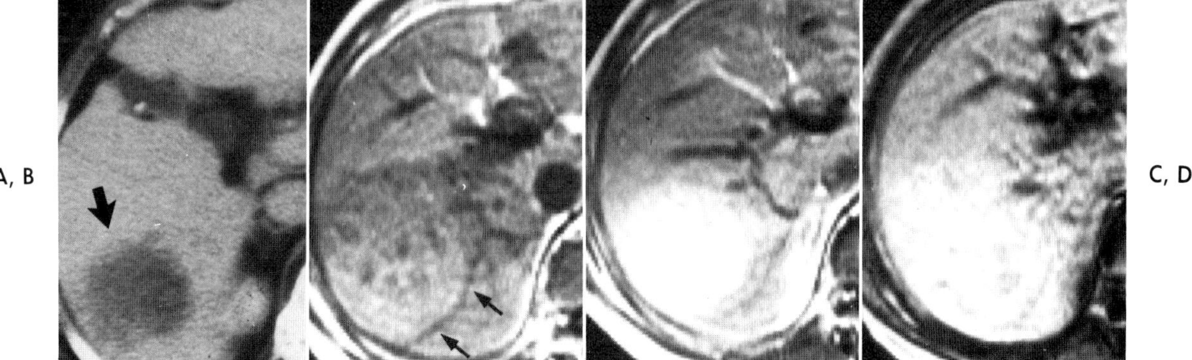

Fig. 11-10 Hepatocellular carcinoma with capsule and intratumoral fat. **A,** Contrast-enhanced CT scan shows a tumor in the right hepatic lobe *(arrow)*. This appearance is nonspecific. **B,** SE 260/18 image at 0.6 T shows a mass in the right lobe displacing normal hepatic vessels. The signal intensity is heterogeneous with mixed areas of increased and decreased intensity (relative to uninvolved liver tissue). A capsule *(arrows)* is seen as a low-intensity line. The increased signal intensity on T1-weighted images is highly suggestive of hepatocellular carcinoma. **C,** SE 2000/30 MR image shows the tumor as an area of increased signal intensity. **D,** SE 2000/30 phase contrast "opposed-phase" image. The tumor is less intense relative to liver, indicating a decrease in tumor signal intensity on the opposed-phase image. This confirms the presence of fat (triglyceride) as a cause for increased tumor signal intensity on the T1-weighted images and strongly suggests hepatocellular carcinoma.

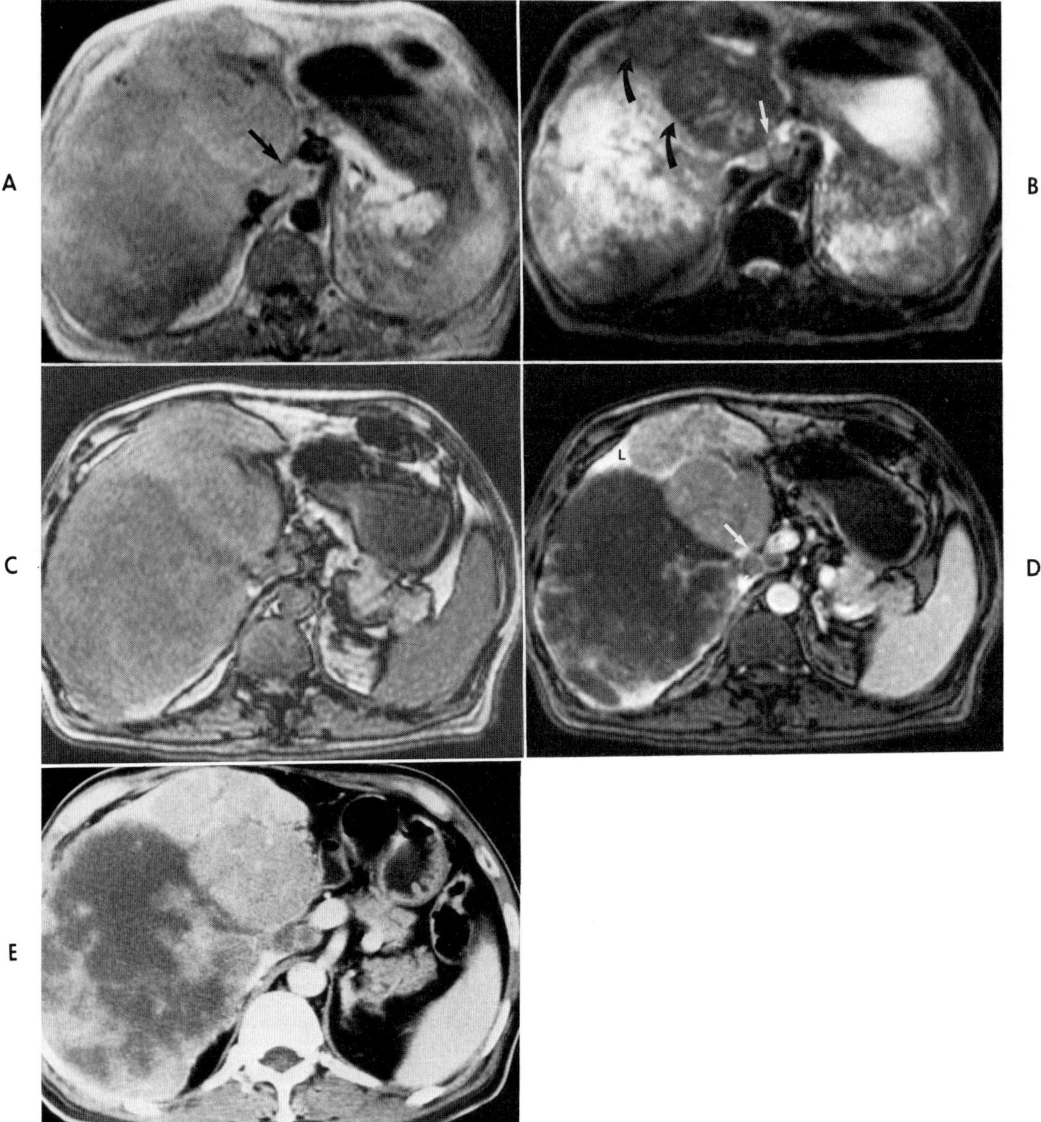

Fig. 11-11 Multifocal hepatocellular carcinoma demonstrating various signal and enhancement characteristics and extrahepatic adenopathy *(arrow)* at 1.5 T. **A,** SE 400/12 image reveals a heterogeneous liver. *Arrow* = lymph nodes. **B,** SE 2500/100 image reveals heterogeneous increased signal posteriorly consistent with tumor. Two masses *(curved arrows)* are present anteriorly with signal similar to that of uninvolved liver except for high-signal streaks. These streaks are evidence against regenerative nodules. **C,** T1-weighted gradient-echo image (140/2.3/90 degrees) is similar to **A. D,** As in **C,** 30 seconds after administration of gadopentatate dimeglumine. The large mass posteriorly does not enhance, suggestive of necrosis. The two anterior masses enhance less than residual liver *(L),* evidence against regenerative nodules. *Arrow* = lymph nodes. **E,** Corresponding CT image during arterial portography reveals findings similar to those in **D.**

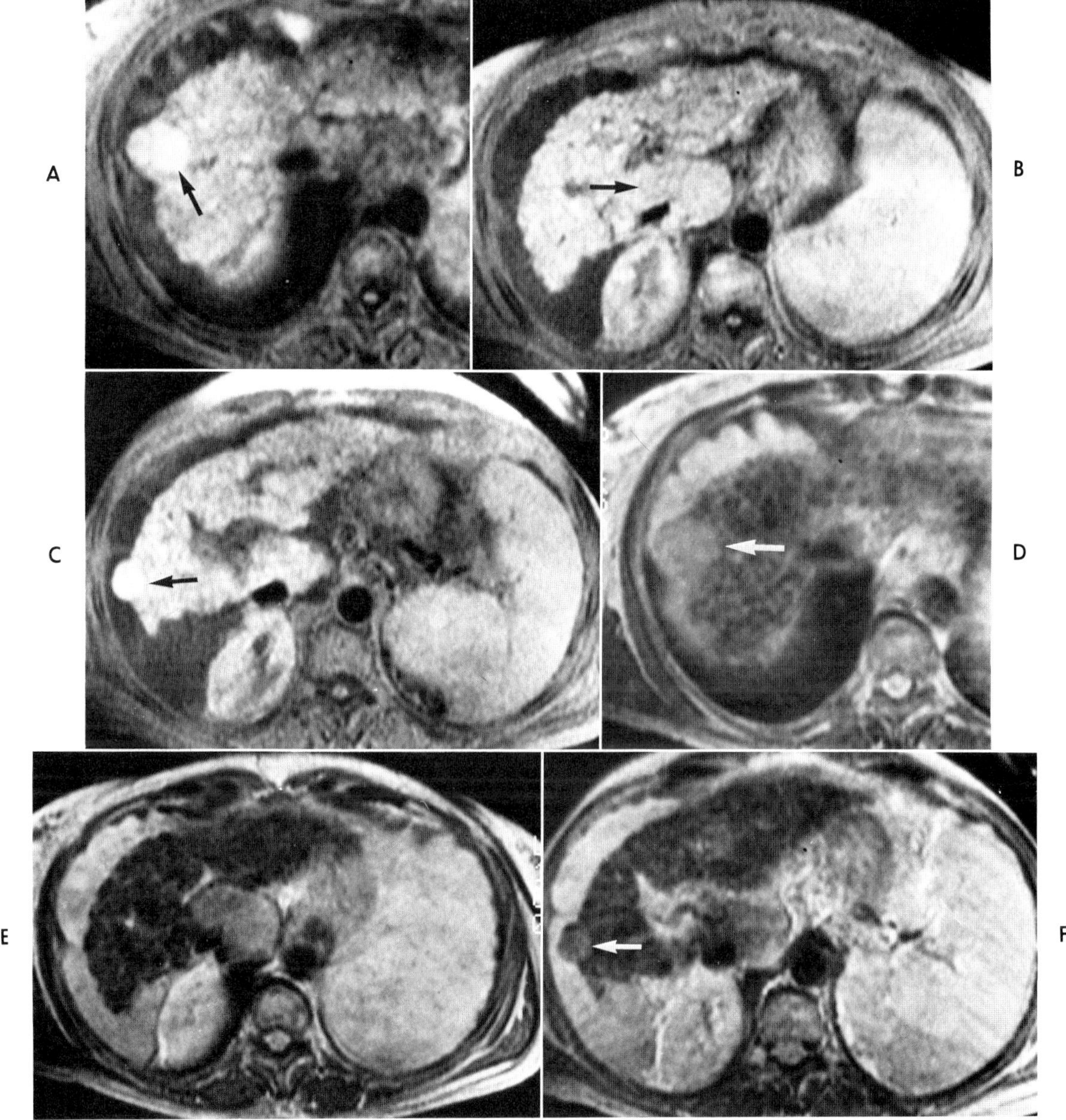

Fig. 11-12 Multiple hepatocellular carcinomas *(arrows)*, most of which are hyperintense on T1-weighted images at 1.5 T. **A** to **C,** T1-weighted images with fat suppression (SE 500/12) depict a hyperintense two-component peripheral mass at the dome of the diaphragm **(A),** a large two-component isointense mass in the caudate lobe **(B)** and a small hyperintense mass laterally. **D** to **F,** Corresponding SE 2500/50 images. All masses have high signal intensity, consistent with hepatocellular carcinoma.

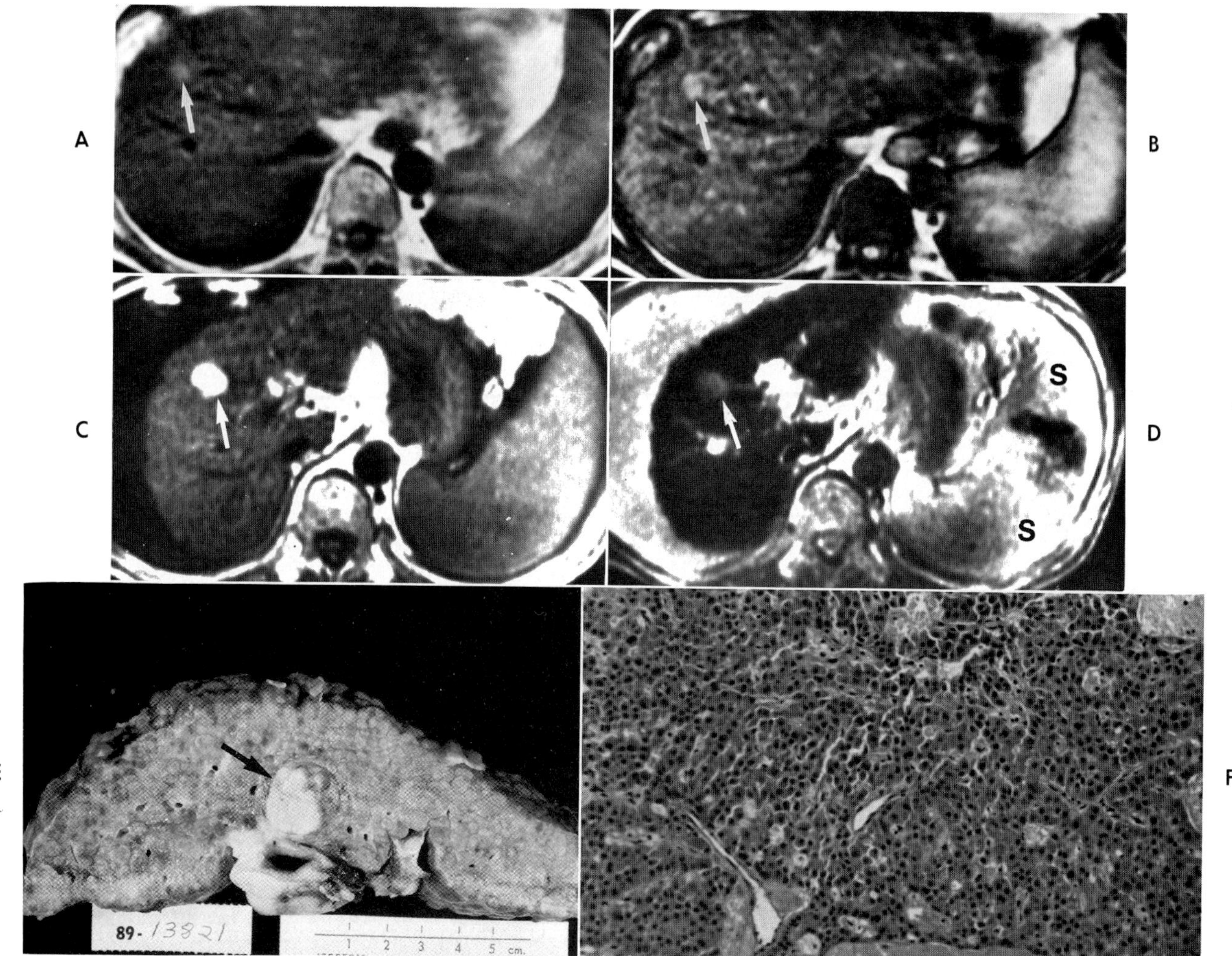

Fig. 11-13 Solitary hyperintense hepatocellular carcinoma in a patient with hemochromatosis, at 1.5 T. **A** and **B,** SE 400/22 axial MR images at the same level. **A** is in phase, whereas **B** is opposed-phase. An 8-mm lesion *(arrows)* is noted that is more intense than the liver, which is heterogeneous and abnormally hypointense. Relative signal intensity on the two images is similar, indicating lack of fat. **C,** Follow-up examination (SE 400/12) 9 months later shows that the mass *(arrow)* has grown. The mass is intermediate in intensity between fat and other soft tissues. Ascites has increased markedly. The liver is heterogeneous and abnormally hypointense. **D,** Corresponding SE 2500/50 image revealing markedly low signal of the liver, except for the lesion *(arrow)*. The spleen *(S)* has a low-signal abnormality anteriorly but otherwise has normal intensity. The pancreas (not shown) was also markedly hypointense. This constellation of findings is typical for hemochromatosis. **E,** Cut section of the liver obtained at surgery for transplantation. A pale, encapsulated mass *(arrow)* is noted within a cirrhotic liver. **F,** Microscopic section, demonstrating well-differentiated hepatocellular carcinoma, with no fat. (From Mitchell, D.G., Palazzo, J., Hann, H-W.Y.L., et al.: J. Comput. Assist. Tomogr. 15:762-769, 1991.)

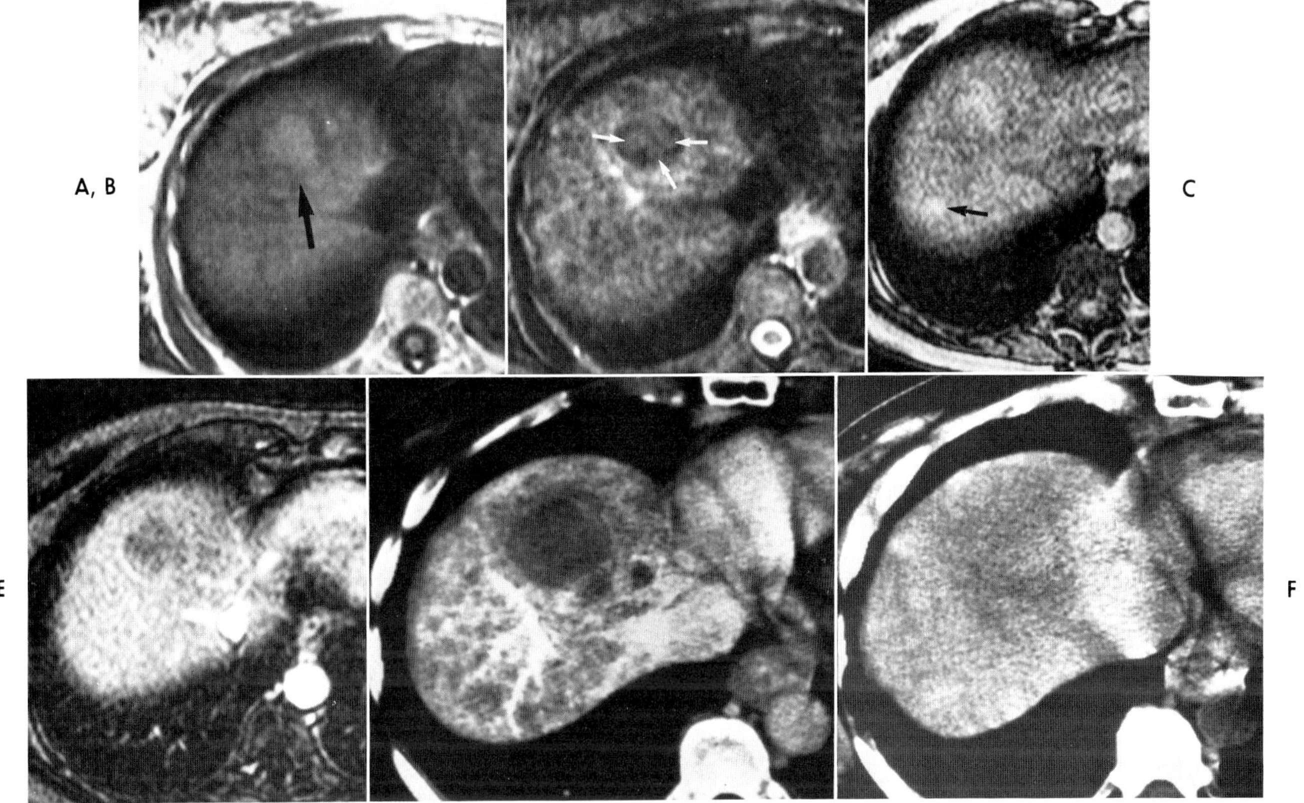

Fig. 11-14   Hepatocellular carcinoma with high signal on T1-weighted images and features of malignancy on T2-weighted and dynamic-enhanced images. **A,** Axial SE 400/12 image at 1.5 T depicts a high-signal mass *(arrow)* near the dome of the diaphragm. **B,** Corresponding SE 2500/100 image reveals foci of increased signal intensity *(arrows),* excluding the possibility of benign regenerative nodule. The remainder of the mass has low signal intensity relative to the liver parenchyma, which is abnormally hyperintense due to active cirrhosis. **C,** T1-weighted gradient-echo image (TR/TE/flip angle = 102/2.3/90 degrees). In spite of limited SNR the lack of respiratory-induced blurring reveals an additional lesion posteriorly *(arrow).* **D,** Snapshot inversion recovery image (TI = 500 msec, centric phase order) acquired 30 seconds after administration of gadopentetate dimeglumine. The lesion is now less intense than liver, further evidence against regenerative liver, which should enhance similar to the rest of the liver during the portal venous phase. **E,** CT with arterial portography. The mass has little if any blood supply from the portal vein. **F,** Delayed CT, 4 hours after **E.** The mass is isodense, indicating that contrast accumulates inside hepatocytes within the tumor. **G,** Capillary phase from hepatic arteriography depicts the mass *(large arrow)* as hypervascular. Additional nodules are noted *(arrows).*

In addition to being hyperintense on T1-weighted images, HCC is unusual in that it may be subtle on T2-weighted images (see Fig. 11-4, 11-5, and 11-14).[235,371] As with high signal on T1-weighted images, low-to-intermediate signal on T2-weighted images is especially likely with small, well-differentiated tumors.

As with metastases, HCC must be distinguished from cavernous hemangioma. In one study, calculated T2 values for HCC and hemangioma were 59 ± 9 versus 102 ± 26 at .35 T, and 49 ± 10 versus 85 ± 21 at 1.5 T ($-p < .001$ for both).[393] Rarely, T2 relaxation may be exceptionally long, such as in the pseudoglandular form of HCC, which is characterized by dense, homogeneous acinar formation.[389]

MORPHOLOGIC FEATURES

MRI is diagnostic of HCC more often than CT, sonography, or scintigraphy because of its demonstration of characteristic morphologic features. T2-weighted spin-echo images may show a "mosaic" or "nodules-in-nodule" pattern of signal intensity, produced by multiple centers of growth interspersed with areas of low signal coagulative necrosis and/or noncancerous regenerative liver tissue (Fig. 11-14).[78,230] Internal heterogeneity is an important feature for distinguishing HCC from regenerative nodule.

A 0.5- to 3.0-mm thick capsule can be identified by T1-weighted MR images in 40% of cases, twice as often as by CT (see Figs. 11-2 to 11-4, and 11-10).[109,230,235] T2-weighted MR images may not demonstrate the capsule, but are more likely to depict the mosaic or nodules-in-nodule patterns.[78] Cavernous hemangioma and cysts do not form capsules or contain intratumoral nodules. Rarely, metastases or hepatic adenoma may have a capsule.

On occasion, HCC has a central scar that may be vascular, inflammatory, or fibrotic (Fig. 11-15).[451,545] Fibrolamellar HCC is especially likely to have a central fibrous scar.[41,150] Fibrolamellar HCC is different from

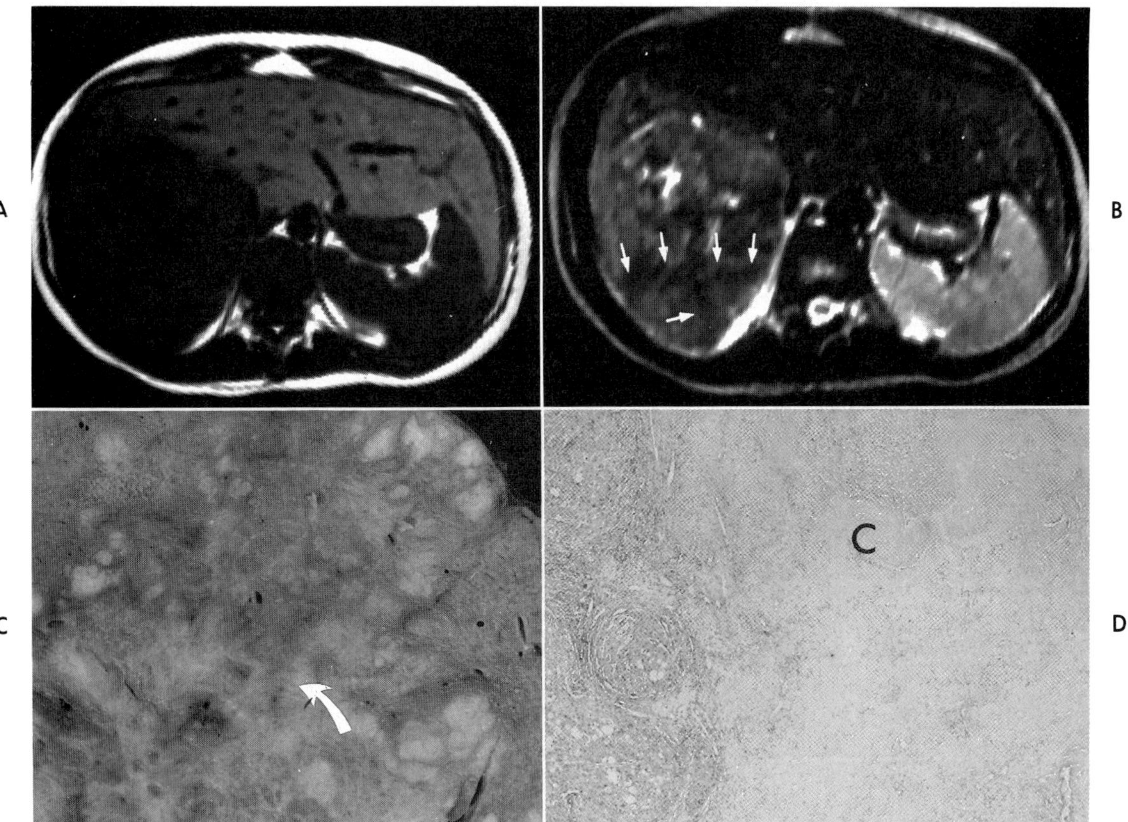

Fig. 11-15 Collagenous scar tissue in hepatocellular carcinoma. **A,** Scar tissue appears isointense relative to the tumor and is therefore not detected on this T1-weighted (SE 260/14) image at 0.6 T. **B,** T2-weighted (SE 2350/120) images display the scar *(arrows)* slightly hypointense relative to surrounding tumor. **C,** Gross pathologic specimen shows pale white collagenous scar tissue (arrow). **D,** Histologic specimen shows dense collagenous (C), hypocellular scar tissue (H & E staining; original magnification, ×31). (From Rummeny, E., Weissleder, R., Sironi, S., et al.: Radiology 171:323-326, 1989.)

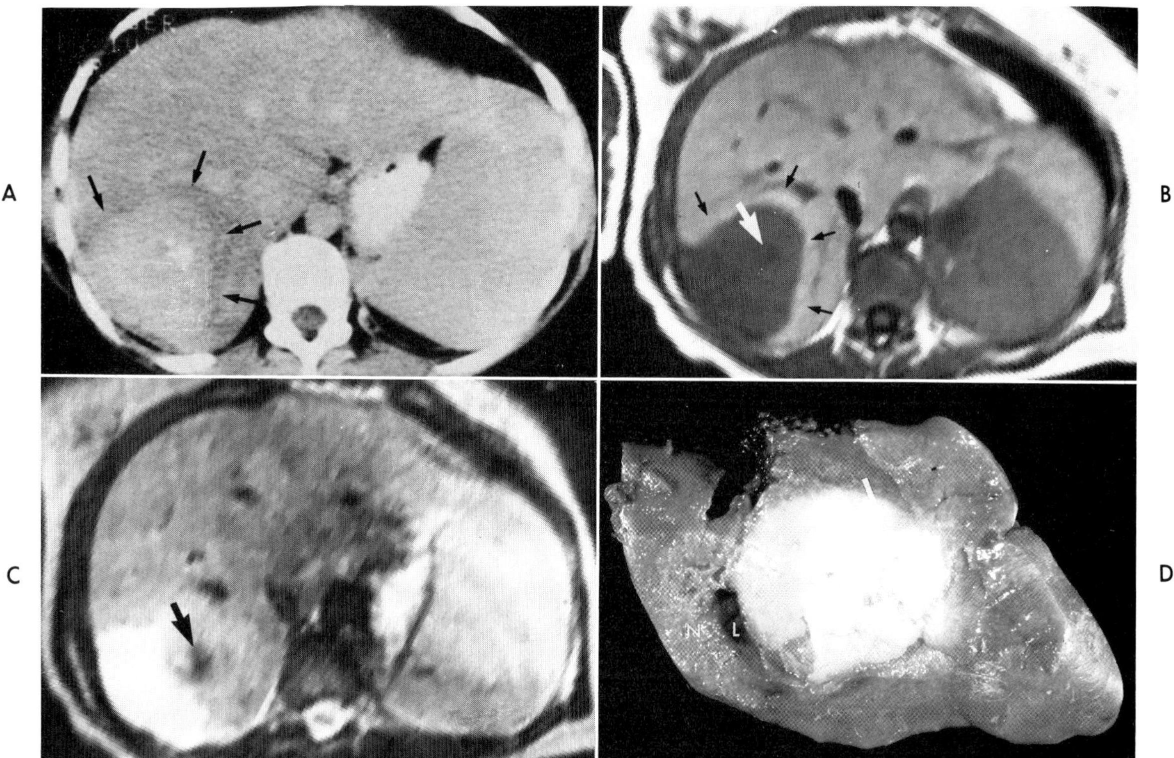

Fig. 11-16   Carcinosarcoma with central scar. **A,** Contrast-enhanced CT scan shows an enhancing mass with a low-attenuation rim. **B,** T1-weighted spin-echo image at 0.6 T (260/14). Tumor is identified as hypointense mass lesion. Central area of reduced intensity is noted *(white arrow)*. Note hyperintense rim *(black arrows)* at tumor-liver border. **C,** SE 2350/120 image shows central hypointensity *(arrow)* and peripheral hyperintensity. **D,** Surgical specimen, sectioned in transverse plane, corresponds to **A** to **C.** Tumor calcification *(arrow)* corresponds to central hypointensity seen on T1- and T2-weighted images. Peripheral hyperintensity in **B** corresponded to histologically evident fatty infiltration of liver adjacent to tumor (not shown). Necrosis *(N)* of liver tissue with liquefaction *(L)* adjacent to tumor is seen. (From Rummeny, E., Weissleder, R., Stark D.D., et al.: AJR 152:63-72, 1989.)

other forms of HCC in most respects. Fibrolamellar HCC is less aggressive and tends to occur in young individuals without cirrhosis or other risk factors for HCC.

Fibrous scars usually have low signal intensity on T1- and T2-weighted images. Vascular and inflammatory scars, however, have high intensity on T2-weighted images because of increased free water.[452] Fibrous scars are more common with HCC; vascular scars are more common with focal nodular hyperplasia. Unfortunately, however, the presence and signal characteristics of scars do not allow reliable distinction between benign and malignant primary hepatic lesions (Fig. 11-16).[452,602]

In some cases, HCC arises within a large regenerative nodule (see Chapter 12).[9] Large regenerative nodules are more likely to have dysplastic or malignant internal foci if they contain iron.[532,533] The presence of a small

HCC tumor within large siderotic regenerative nodules causes a particularly characteristic MRI appearance, consisting of one or more foci of intermediate intensity within a low-signal nodule (see Figs. 11-1 and 11-2).[350,531] Since iron stimulates the growth of tumor cells,[193,194] this may induce malignant change within dysplastic nodules. The appearance of HCC as an iron-negative nodule within a siderotic mass has been described as valuable in making a histologic diagnosis in difficult cases, since HCC does not accumulate iron.[532] We are not aware of any other hepatic lesion that manifests as high intensity within a low-intensity lesion. Therefore this appearance should be considered strongly suggestive of early HCC, even if α-fetoprotein is normal and biopsy does not reveal tumor.

In addition to signal intensity and morphologic features (e.g., capsules, ill-defined margins, or internal heterogeneity), dynamic scanning after administration of gadopentetate dimeglumine may help distinguish HCC from cavernous hemangioma. Even in hypervascular HCC, the arterial supply of the tumor is usually less than the combined portal venous and hepatic arterial supply of hepatic parenchyma. Thus 80% of HCCs show less enhancement than surrounding liver during the first 5-minute period.[307] CT with arterial portography is especially effective at enhancing liver more than HCC,[322] but its utility has not been determined in patients with severely reduced portal flow resulting from massive porto-systemic shunting. CT with arterial portography is likely to be ineffective in patients with reversed portal vein flow.

MRI is more sensitive than CT, sonography, or angiography for detecting intrahepatic vascular invasion.[235] However, interpretation of MR images can be difficult when tumors compress vessels and cause slow flow. Careful comparison between T1-weighted images, flow-sensitive gradient-echo images and multiecho T2-weighted images may be necessary. When vascular invasion is detected, the diagnosis of HCC should be favored because metastases and other hepatic tumors rarely invade vessels.

After therapeutic embolization, MRI may show increased intensity secondary to necrosis, as well as decreased size.[394] Gas bubbles are also common within 2 weeks of embolization.[154,394] MRI appears promising after hepatocellular carcinoma following ethanol injection because signal intensity after successful treatment decreases on T2-weighted images and increases on T1-weighted images. Unsuccessful ethanol ablation is manifested as unchanged signal intensity of the tumor.[407,487]

Benign Hepatocellular Masses

Well-differentiated hepatocellular tumors, whether benign or malignant, resemble normal liver tissue in many respects. These tumors often have relatively short T1, causing them to be isointense or hyperintense relative to liver on T1-weighted images. In some cases, this results from accumulation of lipid within functioning intratumoral hepatocytes. On T2-weighted images, some hepatocellular tumors may be subtle. Certain morphologic features, such as central scars, occur primarily in hepatocellular tumors.

Although benign and malignant hepatocellular tumors share certain MRI features, there are several valuable differential features that help distinguish between them.

HYPERPLASTIC NODULES AND HEPATIC HYPERTROPHY

Although most reports in radiologic literature suggest that large regenerative nodules are entirely benign, recent reports in pathologic literature suggest otherwise. Some large regenerative nodules have dysplastic histology, leading to the term *adenomatoid hyperplasia*.[292,321] Discreet foci of dysplasia or frank malignancy have been noted within dysplastic regenerative nodules (see Figs. 11-1 and 11-2).[*]

Adenomatoid hyperplasia has been described as having high intensity on T1-weighted MR images, although the cause of the high intensity has not been determined. The lack of high signal on T2-weighted images distinguishes these premalignant lesions from most HCCs. Since HCCs may also be hyperintense on T1-weighted images and subtle or hypointense on T2-weighted images, these signal characteristics are not specific. This is consistent with the histologic similarity between hyperplastic nodules and well-differentiated HCC.

Careful analysis of internal morphology is essential for diagnosing HCC. Internal foci of high or low signal suggest centers of more rapid growth and thus indicate a high likelihood of malignancy (see Figs. 11-1, 11-2, and 11-14).

Capsules and irregular margins are important signs of malignancy, the former occurring in early, well-differentiated HCC and the latter with more advanced tu-

mors. Hyperplastic nodules have smooth margins and lack capsules (Figs. 12-1 and 12-2). Enhancement patterns also tend to differ. Hyperplastic nodules are supplied primarily by the portal vein, similar to the remainder of the liver, whereas HCCs are supplied almost exclusively by the hepatic artery. Thus hyperplastic nodules usually enhance similar to the remainder of the liver (see Fig. 12-1), whereas HCC usually enhances less than liver during the early portal venous phase after a bolus of contrast material (see Fig. 11-14).[307] Arterial portography is even more reliable for this differentiation.[322] This distinction is not absolute, however, since early, well-differentiated HCC often retains some portal perfusion, and benign dysplastic nodules have relatively increased arterial perfusion. Additionally, patients with severe cirrhosis often have decreased portal perfusion and increased hepatic arterial perfusion.

Close monitoring with MRI of patients with large regenerative nodules may be prudent. In one series, each of 12 large regenerative nodules, diagnosed by benign histology on initial aspiration, was found to be enlarged on follow-up examination. Malignancy was eventually diagnosed in 10 of the 12.[424] Some investigators recommend percutaneous injection of large dysplastic nodules with ethanol under ultrasound guidance.[292]

Large regenerative nodules that accumulate iron[350,532,533] or fat[534] appear to have greater malignant potential than other nodules. One autopsy series noted malignant foci within 19 of 26 (73%) large iron-accumulative–regenerative nodules.[533] This may be due to the tumor-enhancing effects of iron or to the rapid growth associated with regeneration. HCC occurring within siderotic nodules has a unique MRI appearance, consisting of a predominantly low-signal nodule with a small internal focus of intermediate or high intensity (see Figs. 11-1 and 11-2)[350,531] Fatty dysplastic nodules also can exhibit rapid growth and malignant potential (Fig. 12-3).[534]

Regenerative nodules should be examined carefully for internal foci. If such lesions are found, it might be prudent to proceed directly to surgery if the patient is considered a good surgical risk and if no other lesions are evident. Alternatively, percutaneous treatment might be indicated. We are not aware of any other phe-

---

[*]9, 116, 155, 350, 373, 531-534, 569

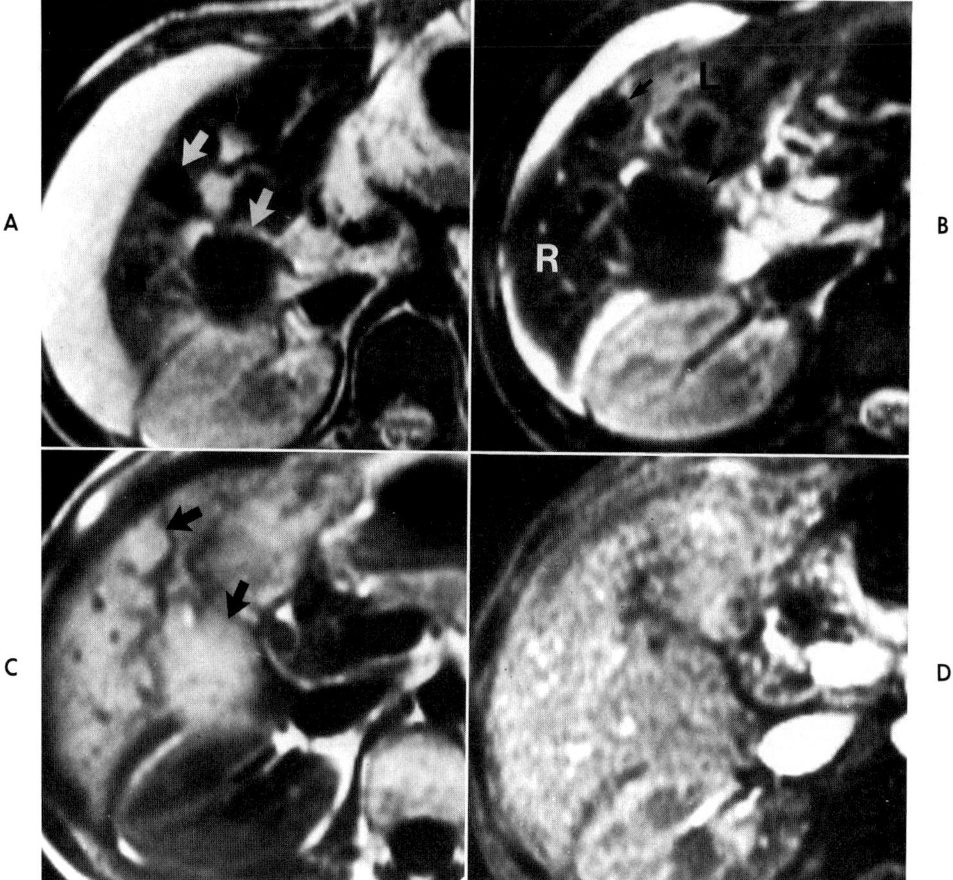

Fig. 12-1 Regenerative nodules in a patient with acute fulminant hepatitis with active cirrhosis. **A,** Transverse T2-weighted image at 1.5 T (SE 2500/100) reveals low-signal masses in the right lobe, consistent with regenerative nodules *(arrows)*. The surrounding hepatic parenchyma is heterogeneous, with abnormally increased signal of the posterior segment of the right lobe *(R)*. **B,** Approximately 1 year later, the regenerative nodules *(arrows)* are essentially unchanged, although the surrounding hepatic parenchyma appears slightly different. There has been regeneration in the posterior segment of the right lobe *(R)*, with increased size and normalization of intensity. The left lobe *(L)* now has heterogeneously increased signal. **C,** On the corresponding T1-weighted image (SE 400/12), the nodules *(arrows)* are slightly hyperintense and are more homogeneous than hepatic parenchyma. **D,** Corresponding GRASS image (25/13, flip angle 20 degrees) shows that the masses are isointense, with no evidence of significant iron.

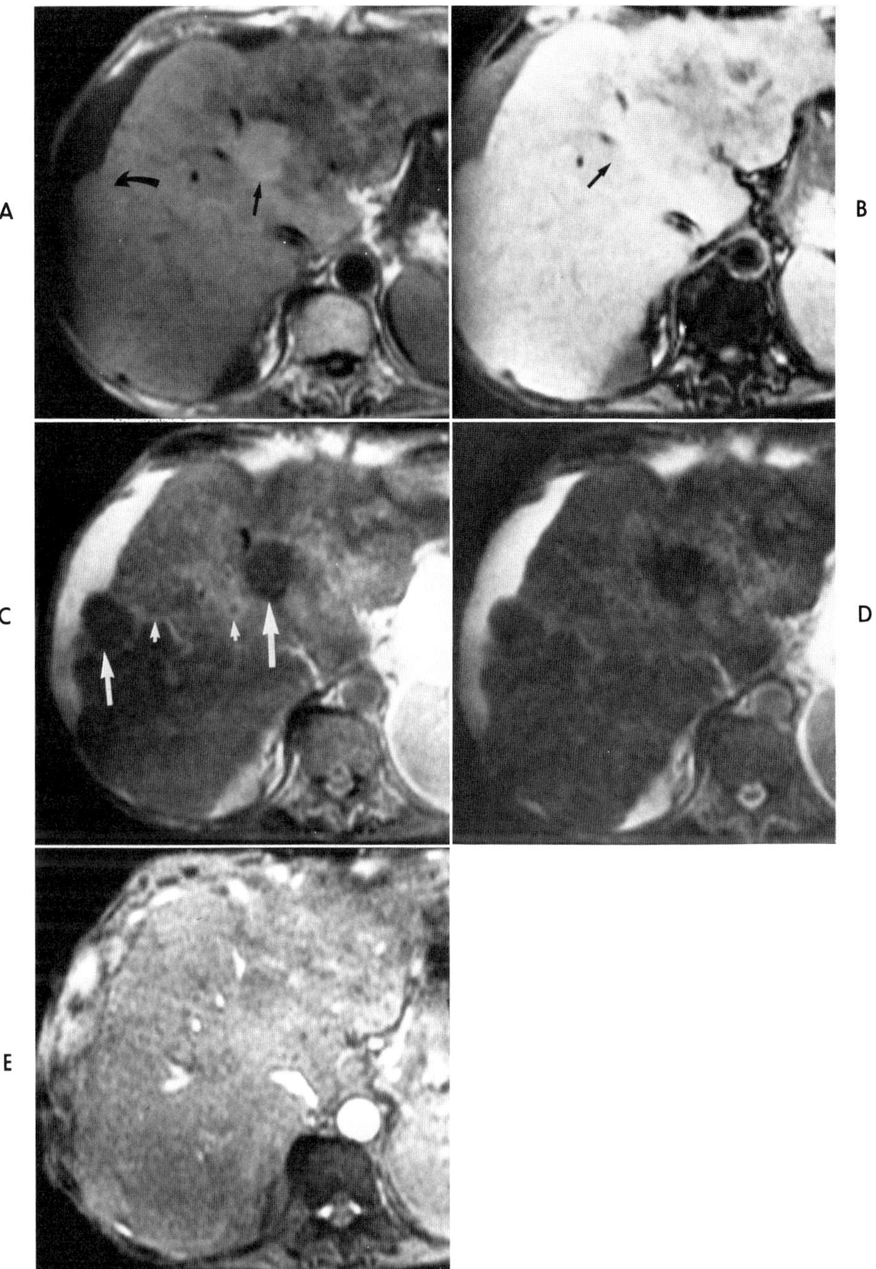

Fig. 12-2   Large regenerative nodules depicted best on spin-echo images at 1.5 T. **A,** SE 400/12 image depicts a nodule in the left lobe *(straight arrow)* as hyperintense relative to the adjacent parenchyma, which has abnormally low signal intensity. A second isointense nodule is depicted as a focal contour abnormality *(curved arrow).* **B,** T1-weighted opposed-phase image (SE 400/14). The nodule in the left lobe remains hyperintense, proving that its high signal intensity is not due to increased fat content. **C,** SE 2500/50 image. The liver has heterogeneous increased signal intensity *(small arrows)* because of inflammatory cirrhosis, causing it to be be brighter than the nodules *(large arrows),* which have relatively normal signal intensity. **D,** SE 2500/100 image. **E,** Corresponding gradient-echo image (TR/TE/flip angle = 25/13/90 degrees). The nodules are barely visible, evidence against increased iron being the cause of their visibility on **C** and **D.**

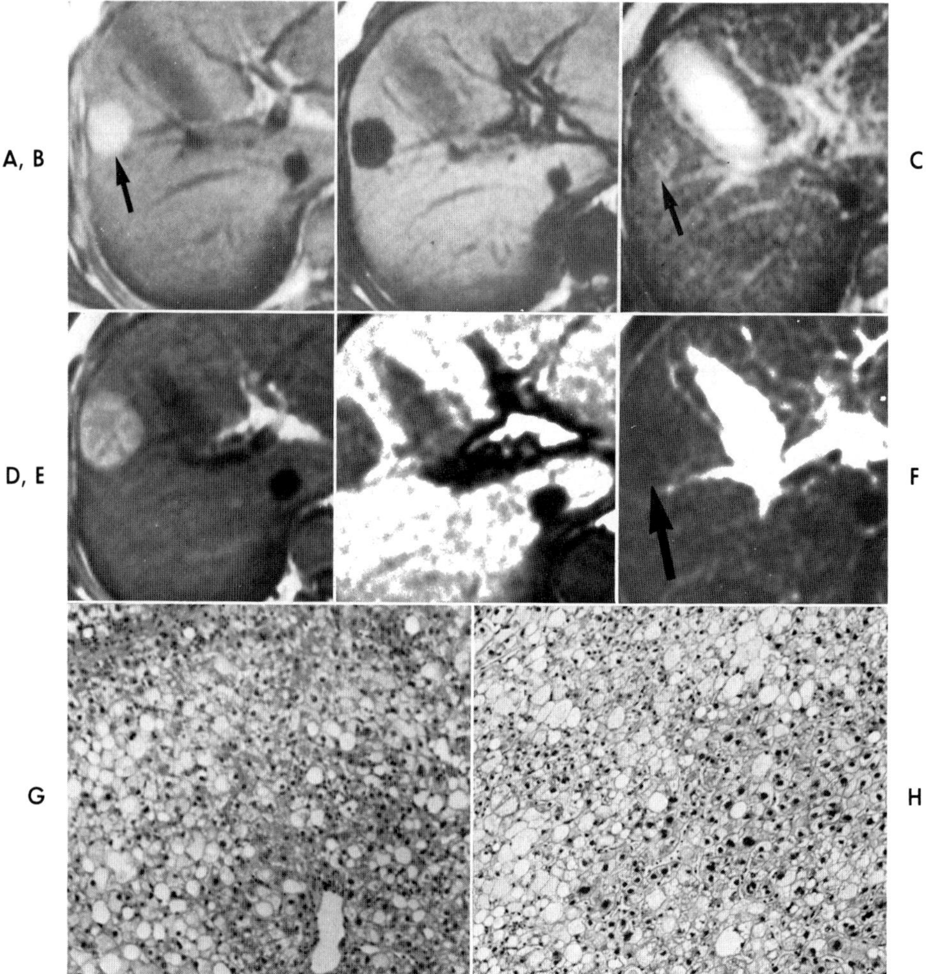

Fig. 12-3   Fatty dysplastic regenerative nodule that grew significantly within 14 months. **A,** SE 400/20 image at 1.5 T reveals a well-marginated, homogeneous high-signal mass *(arrow).* **B,** Corresponding opposed-phase image (400/22) shows a virtual signal void, indicating a composition that includes much fat and water. **C,** On the T2-weighted image (SE 2500/100) the mass is subtle *(arrow)* and slightly more intense than surrounding liver. The liver is heterogeneous, consistent with cirrhosis. **D,** Surgical biopsy reveals a fatty mass with mild dysplasia but no evidence of malignancy. **E,** SE 400/12 image 14 months later reveals marked growth of the mass, which is now less homogeneous than in **A. F,** Corresponding opposed-phase image (400/14), again reveals heterogeneity, with small foci of intermediate intensity. **G,** On the T2-weighted image (SE 2500/100), the mass *(arrow)* is slightly less intense than surrounding liver. **H,** Histologic section from surgical removal (H & E). Dysplasia and non-fatty components have increased, but the histology remains benign. (From Mitchell, D.G., Palazzo, J., Hann, H-W.Y.L., et al.: J. Comput. Assist. Tomogr. 15:762-769, 1991.)

nomenon that causes a high-intensity focus within a low-signal hepatic nodule. An intermediate-intensity focus within a fatty nodule should be viewed with similar suspicion. Since small HCCs are usually well differentiated, biopsy of nodules such as these may fail to disclose tumor, and serologic markers for HCC, such as α-fetoprotein, are usually normal in patients with small tumors.[255,373,521] Since regenerative nodules are delineated and characterized best by MRI, MRI guidance for biopsy may be useful in selected patients.

Massive hepatic regeneration may occur as a response to lobar atrophy or severe heterogeneous hepatic disease (Figs. 12-4 to 12-6).[297] Regenerative liver may mimic a mass, but it should have signal characteristics similar to those of normal hepatic parenchyma, and hepatic vessels may be visible within it. The surrounding hepatic parenchyma may have grossly abnormal signal, however. Awareness of the normal signal of hepatic parenchyma, which is higher than spleen on T1-weighted images and only slightly higher than muscle on T2-weighted images, should allow differentiation between malignancy and regenerative masses. This is important, so that the most pathologic liver can be biopsied.

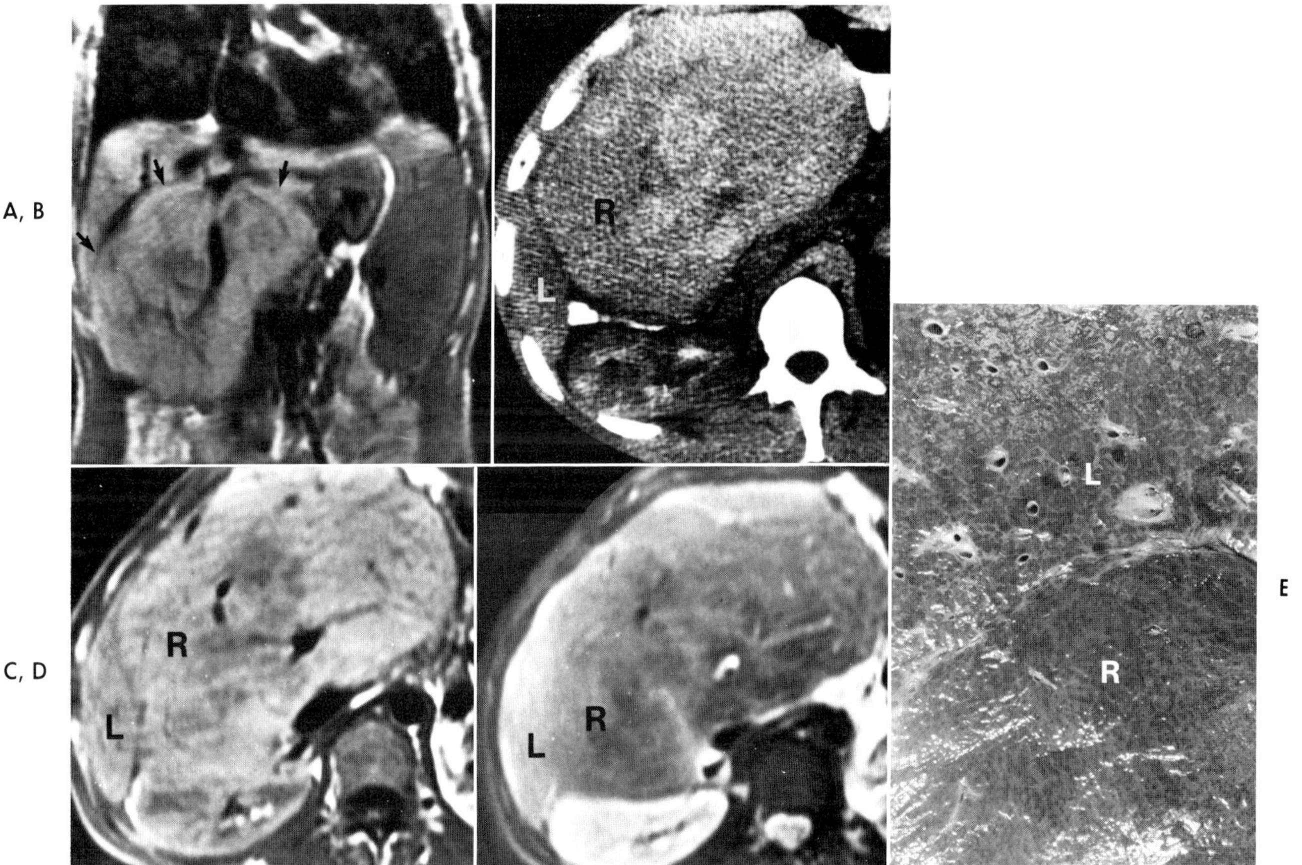

Fig. 12-4   Massive regeneration of the right lobe (same patient as Fig. 11-4). **A,** T1-weighted coronal image at 1.5 T through the posterior portion of the liver depicts the border between a large inferior mass and the right lobe of the liver *(arrows)*. **B,** CT scan 6 hours after contrast enhancement demonstrates slight hyperintensity of the regenerated liver *(R)* relative to the remaining liver *(L)*, consistent with decreased retention of iodinated contrast within hepatocytes of cirrhotic liver relative to those of regenerated liver. **C,** Corresponding axial SE 500/20 image. The regenerated liver is heterogeneous and slightly more intense than the remaining liver. **D,** Corresponding SE 3000/50 image shows that the regenerative mass is heterogeneous and slightly less intense than the adjacent liver. **E,** Autopsy performed 5 weeks later, after death from massive gastrointestinal hemorrhage, revealed massive regeneration in the right lobe, with changes of cirrhosis. Less fibrous tissue is present in the area of regeneration *(R)* than in the remainder of the liver *(L)*. There was no significant iron or fat in either portion.

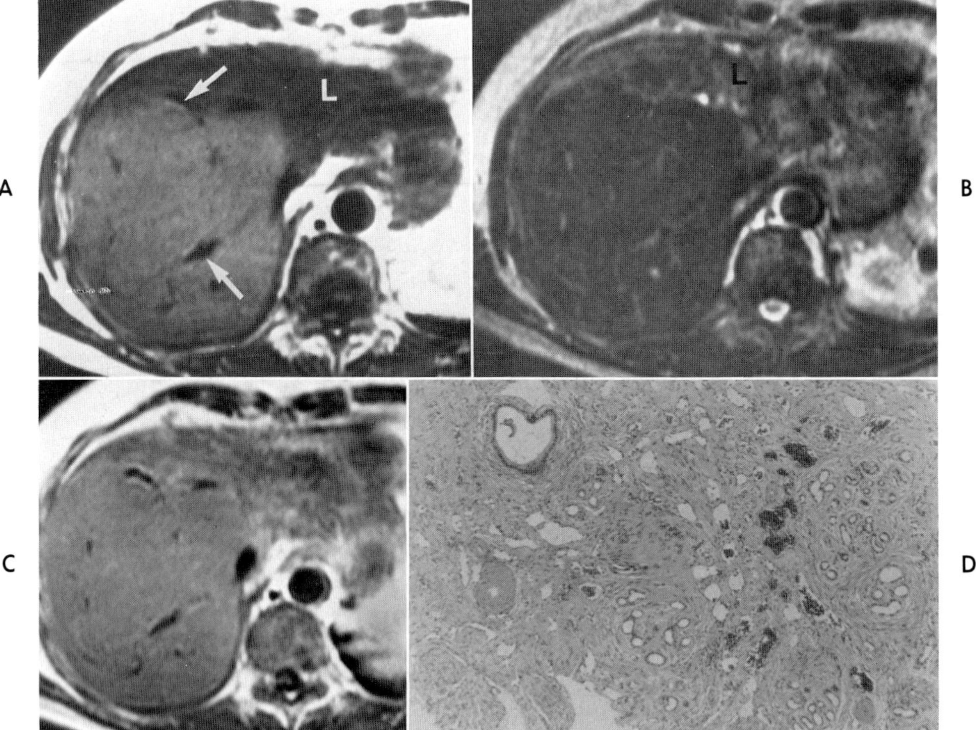

Fig. 12-5 Massive regeneration of the right lobe and atrophy of the left lobe, depicted at 1.5 T. **A,** Axial SE 400/12 image reveals enlargement of the anterior segment of the right lobe with associated displacement of the middle and right hepatic veins *(arrows)*. The left lobe *(L)* is small and hypointense. **B,** Corresponding SE 2500/100 image reveals homogeneous normal intensity of the right lobe but abnormal heterogeneous high signal of the left lobe *(L),* consistent with edema. **C,** Corresponding SE 400/12 image after administration of gadopentetate dimeglumine. The left lobe enhances more than the right (compare with *A*). **D,** Biopsy of the left lobe from surgery (H & E) reveals vascular granulation tissue and proliferative bile ductules with no viable hepatocytes.

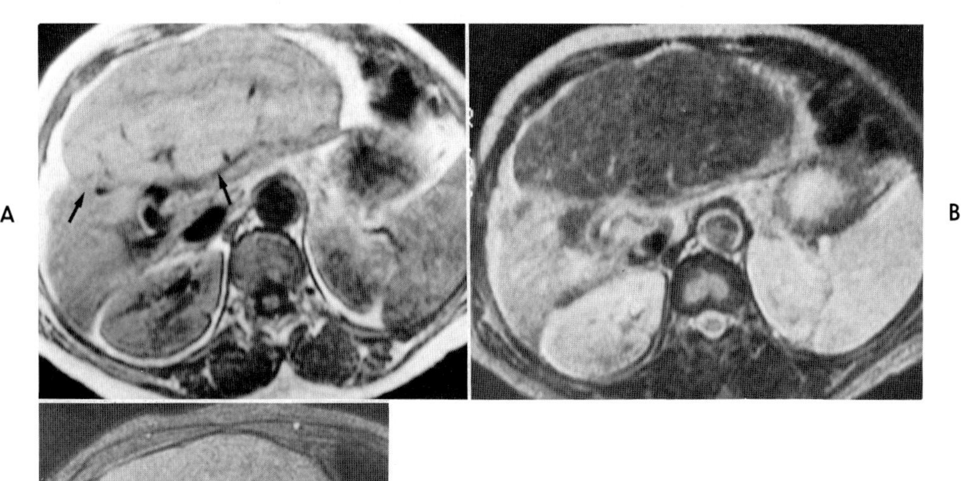

Fig. 12-6 Masslike hypertrophy in a patient with severe active cirrhosis at 1.5 T. **A,** SE 600/20 reveals a large mass in the left lobe *(arrows)*. The right lobe is atrophic and has an abnormally low signal, similar to that of the spleen. **B,** SE 2500/80 depicts the mass as only slightly more intense than muscle, whereas the right lobe is abnormally hyperintense. **C,** Gradient-echo image (TR/TE/flip angle = 33/13/30 degrees) shows both lobes of the liver to have similar intensity, without evidence of increased iron in either. (Courtesy Clare Tempany.)

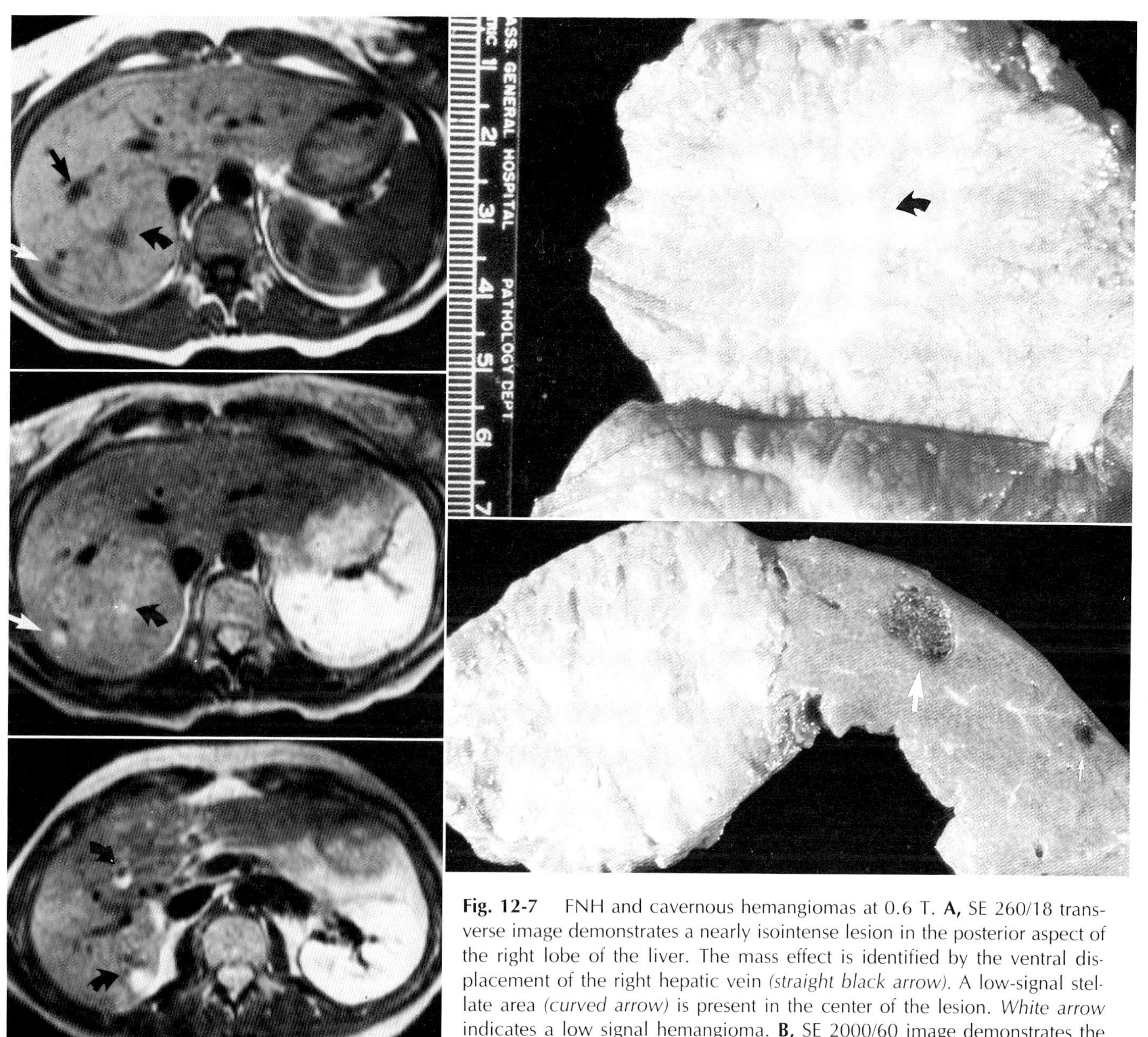

Fig. 12-7   FNH and cavernous hemangiomas at 0.6 T. **A,** SE 260/18 transverse image demonstrates a nearly isointense lesion in the posterior aspect of the right lobe of the liver. The mass effect is identified by the ventral displacement of the right hepatic vein *(straight black arrow)*. A low-signal stellate area *(curved arrow)* is present in the center of the lesion. *White arrow* indicates a low signal hemangioma. **B,** SE 2000/60 image demonstrates the hepatic tumor to have a slightly higher intensity than the adjacent liver. The central stellate region of the FNH *(curved arrow)* and hemangioma *(white arrow)* have increased signal intensity. **C,** SE 2000/60 image inferiorly reveals two additional hemangiomas. **D,** The cut gross specimen demonstrates the central stellate scar of the FNH. **E,** Two small hemangiomas *(arrows)* are seen in liver tissue adjacent to the FNH.

FOCAL NODULAR HYPERPLASIA

Focal nodular hyperplasia (FNH) is a rare benign tumor of the liver that contains hepatocytes, bile duct elements, Kupffer cells, and fibrous tissue. The distinction between FNH and hepatic adenoma (HA) is important because FNH can be treated conservatively, whereas HA is resected due to its propensity for hemorrhage.

Scintigraphy can support the diagnosis of FNH when areas of normal or increased 99mTc-sulfur colloid uptake are identified within the mass, indicating intratumoral Kupffer cells. Unfortunately, 35% of FNH lesions show decreased Kupffer cell activity and therefore cannot be distinguished from cancer. Additionally, hyperplastic nodules may also have increased uptake of sulfur colloid relative to surrounding cirrhotic parenchyma, and HA may contain Kupffer cells and therefore accumulate sulfur colloid.[299]

The CT appearance of FNH varies from hypodense to isodense relative to liver on either noncontrast or contrast-enhanced scans. The finding of a central stellate, low-attenuation region by CT is uncommon. Angiographically, FNH has variable characteristics and can be either hypovascular or hypervascular. Despite the use of scintigraphy, CT, sonography, and angiography, FNH is often difficult to differentiate from benign HA or hepatocellular carcinoma.[256] Surgical exploration is frequently necessary due to its nonspecific imaging findings.

MRI demonstrates FNH by its mass effect and displacement of hepatic vessels, and it can show subtle differences in the signal intensity of FNH compared with adjacent liver (Figs. 12-7 and 12-8). In general, FNH has a signal intensity similar to liver, since both tissues consist of normal hepatocytes and Kupffer cells.[53,277,325,420,469] In many cases, however, FNH is

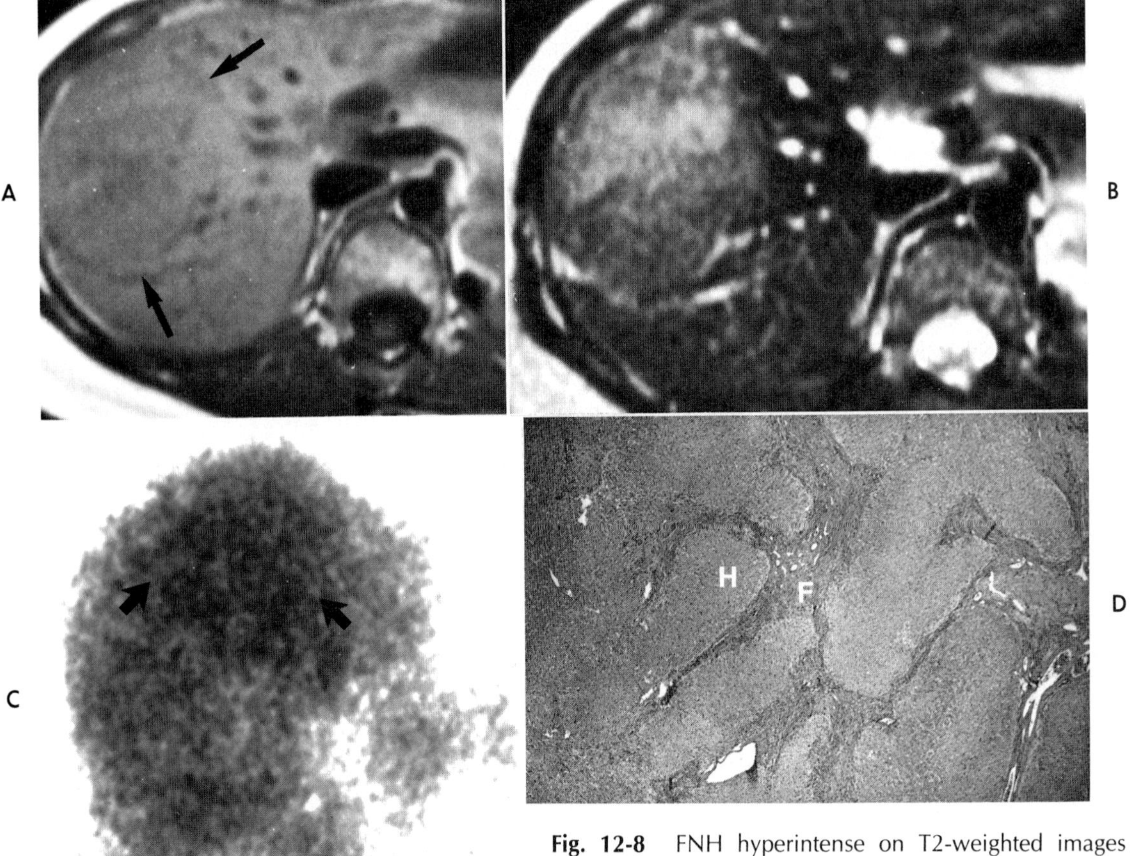

Fig. 12-8 FNH hyperintense on T2-weighted images at 1.5 T. **A,** T1-weighted image (SE 400/12) depicts an isointense mass *(arrows)*, visible because of displacement of hepatic vessels. **B,** Corresponding SE 2500/100 image depicts the tumor as a hyperintense mass. **C,** Right anterior oblique projection of a 99mTC-sulfur colloid scan, demonstrating slightly increased uptake in the region of the mass *(arrows)*, which is diagnostic of FNH. **D,** Microscopic section, demonstrating thick, vascular fibrous bands *(F)* separating regions of benign hepatic tissue *(H)*.

slightly hypointense on T1-weighted images and hyperintense on T2-weighted images, similar to malignant tumors (Figs. 12-8 to 12-10).[319] Since HCC may be nearly isointense with liver on T1- and/or T2-weighted images, the overlap between these two lesions prevents definitive differential diagnosis.[277] In patients with fatty infiltration of the liver, FNH may contain fat (Fig. 12-11).[349]

FNH often contains a central stellate "scar," which usually is bright on T2-weighted images and dark on T1-weighted images.[469] This is because the scar is usually composed of vascular and myxoid tissue, which is rich in free water (Fig. 12-10). The collagen within the scar is usually less organized than the parallel fibers characteristic of tendons in the musculoskeletal system and therefore does not shorten T2 as much. Unfortu-

Text continues on p. 124.

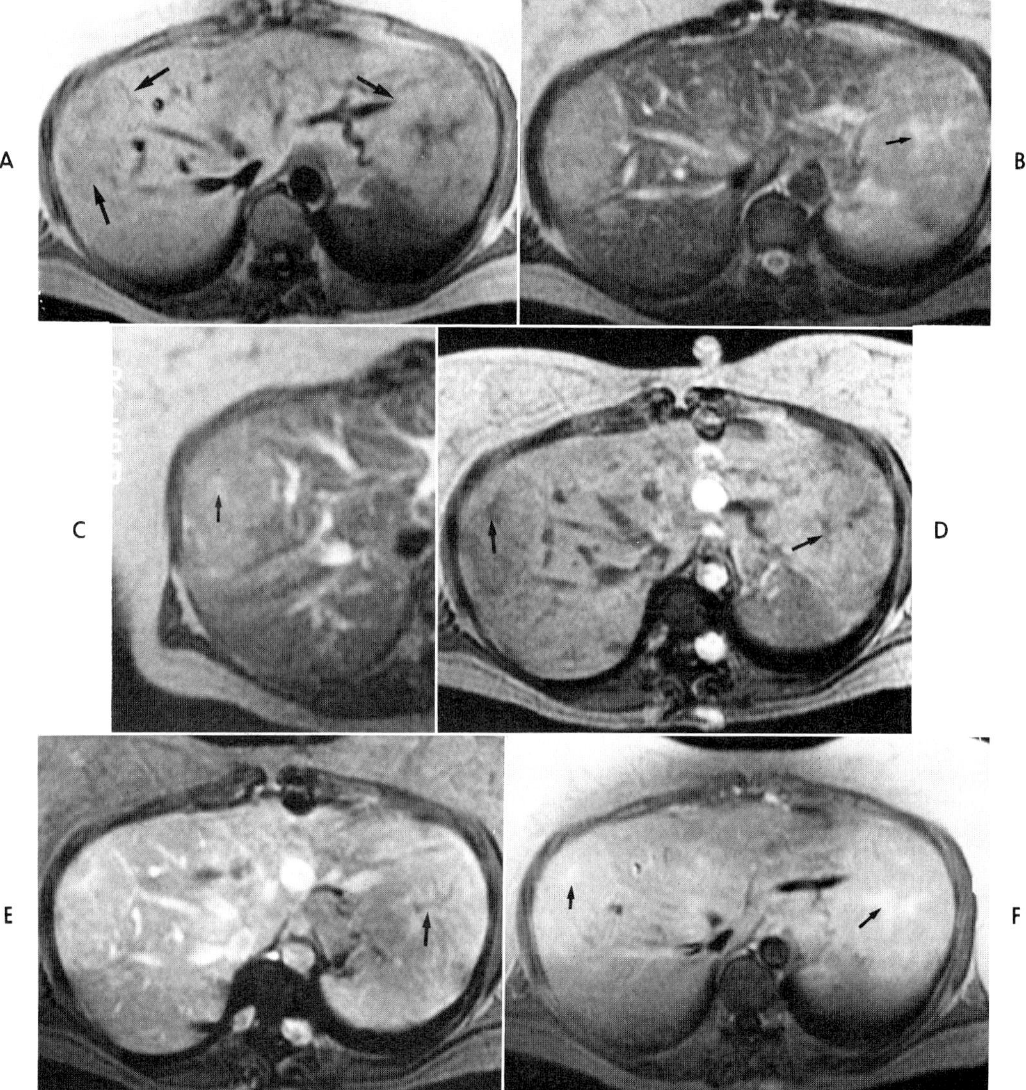

Fig. 12-9 Multiple focal nodular hyperplasias with central scars depicted with and without contrast enhancement at 1.5 T. **A,** SE 400/12 image depicts two lesions *(arrows)* that are nearly isointense with liver. **B** and **C,** Adjacent SE 2500/100 images. The lesions are slightly hyperintense, except for central scars *(arrows)*. **D,** Gradient-echo image (TR/TE = 71/5.3/90 degrees). The central scars *(arrows)* have low signal intensity. **E,** As in **D,** approximately 30 seconds after administration of gadopentetate dimeglumine. The scar in the right lobe has enhanced, whereas the scar in the left lobe *(arrow)* has not. **F,** As in **A,** approximately 3 minutes after administration of gadopentetate dimeglumine. Both scars have enhanced *(arrows)*, and the lesions have enhanced slightly more than the remainder of the liver.

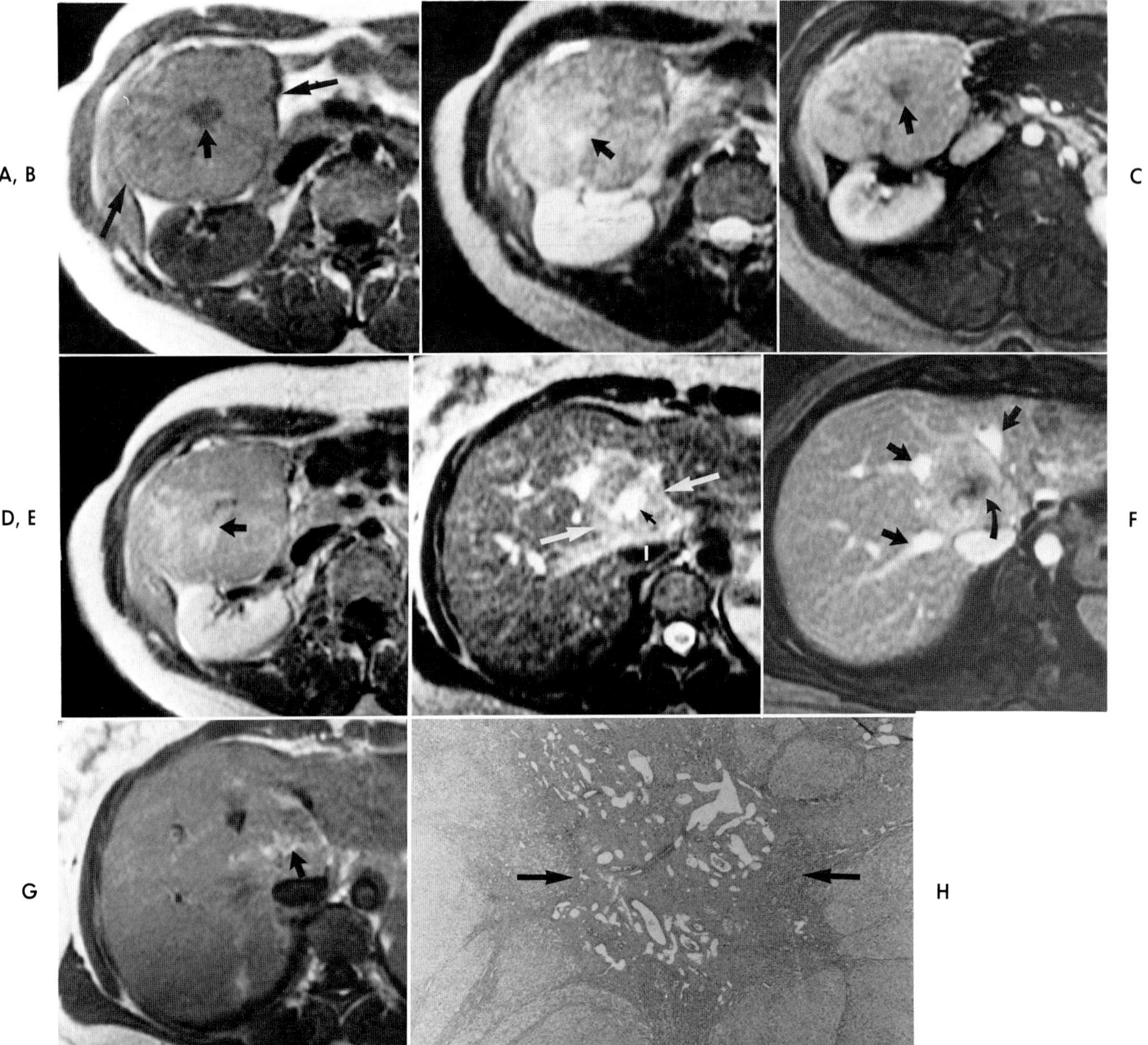

Fig. 12-10 Multiple focal nodular hyperplasias at 1.5 T, demonstrating long T2 and delayed enhancement of central scars. **A,** SE 450/11 image demonstrates a large isointense mass *(large arrows)* projecting from the inferior surface of the liver. There is a central low-signal scar *(small arrow)*. **B,** SE 2500/100 image demonstrates high signal of the mass and the scar *(arrow)*. **C,** T1-weighted gradient-echo image (TR/TE/flip angle = 71/2.3/90 degrees) approximately 30 seconds after administration of gadopentetate dimeglumine demonstrates nonenhancement of the central scar *(arrow)*. **D,** SE 450/11 image approximately 5 minutes after administration of gadopentetate dimeglumine demonstrates enhancement of the scar *(arrow)*. **E,** SE 2500/100 image depicts a second mass *(large arrows)* anterior to the inferior vena cava *(I)*. There is a central high-signal scar *(small arrow)*. **F,** T1-weighted gradient-echo with bolus enhancement (as in **C**), demonstrating nonenhancement of the scar *(curved arrow)*. Because of the proximity of the mass to the three hepatic veins *(straight arrows)*, it was not removed. **G,** SE 450/11 delayed postbolus image (as in **D**) demonstrates enhancement of the scar *(arrow)*. **H,** Histologic section (H & E) of the mass in **A** to **D**, showing the central scar *(arrows)*, which contains abundant large vascular spaces analogous to those seen in cavernous hemangiomas.

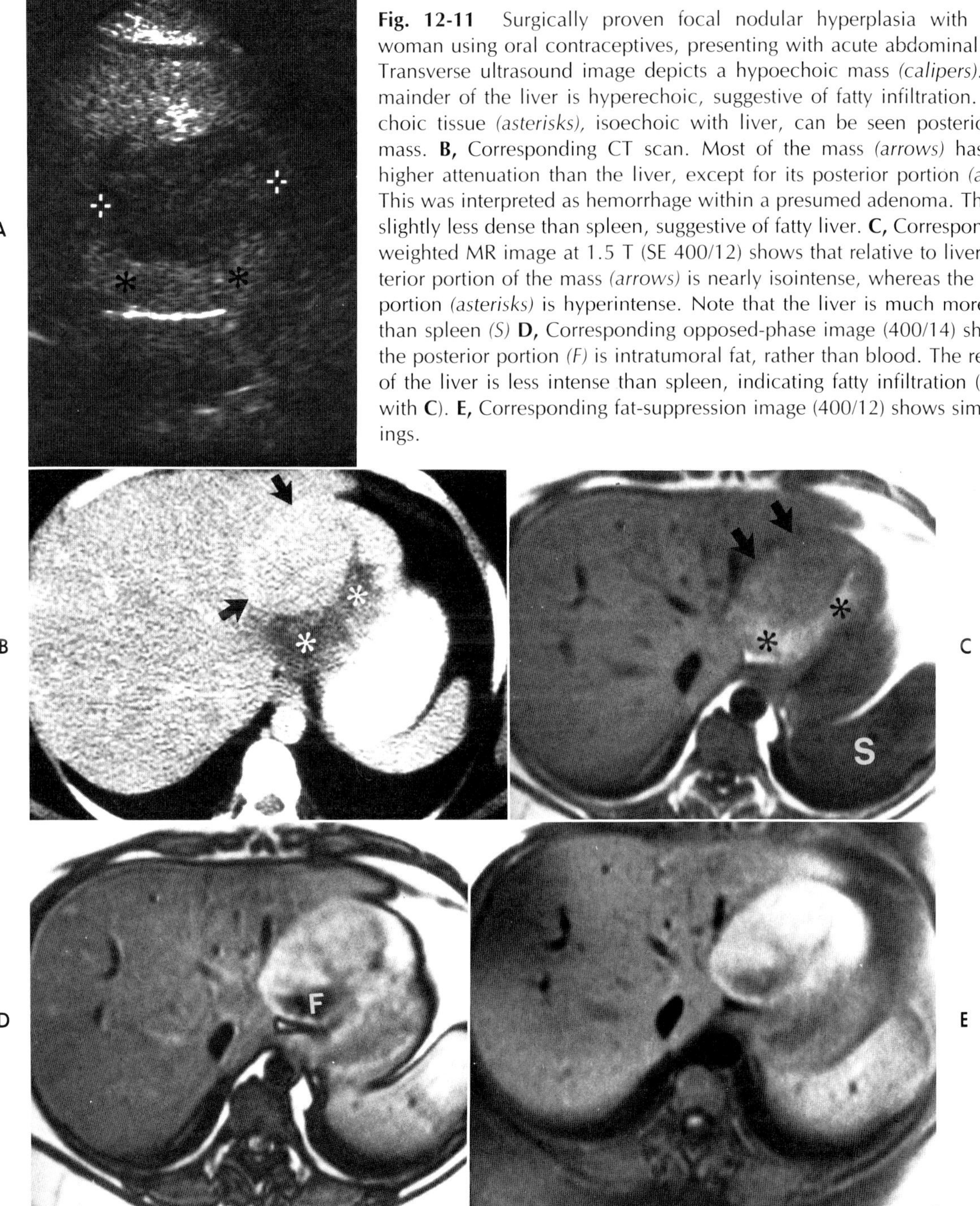

Fig. 12-11 Surgically proven focal nodular hyperplasia with fat in a woman using oral contraceptives, presenting with acute abdominal pain. **A,** Transverse ultrasound image depicts a hypoechoic mass *(calipers).* The remainder of the liver is hyperechoic, suggestive of fatty infiltration. Hyperechoic tissue *(asterisks),* isoechoic with liver, can be seen posterior to the mass. **B,** Corresponding CT scan. Most of the mass *(arrows)* has slightly higher attenuation than the liver, except for its posterior portion *(asterisks).* This was interpreted as hemorrhage within a presumed adenoma. The liver is slightly less dense than spleen, suggestive of fatty liver. **C,** Corresponding T1-weighted MR image at 1.5 T (SE 400/12) shows that relative to liver, the anterior portion of the mass *(arrows)* is nearly isointense, whereas the posterior portion *(asterisks)* is hyperintense. Note that the liver is much more intense than spleen *(S)* **D,** Corresponding opposed-phase image (400/14) shows that the posterior portion *(F)* is intratumoral fat, rather than blood. The remainder of the liver is less intense than spleen, indicating fatty infiltration (compare with **C**). **E,** Corresponding fat-suppression image (400/12) shows similar findings.

Figure continues.

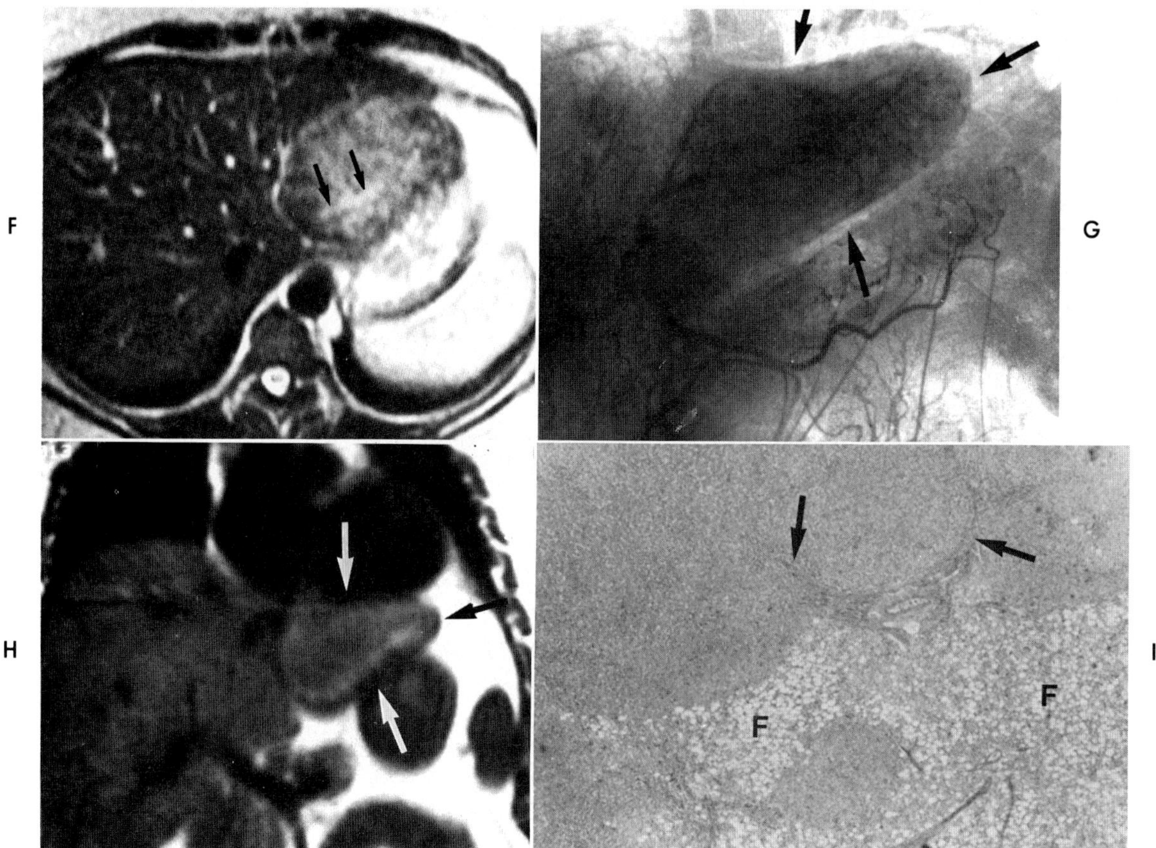

Fig. 12-11, cont'd.   **F,** Corresponding T2-weighted image (SE 2500/100) shows the whole mass to be hyperintense to liver. Note the bright band between the fatty and nonfatty components *(arrows),* representing chemical shift misregistration artifact. **G,** Arterial phase of angiogram showing hypervascularity. **H,** Coronal MR image (SE 600/20), for comparison with **G. I,** Histologic section at the border between the fatty *(F)* and relatively nonfatty portions of the mass. Fibrous bands *(arrows)* separating regions of benign hepatic tissue were diagnostic of FNH. (From Mitchell D.G., Palazzo, J., Hann, H-W.Y.L., et al.: J. Comput. Assist. Tomogr. 15:762-769, 1991)

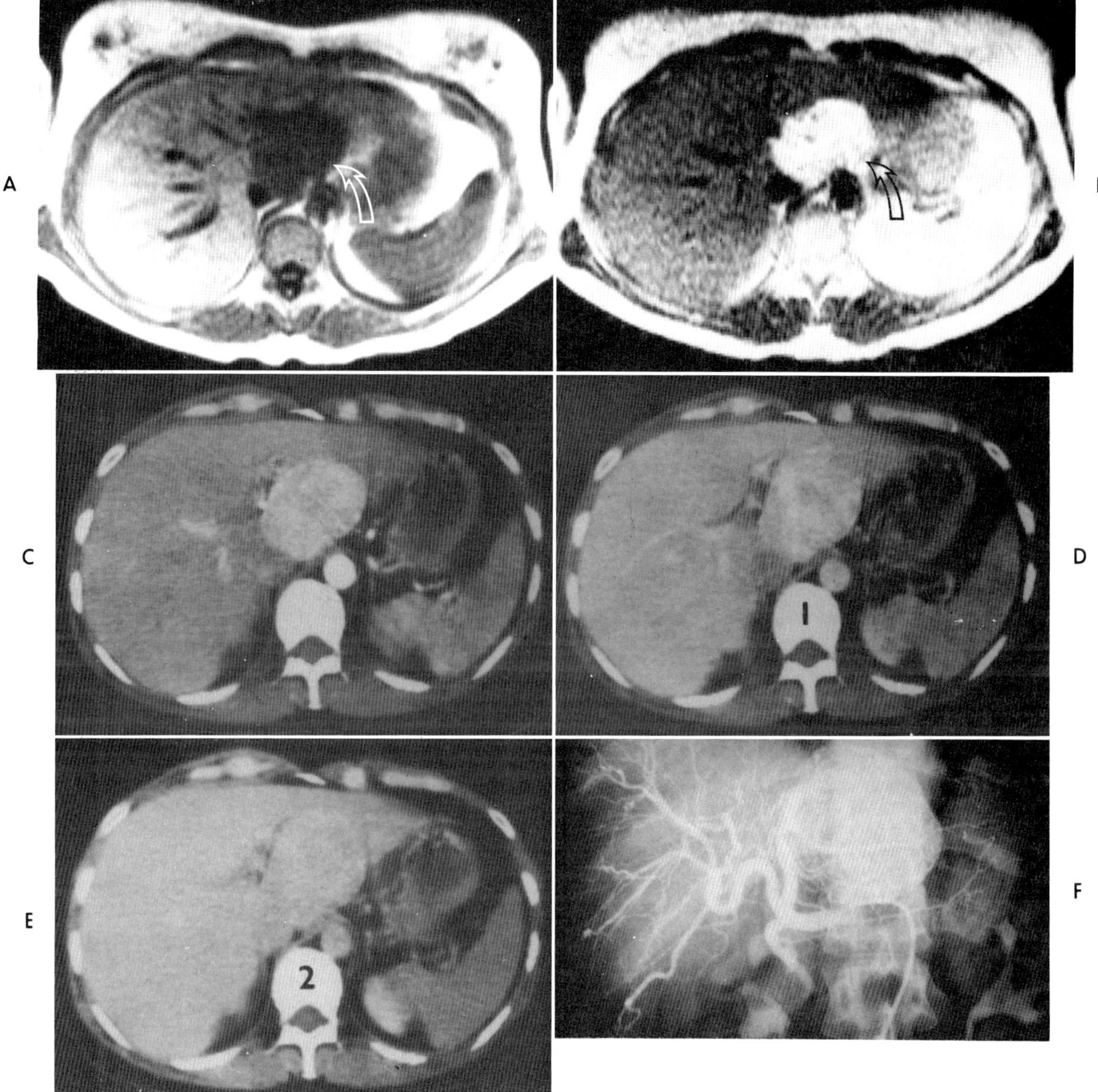

Fig. 12-12   Hepatic adenoma. **A,** IR 1500/450/30 image at 0.6 T shows a low-intensity mass *(arrow)* in the left hepatic lobe. **B,** SE 1500/100 MR image shows high signal of the lesion. **C to E,** Dynamic bolus contrast-enhanced CT shows early enhancement with rapid washout of contrast at 1 minute; by 2 minutes the lesion was isointense to liver. **F,** Angiogram confirms the hypervascular nature of this lesion.

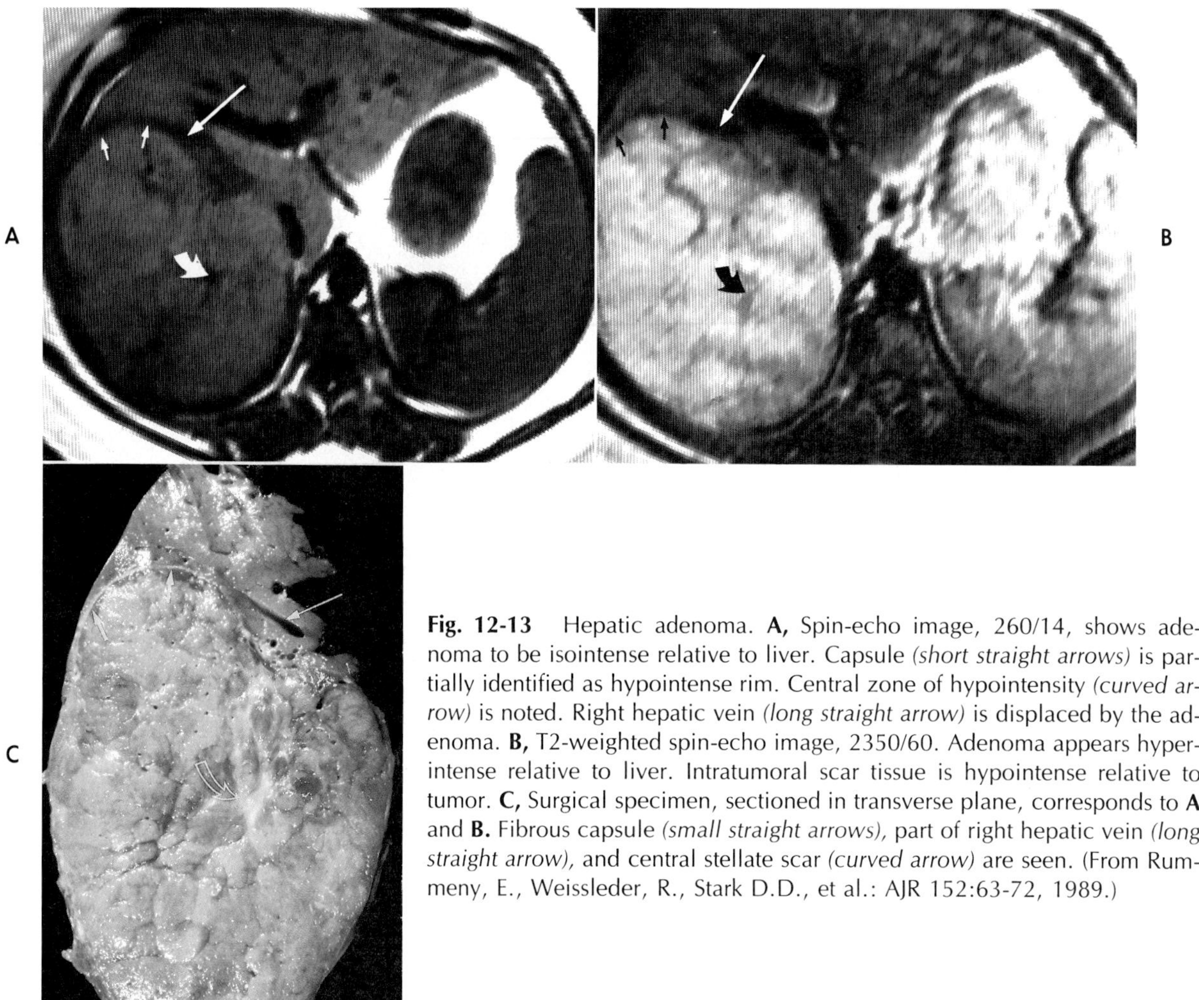

Fig. 12-13 Hepatic adenoma. **A,** Spin-echo image, 260/14, shows adenoma to be isointense relative to liver. Capsule *(short straight arrows)* is partially identified as hypointense rim. Central zone of hypointensity *(curved arrow)* is noted. Right hepatic vein *(long straight arrow)* is displaced by the adenoma. **B,** T2-weighted spin-echo image, 2350/60. Adenoma appears hyperintense relative to liver. Intratumoral scar tissue is hypointense relative to tumor. **C,** Surgical specimen, sectioned in transverse plane, corresponds to **A** and **B.** Fibrous capsule *(small straight arrows)*, part of right hepatic vein *(long straight arrow)*, and central stellate scar *(curved arrow)* are seen. (From Rummeny, E., Weissleder, R., Stark D.D., et al.: AJR 152:63-72, 1989.)

nately, the presence and characteristics of the scar do not allow reliable differential diagnosis, and histologic diagnosis remains necessary in most cases.[277,452]

The peripherally radiating septae of FNH contain large vascular channels and bile ducts. Delayed and persistent enhancement of the scar, analogous to that seen with cavernous hemangiomas, may occur after administration of gadopentetate dimeglumine (see Figs. 12-9 and 12-10). In other cases the lesion and scar may both enhance rapidly. It is uncertain whether contrast enhancement can improve diagnostic specificity.

HEPATOCELLULAR ADENOMA

The incidence of hepatocellular adenoma (HA) is greatest in women of childbearing age, especially those who use oral contraceptives. Pathologically, the typical features of HA are a thin pseudocapsule, intracellular glycogen deposition, lack of architecture, paucity of bile ducts, and degenerative necrosis.[256] Necrosis and

hemorrhage are common causes of pain, and life-threatening hemorrhage into the peritoneum can occur. Malignant potential has not been established, but if HA fails to regress on cessation of oral contraceptive use, surgical excision is indicated.

As with FNH, MRI tissue characteristics vary, and HA may be indistinguishable from malignant tumors (Figs. 12-12 and 12-13). As with other hepatocellular masses, HA may be hyperintense on T1-weighted images and hypointense on T2-weighted images relative to liver.[156] Rarely, T1-weighted MR images may show low-intensity pseudocapsules, similar to HCC (see Fig. 12-13).[156] A central scar similar to that seen with HCC and FNH can also occur.[452] HA may also undergo central necrosis and calcify, which manifests as low signal intensity on T2-weighted images (see Fig. 12-13). Central foci suggesting separate internal centers of growth, as seen with HCC, are not expected to occur with HA.

Other Focal Hepatic Pathology

LYMPHOMA

Primary hepatic lymphoma is rare, but secondary involvement occurs in 20% of patients with Hodgkin's disease.[540,584,629] Non-Hodgkin's lymphoma may involve the liver in as many as 50% of patients evaluated at autopsy. CT is quite insensitive, detecting hepatic involvement in only 4% of patients.[629] Percutaneous biopsy is unreliable because of sampling error, since patchy periportal infiltration is common.

Although focal lymphoma has been detected by unenhanced MRI (Figs. 13-1 to 13-3), these lesions may be isointense.[436,584,594] This probably depends on the proportion of lymphoma cells and edema relative to liver tissue.

Detection of diffuse lymphoma has been even more elusive. In some cases the lymphoma may incite an inflammatory response, causing a nonspecific diffuse or periportal signal increase on T2-weighted images. Contrast agents that are taken up by reticuloendothelial cells selectively are likely to improve the accuracy of MRI for detecting hepatic, as well as splenic, lymphoma (Fig. 13-4).[592] The accuracy of CT for detecting hepatic lymphoma has been improved by use of EOE-13 (ethiodized-oil emulsion), but adverse reactions have prevented approval of these agents for clinical use.[540]

ABSCESS

Pyogenic liver abscess occurs most commonly in older patients with cancer or biliary disease (Fig. 13-5 and 13-6). The symptoms and signs of hepatic abscess are often nonspecific, delaying diagnosis and therapy. Hepatic abscesses can be detected by scintigraphy and sonography, but CT is more sensitive.[190] The clinical role of MRI relative to CT for diagnosing hepatic abscesses has not been resolved. Hepatic abscesses have high contrast with the liver due to their long T1 and T2 relaxation times. Imaging findings are nonspecific, however, since necrotic tumors can have similar findings. Intracavitary gas (Fig. 13-5), a specific finding, is present in less than 20% of cases.

Two separate groups of investigators have administered gadopentetate dimeglumine to rats with liver abscesses, noting that lesion conspicuity on spin-echo images increased.[473,591] In abscesses that were 2 to 7 days old, the wall of the abscess enhanced. Conspicuity of small abscess decreased on delayed images 30 to 60 minutes after injection, however, because of delayed leakage into the abscess. Iron oxide particles increased the conspicuity of small lesions, alone or in combination with gadopentetate dimeglumine.[591]

Small disseminated candida abscesses may develop in the liver and spleen in immunocompromised patients, causing high-signal foci on T2-weighted images. Their identification can be facilitated by fortuitous decreased hepatic and splenic signal on these images secondary to transfusional siderosis (Figs. 13-7 and 13-8).[76]

Amebic liver abscess (Figs. 13-9 and 13-10) is common in the southwestern United States and is endemic in Latin America. MRI appears to be as sensitive as CT for detecting amebic liver abscesses.[122,422] Regional hepatic edema can be quite prominent on T2-weighted images. Antibiotic therapy and/or abscess drainage can rapidly reduce this edema, allowing MR to evaluate therapy.[122] Although it may take months for a sterile abscess cavity to resolve, collagen and other reactive changes can be seen in the maturing abscess wall.

Echinococcal (hydatid) disease is the most common human larval cestodiasis and a cause of significant morbidity and mortality. Clinical management is complex, including surgical removal if possible and medical treatment for patients with recurrent or nonoperative disease. Recently, ultrasound guided drainage has been used for selected patients.[257]

Several investigators have found MRI effective for detecting and characterizing echinococcal disease.[80,213,363,609] A thin, low-intensity rim may be seen with advanced disease (Figs. 13-11 to 13-14). In some cases, septations and daughter cysts may be seen better with MRI than with CT or ultrasound.[80,609] The inability of MRI to show microcalcifications limits its specificity, however.

HEMORRHAGE

Acute parenchymal or perihepatic hemorrhage usually has low signal on T1- and T2-weighted images because of heterogeneous susceptibility produced by intracellu-

Text continued on p. 138.

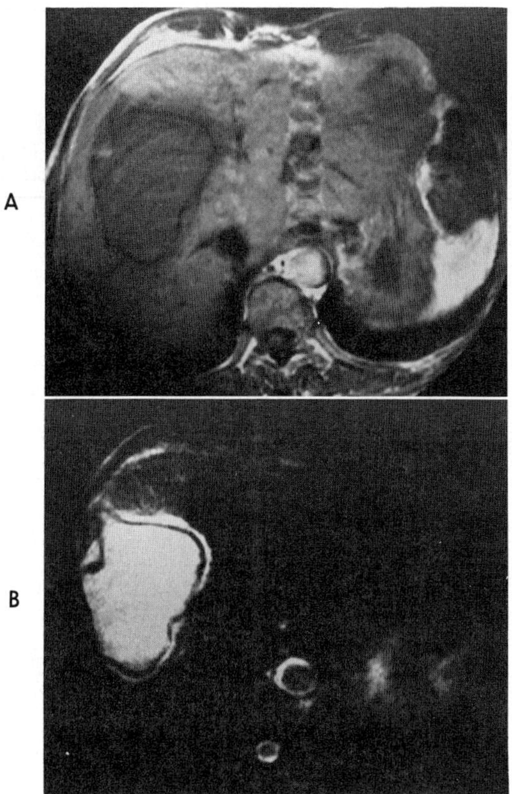

Fig. 13-11   Unilocular hydatid cyst. **A,** SE 700/20 image. **B,** SE 2000/100 (Courtesy L. te Strake.)

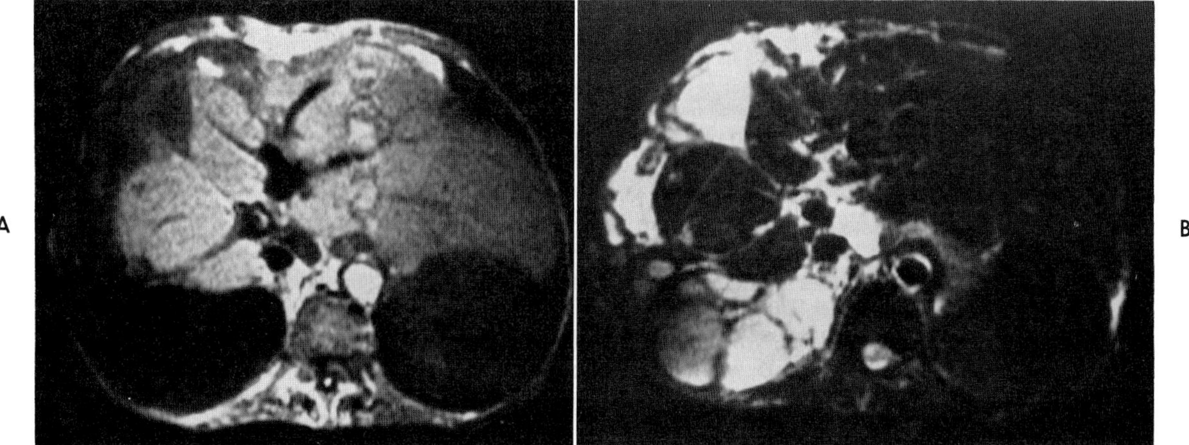

Fig. 13-12   Multilocular hydatid cyst. **A,** SE 500/20 image. **B,** SE 2000/100 (Courtesy L. te Strake.)

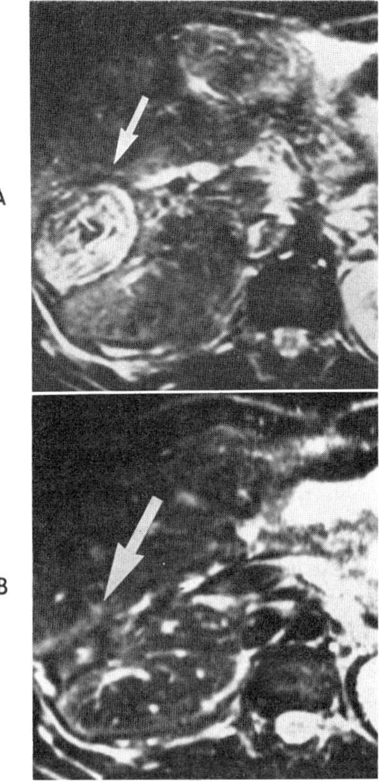

Fig. 13-13   Hydatid cyst (SE 2000/100) before **(A)** and after **(B)** Albendazole treatment. (Courtesy L. te Strake.)

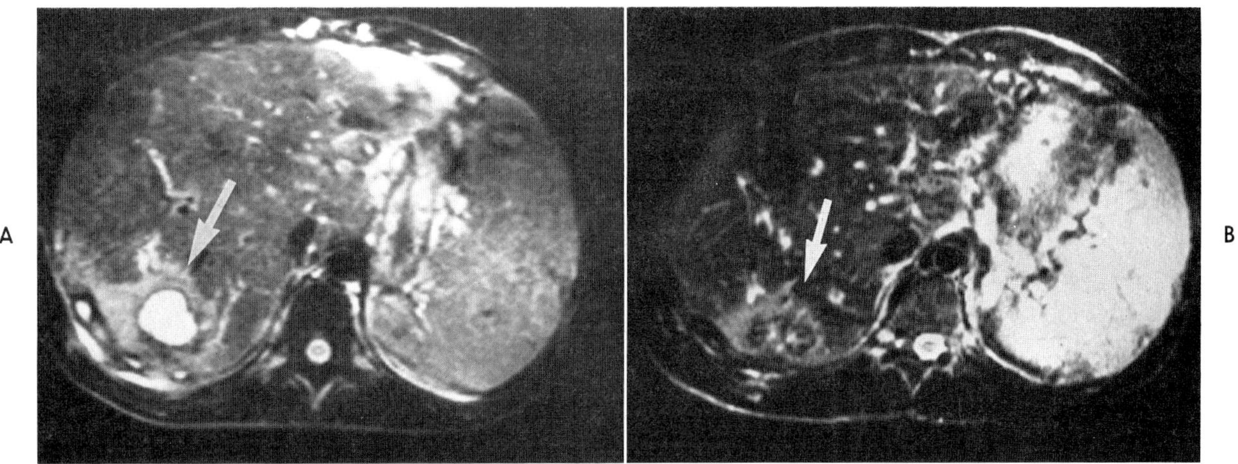

Fig. 13-14   Hydatid cyst (SE 2000/100) before **(A)** and after **(B)** Albendazole treatment. (Courtesy L. te Strake.)

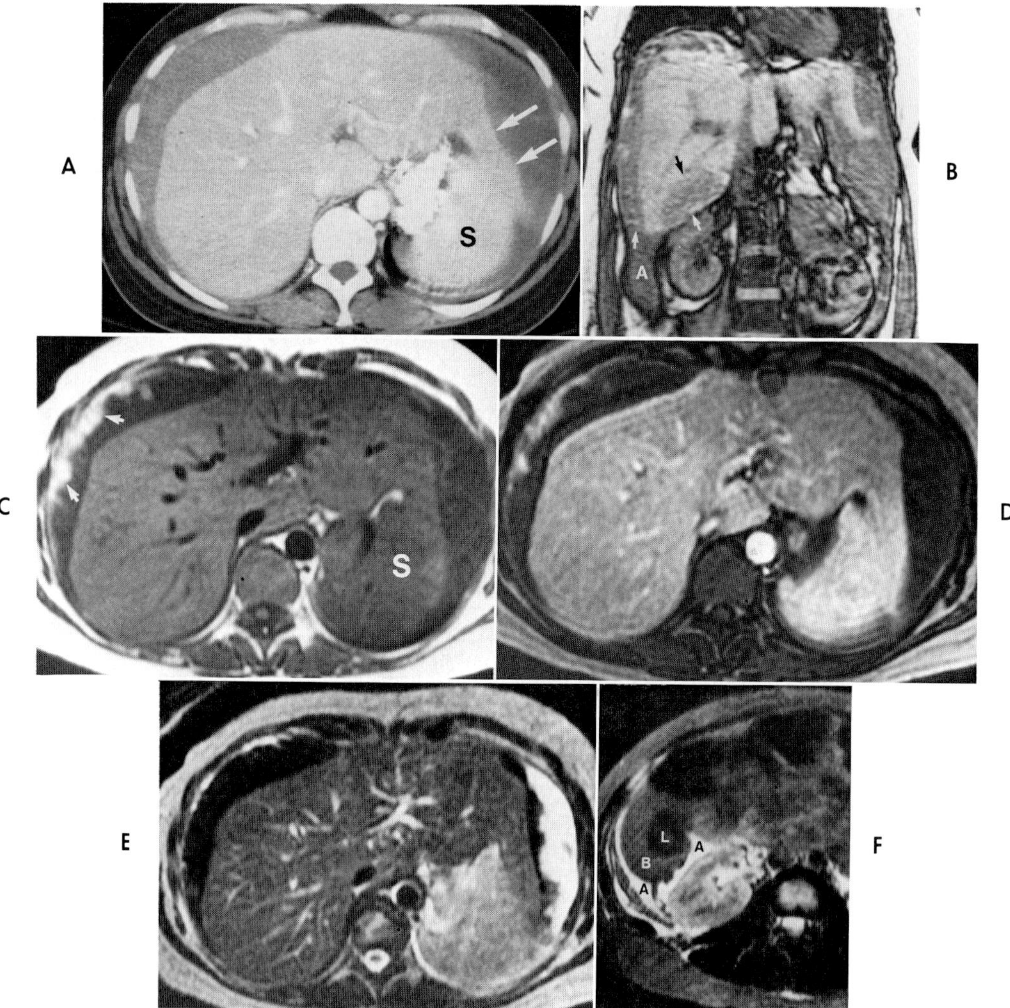

Fig. 13-15 Massive acute perihepatic subcapsular hemorrhage in a woman with eclampsia. **A,** Contrast-enhanced CT scan after delivery demonstrates perihepatic fluid. Note that the left lobe (arrows) extends lateral to the spleen *(S)*. **B,** Coronal T1-weighted gradient-echo image (TR/TE/flip angle = 101/2.3/90 degrees). Note differentiation between intermediate-signal subcapsular fluid *(small arrows)* and low-signal ascites *(A)*. **C,** T1-weighted SE image (TR/TE = 550/12). Note high signal from methemoglobin anterolaterally *(arrows)*. S = spleen. **D,** Axial T1-weighted gradient-echo image (TR/TE/flip angle = 101/2.3/90 degrees) obtained 30 seconds after administration of gadopentetate dimeglumine, demonstrating homogeneous enhancement of liver, excluding the possibility of large hepatic infarct or hemorrhage. No focal cause of the subcapsular hemorrhage was found. Note heterogeneous enhancement of the spleen, a normal finding within 1 minute of contrast administration. **E,** Corresponding SE 3000/100 image. Blood surrounding the right lobe has low signal intensity, presumably because of intact red blood cells. Blood lateral to the left lobe has high signal intensity, suggesting lysis of red blood cells. **F,** SE 3000/100 image at the inferior tip of the liver *(L)* demonstrating subcapsular blood *(B)* and ascites *(A)*.

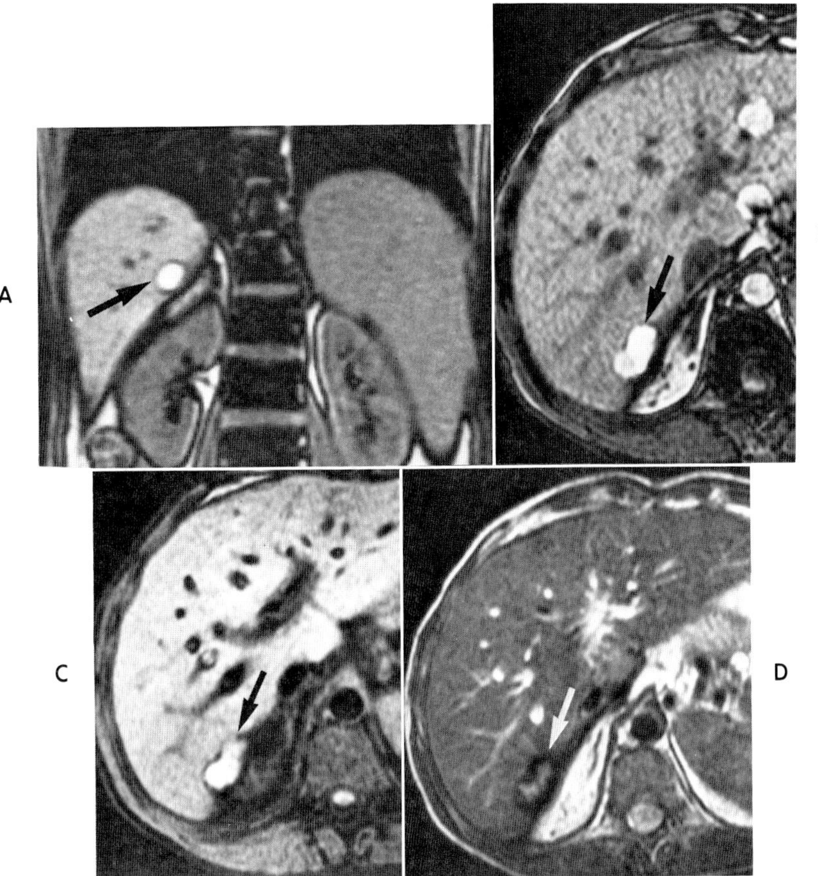

Fig. 13-16   Small perihepatic hematoma secondary to hepatic transplantation depicted at 1.5 T. **A,** Coronal T1-weighted gradient-echo (TR/TE/flip angle = 103/2.3/90 degrees) reveals a focal high-signal collection *(arrow)* at the posterior aspect of the right hepatic lobe. **B,** Comparable axial image. **C,** SE 400/14 image with fat suppression depicts the hyperintense lesion, and a low signal rim separating it from hepatic parenchyma **D,** SE 2500/50 image depicts the hematoma as high signal, with increased thickness of the peripheral low signal rim, due to increased sensitivity to iron within hemosiderin.

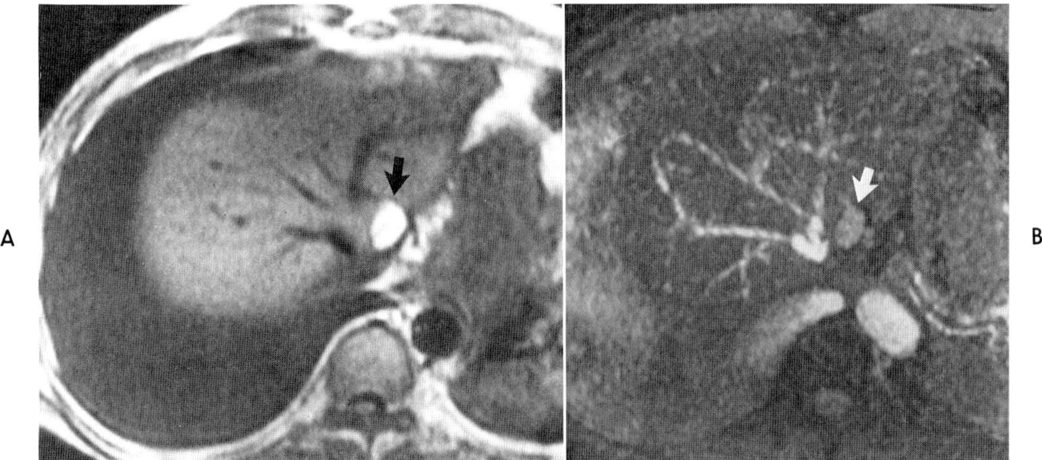

Fig. 13-17   Small perihepatic hematoma secondary to hepatic transplantation, depicted on spin-echo and MR angiographic images at 1.5 T. **A,** SE 400/12 image depicts a focal hematoma *(arrow)* adjacent to the superior aspect of the caudate lobe. **B,** MR angiographic slab at the level of the hepatic veins. The hematoma *(arrow)* has high signal because of the high T2/T1.

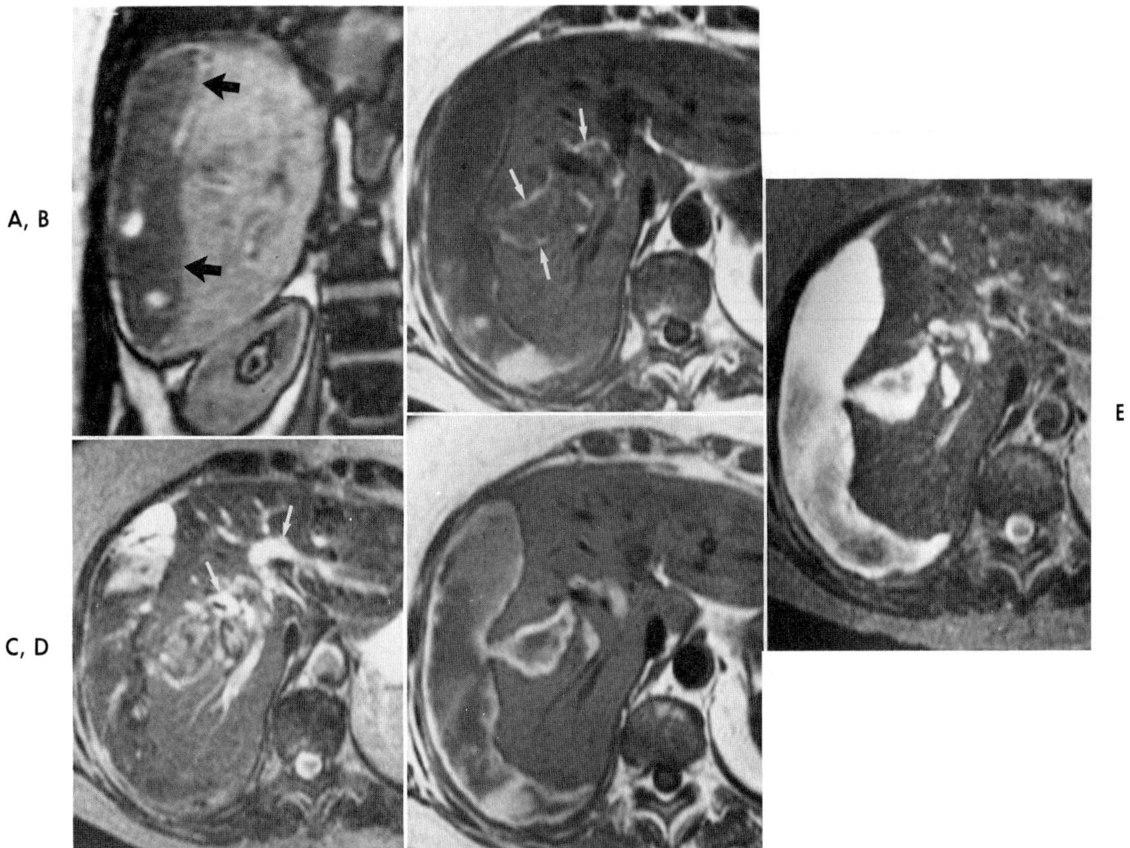

Fig. 13-18 Massive hepatic parenchymal and subcapsular hemorrhage secondary to liver biopsy. **A,** Coronal gradient-echo image (TR/TE/flip angle = 103/2.3/90 degrees) reveals a low-signal collection lateral to the liver *(arrows),* without any evidence of peritoneal fluid. There are high-signal foci within the collection consistent with methemoglobin. **B,** SE 400/12 image reveals the collection to be primarily low signal, except for the posterior portion. *Arrows* indicate the intraparenchymal component. **C,** SE 2500/100 image shows that most of the collection has low signal, consistent with intact red cells. Based on the low signal in **A** and **B,** these red cells contain deoxyhemoglobin. *Arrows* indicate dilated bile ducts. **D,** SE 400/12 image 1 week after **B.** The peripheral signal intensity of the hematoma is increasing, indicating increased oxidation to methemoglobin. **E,** Corresponding SE 2500/100 image (compare with **C**). Increased signal intensity indicates lysis of red blood cells.

lar deoxyhemoglobin (Fig. 13-15). A hyperintense rim may be noted on T1- and T2-weighted images, consistent with extracellular methemoglobin.[184,187] With time, signal intensity increases within the center of the lesion as red blood cells continue to lyse and deoxyhemoglobin is oxidized, forming methemoglobin (Figs. 13-16 to 13-18). The signal intensity may vary in different components of the hemorrhage because of gravity and variable effects of motion on red blood cell lysis and clot retraction.

Postpartum perihepatic hemorrhage can occur in association with preeclampsia (Fig. 13-15). Hemorrhage may be massive, but these patients can be managed nonoperatively, especially if they are young primipa-

ras.[305] This hemorrhage may be part of the HELLP (hemolytic anemia, elevated liver enzymes, low platelets) syndrome. Hepatic infarction may be seen in these patients, manifested as a segmental zone of low signal on T1-weighted images and high signal on T2-weighted images.[264]

Hepatic infarction is otherwise rare because of the dual blood supply of the liver via hepatic arteries and portal veins. Additionally, there are extensive collateral anastamoses for both of these vascular systems between lobes and segments. Occasionally, infarctions can occur resulting from occlusion of portal veins and hepatic arteries by different pathologies or extensive malignant involvement of portal tracts.

P A R T

III

DIFFUSE LIVER DISEASE

Initial attempts at characterizing liver disease by measuring T1 and T2 were unsuccessful.[169] These measurements are affected by numerous technical factors, some of which cannot be controlled by the operator. Relaxation times of healthy liver also vary. T1 relaxation time appears to decrease with age and, in women, increases during medication with oral contraceptives.[435] More recently, chemical shift imaging techniques have proven valuable for detecting hepatic lipid, and improved image quality has allowed a more detailed assessment of hepatic texture and morphology. In this section, we review the unique contributions MRI can make towards diagnosis of diffuse liver disease and the evaluation of focal abnormalities in these patients.

Fatty Liver

Fat may accumulate within hepatocytes after exposure to ethanol or other chemical toxins or in patients with diabetes mellitus and obesity. Patients with advanced malignancy commonly have fatty livers, possibly because of poor nutrition and the hepatotoxic effects of chemotherapy. Fatty liver is often associated with elevated hepatic transaminases.[383,573]

Fatty change is frequently patchy or even focal, most likely reflecting regional differences in perfusion; areas of decreased portal flow tend to accumulate less fat than better perfused areas, probably because less dietary lipid reaches the hepatocytes.[8] There are certain regions of the liver that are commonly involved by fatty infiltration, such as the medial segment of the left lobe adjacent to the falciform ligament.[620] The other side of the medial segment, adjacent to the portal vein, is commonly spared when the remainder of the liver is fatty.[28,465,599]

OTHER MODALITIES AND CONVENTIONAL MRI

Liver imaging with CT, sonography, and scintigraphy is complicated by patchy or focal fatty infiltration. Fatty liver may appear heterogeneous on scintigraphic planar or single photon emission computed tomographic (SPECT) images.[221] Diffuse fatty infiltration can mimic cirrhosis or chronic hepatitis on ultrasound images.[288,376] On CT images, metastases may be isodense with fatty liver, thus eluding detection.[284,293] Focal fatty infiltration can mimic low-attenuation masses on CT and hyperechoic masses on ultrasound (Figs. 14-1 to 14-4) and can produce scintigraphic heterogeneity that mimics diffuse and/or focal malignancy.[232,617]

Focal areas of relative sparing within diffusely fatty livers mimic typical hypoechoic lesions on ultrasound (Fig. 14-5).[599] Since metastases may be denser than fatty liver, focal sparing may mimic masses on CT as well.[284]

Although certain portions of the liver are especially likely to be affected by focal fat or focal sparing, and a wedge shape is characteristic, the findings are not specific enough to prevent diagnostic dilemmas. Lack of mass effect and the presence of normal vascular structures within regions of focal fat are helpful signs but only for very large fatty regions. After cavernous hemangioma, patchy or focal fatty infiltration of the liver is the most common problem in differential diagnosis of hepatic lesions. Fortunately, fatty infiltration is not a diagnostic problem for MRI.

Conventional spin-echo pulse sequences are relatively insensitive to fatty infiltration.[492,494,596] Commonly used spin-echo–pulse sequences show only 5% to 15% difference in signal intensity between normal liver and those containing 10% fat (triglyceride) by weight. In isolated cases, however, fatty masses or marked focal fatty infiltration can be depicted on T1-weighted spin-echo images (Figs. 14-3 and 14-5).[232,596]

T2-weighted images are especially insensitive to fatty infiltration. Thus if a suspicious zone of decreased attenuation seen on CT scan is normal on T2-weighted MR images, it is unlikely to represent cancer, especially if the area is slightly bright on T1-weighted images.

Diagnosis of focal fat on conventional spin-echo images represents a conclusion based on not making a finding. Fortunately, chemical shift techniques allow definitive unambiguous diagnosis of fatty hepatic abnormalities.

CHEMICAL SHIFT IMAGING

Chemical shift imaging techniques allow separation of the signal from fat and water protons based on differences in resonance frequency (i.e., chemical shift) (see Chapter 5, Chemical Shift Imaging). These techniques allow an absolute diagnosis of focal or diffuse fatty infiltration.[99,198,415,443]

The most effective technique for detecting regions of fatty liver is the opposed-phase image, originated by Dixon.[99] Intensity in these images is the absolute value of water intensity minus fat intensity. Whereas most tissues appear similar on in-phase and opposed-phase images, fatty liver will be noticeably darker.*

Opposed-phase images are more sensitive to fatty liver than fat-suppressed images.[348] As an example, consider a fatty liver where fat accounts for 10% and water 90% of the signal on a conventional in-phase image. On the comparable opposed-phase image with

---

*198, 276, 280, 348, 443, 468

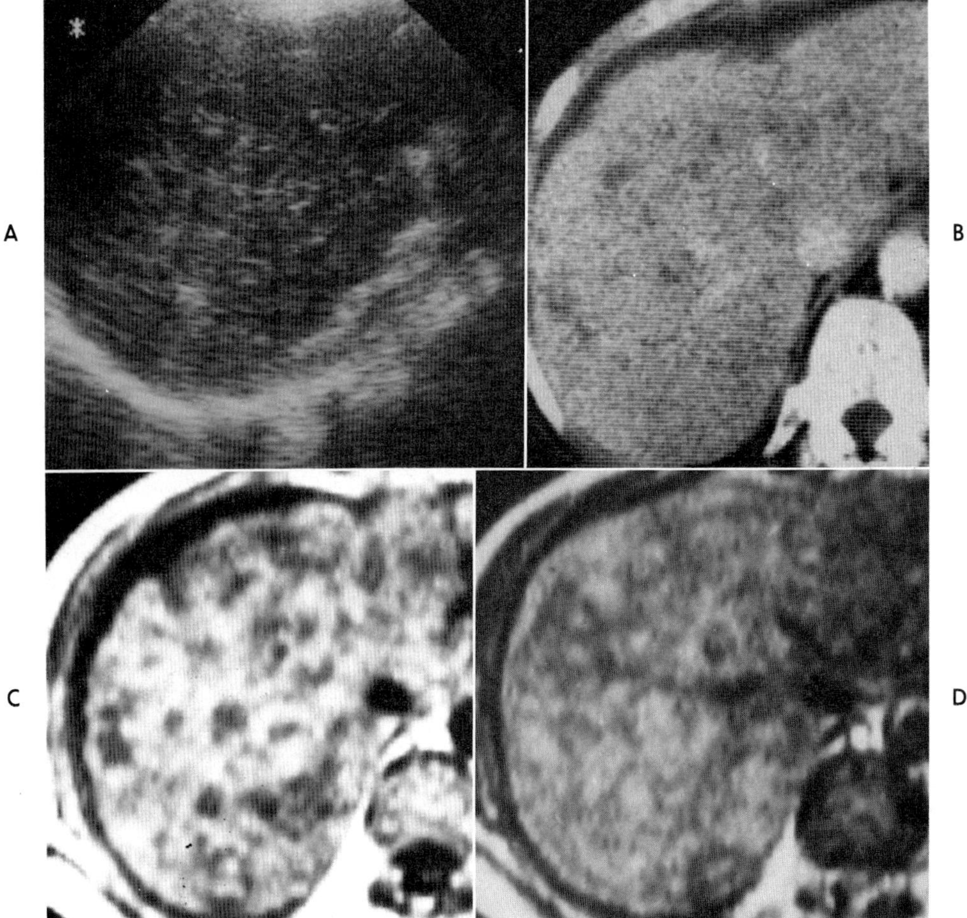

Fig. 14-1   Fatty liver versus diffuse metastases in a 48-year-old alcoholic woman with breast cancer resolved by MRI at 0.6 T. **A,** Sonography shows diffuse echogenicity of the liver. **B,** A CT scan shows ascites and diffuse hypodense areas in the right hepatic lobe. Sonography and CT are nondiagnostic because of the similar appearance of diffuse fat and diffuse breast cancer. Percutaneous biopsy was contraindicated by ascites and coagulopathy. **C,** SE 260/15 image shows multiple low–signal-intensity nodular lesions. Since fat shows increased signal intensity on T1-weighted images, this image is diagnostic of metastatic cancer. The nodular morphology of metastatic cancer is more apparent with MR than with CT or sonography. **D,** SE 2000/60 image at the same level shows nodules of metastatic cancer to have a slightly increased signal intensity relative to surrounding liver. Autopsy confirmed the MR diagnosis of metastatic cancer.

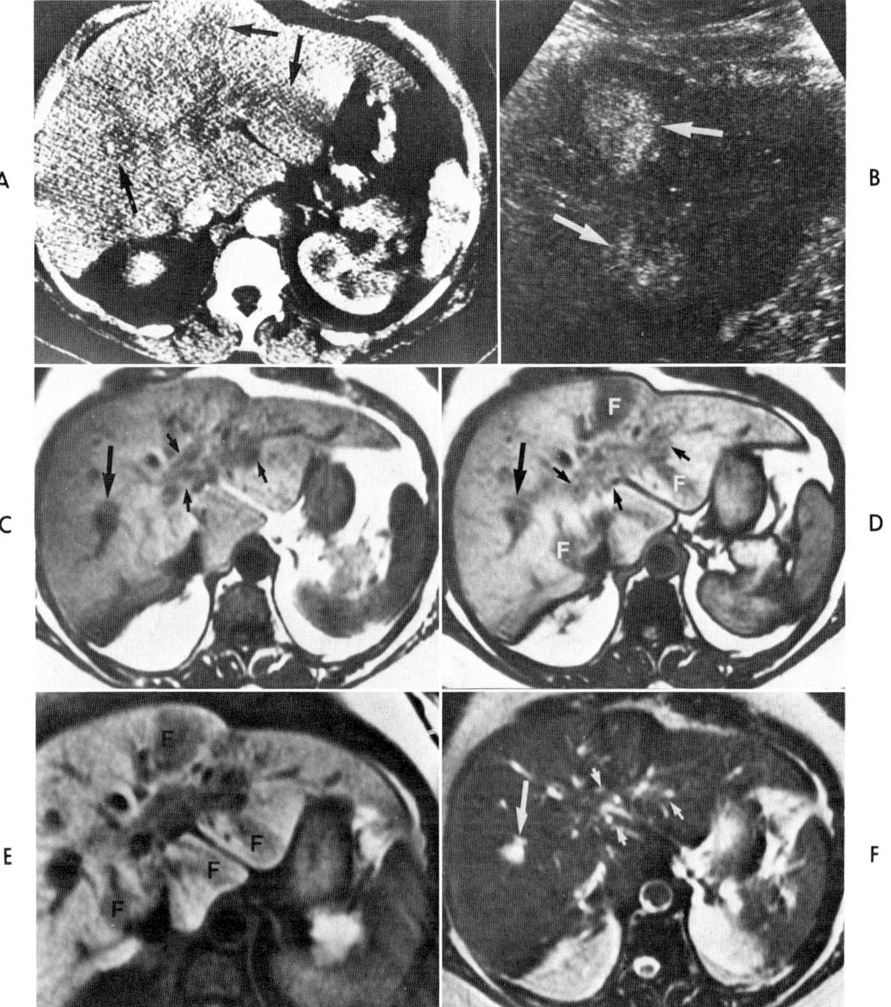

Fig. 14-2 Patchy fatty infiltration, periportal infiltration, and a benign lesion in a patient with sclerosing cholangitis. **A,** Contrast-enhanced CT scan reveals numerous low-attenuation regions *(arrows)* that are suspicious for metastatic lesions. **B,** Transverse ultrasound image of the left lobe shows two hyperechoic lesions *(arrows)*. Additional lesions were noted on other images. **C,** Axial SE 400/20 image at 1.5 T, corresponding to **A.** A discreet low-signal right-lobe lesion *(large arrow)* and low-attenuation left periportal tissue *(small arrows)* are noted. There is no lesion visible in the other regions of abnormality seen by ultrasound or CT. **D,** Opposed-phase image (400/22) corresponding to **C.** Most of the hepatic parenchyma remains brighter than the spleen, but there are numerous low-signal areas, indicating focal fatty infiltration *(F)*. Note that the lesion in the right lobe *(large arrow)* and the left-periportal low signal *(small arrows)* are unchanged. **E,** Corresponding fat-suppression image (400/20) shows the same findings as in **D,** but there is less contrast between fatty and nonfatty liver. Note that the areas of focal fat are more intense than the other signal defects, whereas in **D** they are similar or less intense. **F,** Axial T2-weighted image (SE 2500/100) shows a benign lesion in the right lobe *(large arrow)* and minimal periportal increased intensity *(small arrows)*, but the areas of focal fat are not visible. (From Mitchell, D.G., Kim, I., Chang, T.S., et al.: Invest. Radiol. 26:1041-1052, 1991.)

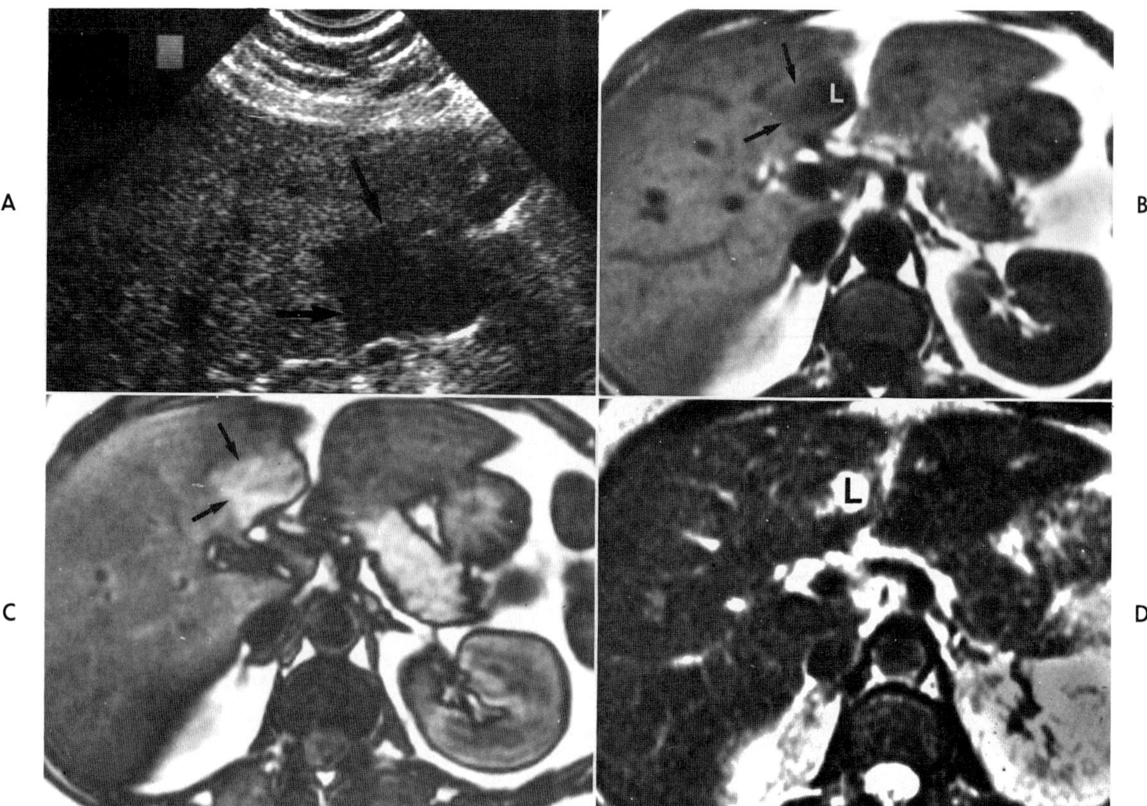

Fig. 14-5 Diffuse fatty infiltration with areas of relative sparing, one of which contains a benign lesion. **A,** Transverse ultrasound image shows the liver to be hyperechoic with obscured portal vein walls, suggestive of fatty infiltration. There is a focal hypoechoic region in the posterior portion of the medial segment of the left lobe *(arrows).* **B,** Axial in-phase SE 400/22 image at 1.5 T depicts this as slightly decreased signal intensity *(arrows),* within which is a lower-signal lesion *(L).* Note that liver is much more intense than kidney and is isointense to pancreas. **C,** Opposed-phase image (400/22). Except for the spared area *(arrows),* the remainder of the liver has become less intense than kidney and pancreas, indicating fatty infiltration. The focal region is heterogeneous and nearly isointense with pancreas. **D,** T2-weighted image depicts a benign lesion *(L)* within the region of focal sparing. The rest of this region is isointense relative to the remainder of the liver.

identical TR and TE, liver will only have 80% as much signal (90 minus 10) as on the in-phase image. On a fat-suppressed image, however, fatty liver will have approximately 90% of its total signal, assuming the 10% from lipid is totally suppressed. An additional disadvantage of current fat-suppression images is that they are more sensitive to magnetic field heterogeneity than are opposed-phase images.

Theoretically, a fat image, produced by suppressing signal from water, should be even more sensitive to fatty liver, since the residual fat signal should have extreme contrast compared with the signal void of normal liver or other water tissues. The superiority of water suppression in this respect has been confirmed in an animal model using small fields of view and sacrifice of the animals before imaging to eliminate motion-induced artifacts (Figs. 14-6 to 14-9.)[348] In clinical practice, however, water-suppressed images are dominated by fat and the motion artifact from it. Additionally, it may be difficult to differentiate small amounts of fat from imperfect suppression of water signal because of magnetic field heterogeneity or radiofrequency imperfections.

Because of the high signal of fat on short TR/TE images, short TR/TE opposed-phase images are most sen-

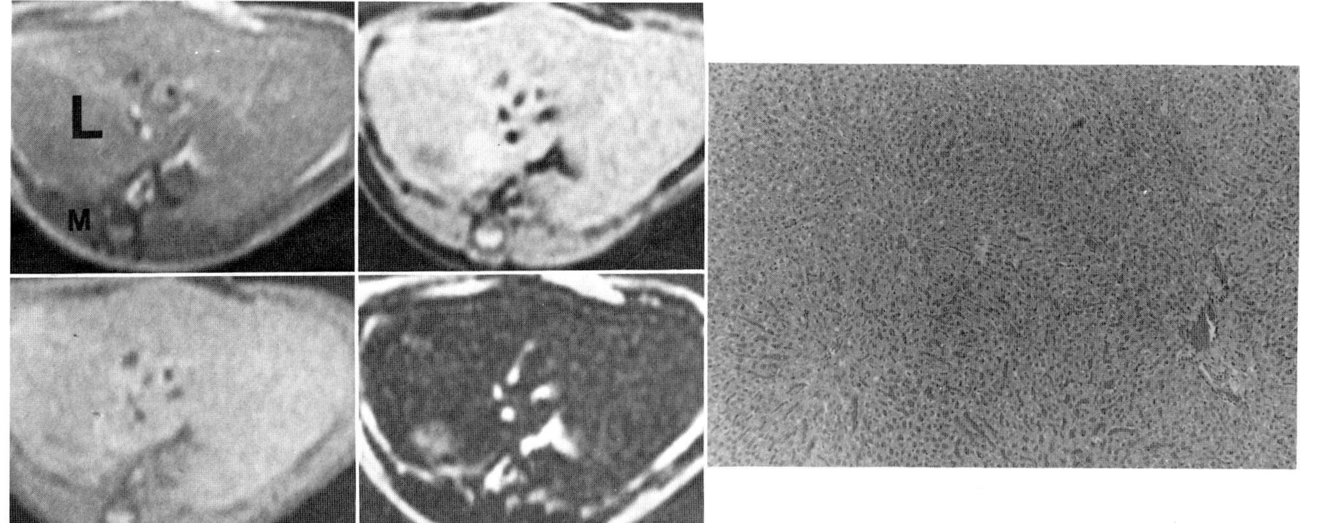

Fig. 14-6 Control rat liver at 1.5 T (TR = 1500 msec, TE = 15 msec). **A,** In-phase image. Signal of the liver *(L)* is intermediate between paraspinal muscles *(M)* and adipose tissue. **B,** Opposed-phase image. The relative intensity of the liver parenchyma and paraspinal muscles is similar to that in the in-phase image because the normal liver contains only a small amount of fat. **C,** Water image. The relative intensity of the liver and paraspinal muscle is unchanged. **D,** Fat image. The liver and paraspinal muscle are signal voids, indicating that fat contributes virtually no signal to the in-phase image in this control rat. **E,** Histologic specimen (H & E). There is no evidence of fat. (From Mitchell, D.G., Kim, I., Chang, T.S., et al.: Invest. Radiol. 26:1041-1052, 1991.)

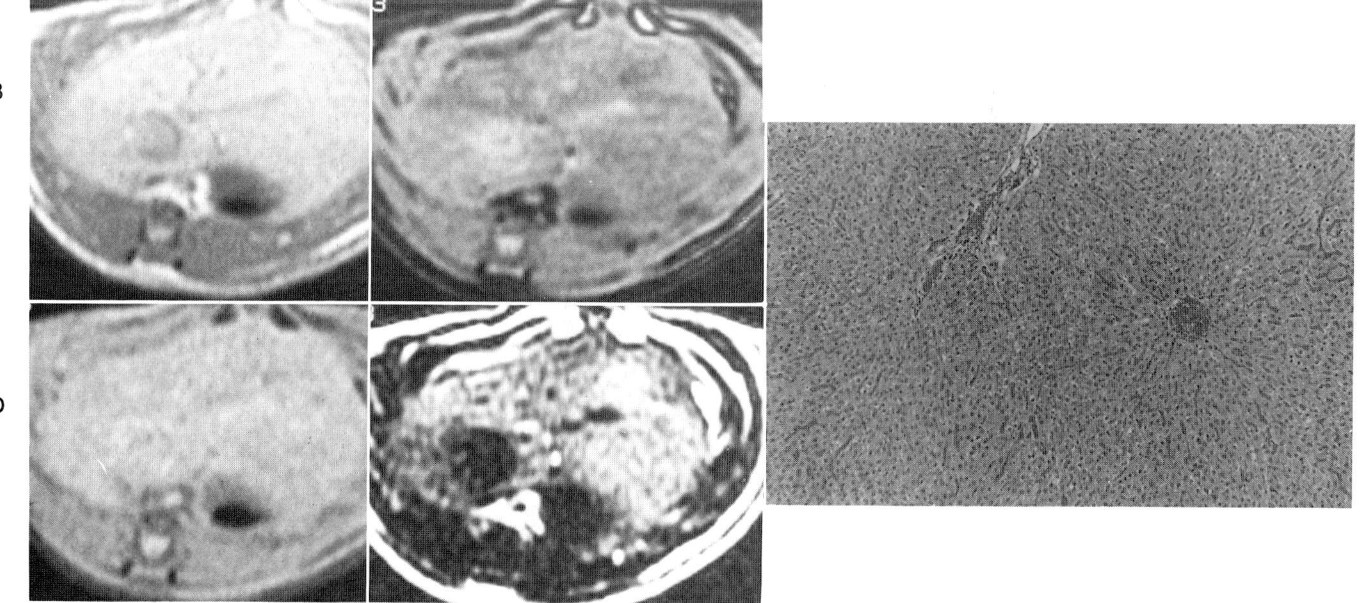

Fig. 14-7 Mild fatty infiltration of the liver of an alcohol-fed rat at 1.5 T (TR = 1500 msec, TE = 15 msec). **A,** In-phase image. Signal intensity of the liver is greater than that of the paraspinal muscle, similar to 14-6, *A. B,* Opposed-phase image. Signal intensity of the liver is low and is similar to that of the paraspinal muscle because in this image the fat signal has been subtracted from the water signal. **C,** Water image. The signal of liver relative to paraspinal muscle is similar to that in 14-7, *B.* Water image does not help in the diagnosis of mild fatty liver. **D,** Fat image. The liver has a higher signal intensity than paraspinal muscles, indicating fatty liver. **E,** Histologic specimen (H & E). Occasional small lipid droplets can be seen. (From Mitchell, D.G., Kim, I., Chang, T.S., et al.: Invest. Radiol. 26:1041-1052, 1991.)

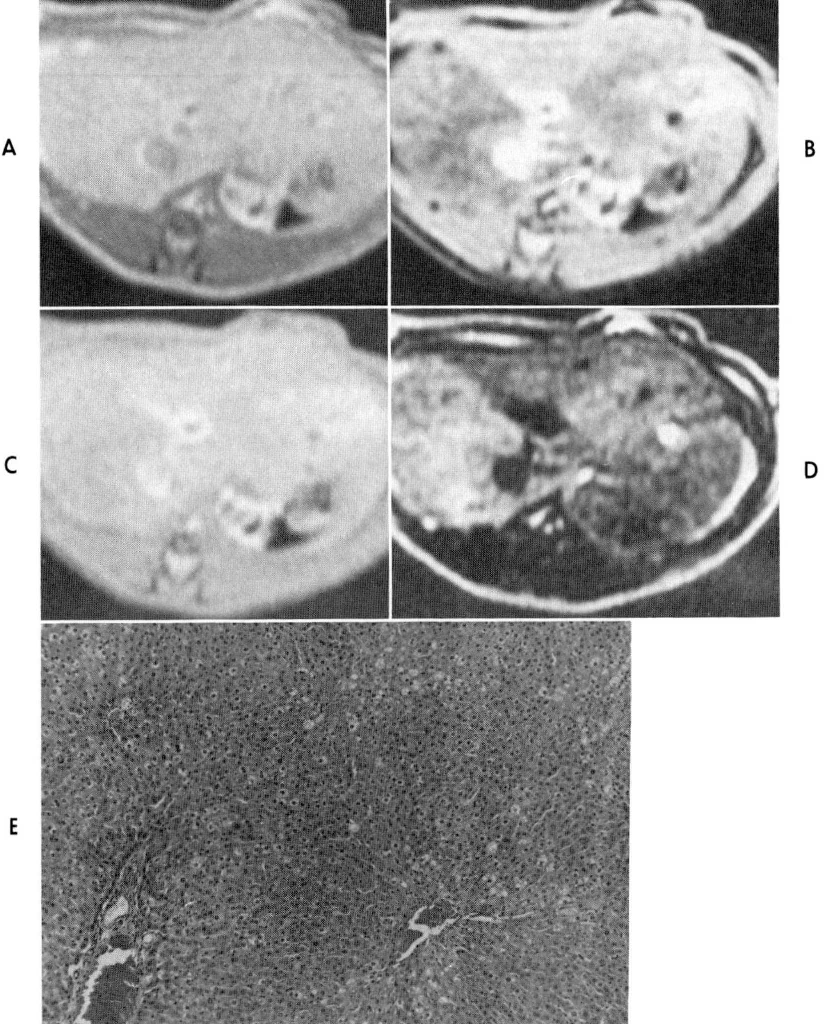

Fig. 14-8 Moderate fatty infiltration of the liver of an alcohol-fed rat at 1.5 T (TR = 1500 msec, TE = 15 msec). **A,** In-phase image. Signal intensity of the liver is greater than that of the paraspinal muscle, similar to 14-6, *A* and 14-7. **B,** Opposed-phase image. Signal intensity of the liver is lower than paraspinal muscle. **C,** Water image. The liver is only slightly brighter than paraspinal muscle, indicating fatty infiltration. **D,** Fat image. The liver has a markedly higher signal intensity than the paraspinal muscles. **E,** Histologic specimen (H & E). Lipid-rich hepatocytes are more frequent than in 14-7, *E*. (From Mitchell, D.G., Kim I., Chang, T.S., et al.: Invest. Radiol. 26:1041-1052, 1991.)

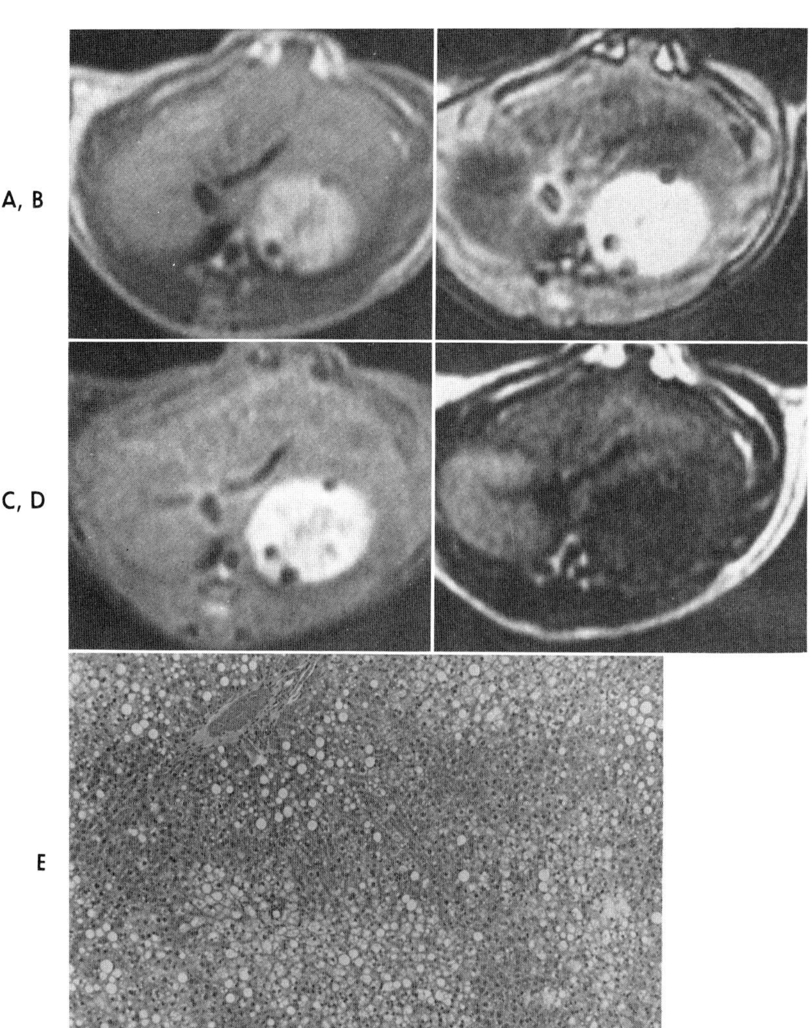

Fig. 14-9   Severe fatty infiltration of the liver of an alcohol-fed rat at 1.5 T (TR = 1500 msec, TE = 15 msec). **A,** In-phase image. Signal intensity of the liver relative to paraspinal muscle is similar to 14-6, *A*; 14-7, *B*; and 14-7, *E*. **B,** Opposed-phase image. Signal intensity of the liver is markedly less than that of paraspinal muscle. **C,** Water image. Liver is slightly more intense than muscle. **D,** Fat image. The liver has a markedly higher signal intensity than the paraspinal muscles. **E,** Histologic specimen (H & E) shows abundant clear lipid droplets. (From Mitchell, D.G., Kim, I., Chang, T.S., et al: Invest. Radiol. 26:1041-1052, 1991.)

sitive to fatty infiltration. These sequences can be obtained in less than 5 minutes on most systems. For diagnosis of fatty infiltration, the opposed-phase image is most effective if it is paired with an in-phase image with similar TR, TE, and other parameters. By so doing, even subtle changes in relative contrast between liver and spleen can be detected (Fig. 14-10).

Although less sensitive to fatty infiltration than the corresponding T1-weighted sequence, opposed-phase T2-weighted images can be useful for detecting focal hepatic lesions, since they outperform the corresponding T2-weighted in-phase images in patients with fatty liver.[276,502] On occasion, however, HCCs with fatty degeneration may be obscured on these images.

The spin-echo opposed-phase technique is not commercially available from most manufacturers, since companies have not perceived a great demand for these sequences from the general community. This is in part because MRI vendors have not stimulated this interest through their advertising.

Gradient-echo images with appropriate TE (approximately 2.1 msec at 1.5 T) are also effective opposed-phase images (Fig. 14-11 and 14-12). With TE = 4.2 msec, fat and water are in-phase. The effectiveness of gradient-echo chemical shift imaging by modulating TE is uncertain at lower field strengths, since larger variations of TE are necessary.

The phases of fat and water are at least partially opposed to each other on most gradient-echo images. Therefore fatty liver can be a cause of decreased signal on these images, potentially mimicking iron overload (Fig. 14-13). These two forms of diffuse liver disease can be differentiated by comparison with T2-weighted SE images; the signal of fatty liver will be normal or sligtly increased with fatty liver but decreased with iron overload.

Although hypoechoic areas within fatty liver usually represent focal sparing, occasionally this appearance is caused by foci with similar quantities of fat located inside fewer but larger intracellular lipid droplets.[63] This

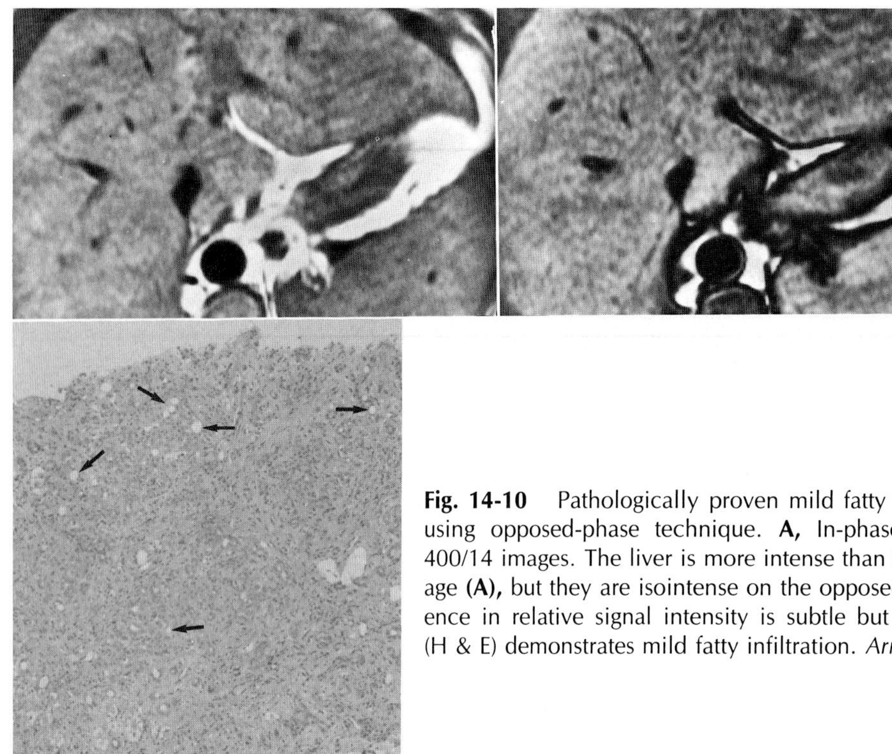

Fig. 14-10 Pathologically proven mild fatty infiltration detected at 1.5 T, using opposed-phase technique. **A,** In-phase and **B,** opposed-phase SE 400/14 images. The liver is more intense than the spleen in the in-phase image **(A),** but they are isointense on the opposed-phase image **(B).** The difference in relative signal intensity is subtle but real. **C,** Microscopic section (H & E) demonstrates mild fatty infiltration. *Arrows* indicate vessicular fat.

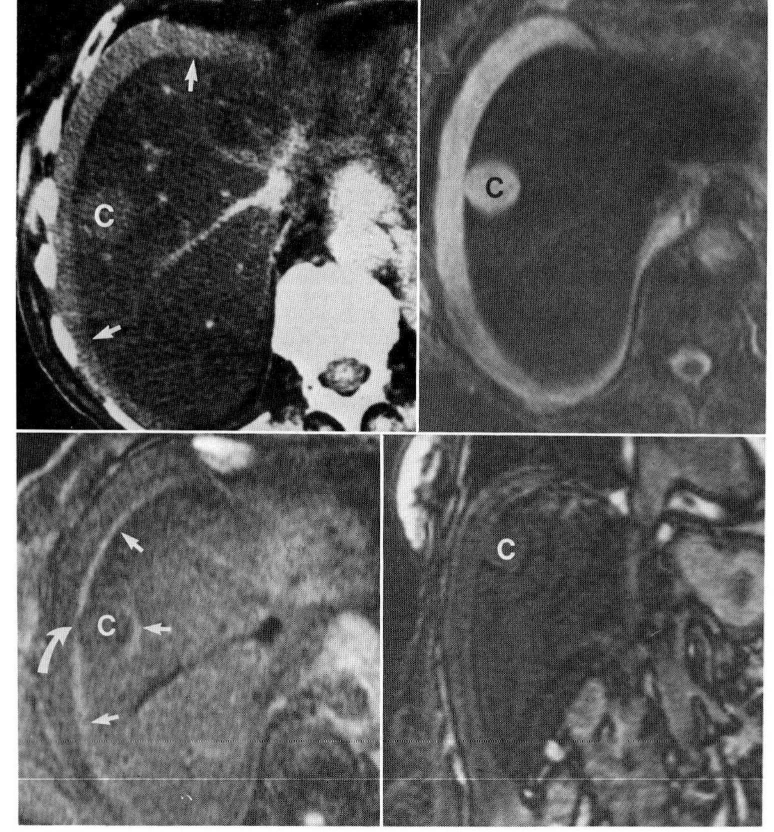

Fig. 14-11 Severely fatty liver hypointense or isointense relative to ascites and an hepatic cyst (C) on fat suppressed and opposed-phase images at 1.5 T and on CT scan. **A,** Axial enhanced CT scan. Ascites *(small arrows)* and cyst are both denser than liver. **B,** SE 2500/100 image depicts the cyst as isointense to ascites. **C,** SE 400/12 image with fat suppression. The liver, cyst, and ascites are now isointense. In spite of fat suppression, substantial hepatic fat signal persists. This can be determined by noting the high-signal chemical-shift artifact from misregistration of hepatic lipid relative to ascites and cyst *(arrows).* Note that there is no bright band at the interface between cyst and ascites *(curved arrow).* **D,** Coronal opposed-phase gradient-echo image (TR/TE/flip angle = 103/2.3/90 degrees). There is little signal from the liver.

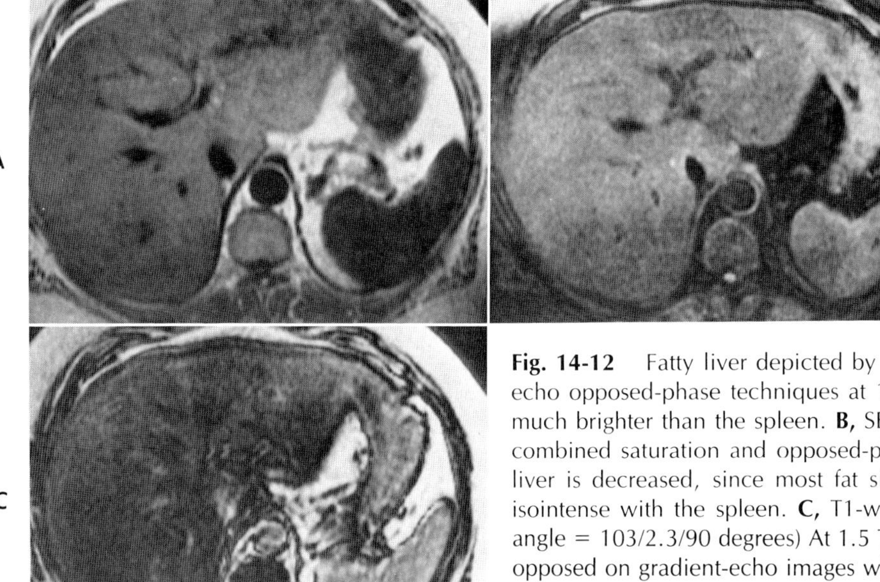

Fig. 14-12 Fatty liver depicted by spin-echo fat-suppression and gradient-echo opposed-phase techniques at 1.5 T. **A,** SE 400/12 image. The liver is much brighter than the spleen. **B,** SE 400/14 image with fat suppression (by combined saturation and opposed-phase techniques). Relative signal of the liver is decreased, since most fat signal has been eliminated. The liver is isointense with the spleen. **C,** T1-weighted gradient-echo image (TR/TE/flip angle = 103/2.3/90 degrees) At 1.5 T the phases of water and fat protons are opposed on gradient-echo images with TE = 2.3 msec. Water and fat signal in hepatic voxels interferes destructively, causing liver to be markedly less intense than spleen. The signal void at interfaces between fat and water results from fat-water signal cancellation within these voxels.

Fig. 14-13 Low signal of fatty liver on gradient-echo "MR angiographic" image at 1.5 T, mimicking iron overload (same patient as Fig. 7-4). **A,** Axial gradient-echo image obtained for vascular imaging (TR/TE/flip angle = 25/13/20 degrees) reveals decreased signal of the liver relative to kidneys, muscle, and spleen *(S)*, mimicking iron overload such as from hemochromatosis. **B,** SE 2500/100 image reveals slightly increased hepatic signal (much brighter than background and muscle, even with this long TE), probably from fatty infiltration. If there were iron overload, hepatic signal would be decreased. **C,** SE 400/12 image. The liver is much brighter than spleen. **D,** SE 400/12 image with fat suppression. The liver is slightly less intense than spleen, confirming fatty liver (compare with C).

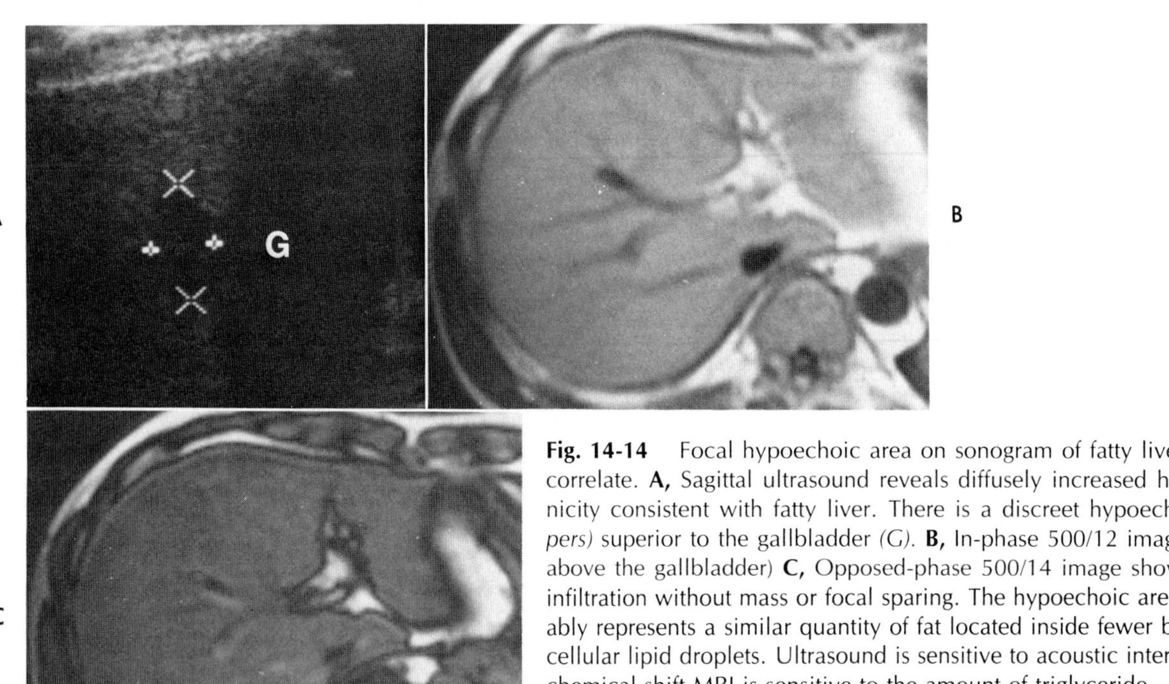

Fig. 14-14 Focal hypoechoic area on sonogram of fatty liver without MRI correlate. **A,** Sagittal ultrasound reveals diffusely increased hepatic echogenicity consistent with fatty liver. There is a discreet hypoechoic area *(calipers)* superior to the gallbladder *(G)*. **B,** In-phase 500/12 image immediately above the gallbladder) **C,** Opposed-phase 500/14 image shows diffuse fatty infiltration without mass or focal sparing. The hypoechoic area in **A** presumably represents a similar quantity of fat located inside fewer but larger intracellular lipid droplets. Ultrasound is sensitive to acoustic interfaces, whereas chemical shift MRI is sensitive to the amount of triglyceride.

is because echogenicity does not directly reflect the amount of fat but reflects the density of acoustic interfaces, which in turn depends on the size and number of droplets. Chemical shift techniques, however, are sensitive to the amount, rather than the distribution, of lipid within voxels. In cases where different lipid droplet size is the cause of a focal hypoechoic area, even chemical shift imaging will not demonstrate a focal abnormality (Fig. 14-14). The lack of a lesion on good quality T1- and T2-weighted images is strong presumptive evidence against a malignancy, however. Additionally, a metastasis that is isointense to fatty liver on in-phase images is likely to be more intense than fatty liver on opposed-phase images.

The morphology of focal fatty infiltration must be examined to differentiate it from fat within HCC or benign tumors such as adenoma, focal nodular hyperplasia, regenerative nodule, or lipomatous tumors (Figs. 12-3 and 12-11).* HCC tends to be more well defined than focal fatty infiltration, and usually contains some elements with high signal on T2-weighted images (Fig. 11-7).

---

*137, 232, 252, 314, 438, 526, 534

Inflammatory Disease

VIRAL HEPATITIS

Viral hepatitis can produce significant acute morbidity. Hepatitis B and C viruses are transmitted parenterally and can cause chronic hepatitis and cirrhosis, as well as acute disease. Hepatitis C has been a particular problem in recipients of blood transfusions. A specific serologic test for hepatitis C, which accounts for most cases of parenterally transmitted non-A, non-B hepatitis, has recently been developed.[266] Non-A, non-B, non-C hepatitis is now referred to as *hepatitis-delta.* Recently, interferon has been used to decrease hepatic injury from chronic active hepatitis.[34,97]

Acute hepatitis can be diagnosed by clinical and serologic studies, and imaging is not part of the standard initial work-up. In patients with chronic hepatitis, however, imaging studies can be used to detect cirrhosis or ascites and to exclude HCC. On T2-weighted images of patients with acute or chronic active hepatitis, a collar of high signal intensity can often be noted surrounding portal vein branches, corresponding to inflammation. This finding is nonspecific, however.[323]

In hepatitis models of animals and some patients with acute or chronic active hepatitis with focal inflammatory changes, diffuse or regional high signal can be identified on T2-weighted MR images (Figs. 15-1 to 15-3).[492,494] Use of MRI to guide biopsy of these selected areas may reduce sampling error, a significant problem with current methods of histologic diagnosis by blind biopsy. MRI might also prove useful for monitoring the effectiveness of interferon therapy for chronic active hepatitis (Fig. 15-3).

Enlarged periportal lymph nodes are common in patients with viral hepatitis. These nodes may be discreet or confluent, but the portal vein and other structures usually maintain their shapes and are not compressed (Fig. 15-4).

RADIATION-INDUCED HEPATITIS

Portions of the liver are often included in radiation portals for a variety of malignancies. Within 6 months of radiation injury, edema can be noted, depicted as decreased intensity on T1-weighted images and increased intensity on T2-weighted images (Fig. 15-5).[554,616] In patients with fatty liver, fat is usually decreased within the radiation portal,[87,157,554] presumably because of decreased delivery of triglycerides from diminished portal flow.

SCLEROSING CHOLANGITIS

Although sclerosing cholangitis is usually considered a disease of the biliary system, it is included here because it can manifest as a periportal disease. Intense inflammatory fibrosis involves the intrahepatic and extrahepatic biliary systems and expands the portal tracts.[67,271,476,601] Enlarged portal lymph nodes may be present. The hepatic parenchyma is often normal, even in patients with liver failure and portal hypertension. However, the disease may progress to secondary biliary cirrhosis. Unlike primary biliary cirrhosis, which predominates in women, approximately 70% of patients with sclerosing cholangitis are male.[601]

The etiology of primary sclerosing cholangitis is not known, although many patients have inflammatory bowel disease, particularly ulcerative colitis. Secondary sclerosing cholangitis may occur as a sequela of biliary surgery or choledocholithiasis[601] or after hepatic arterial FUDR chemotherapy.[480]

Cholangiographic findings include beaded dilatation of intrahepatic and extra-hepatic bile ducts, with similar findings noted by contrast-enhanced CT.[421,475,529] Bile duct thickening has been described,[475] although it is uncertain if bile wall thickening can be distinguished from periportal inflammation.

With MRI, scattered areas of biliary dilatation can be seen, along with marked periportal inflammation. The biliary dilatation can best be distinguished from periportal inflammation on heavily T2-weighted images with sufficient spatial resolution and SNR, on which it is depicted as fluid-equivalent signal, paralleling portal vein branches. Periportal inflammation is manifested as low signal intensity on T1-weighted images and a signal intermediate between that of liver and bile on T2-weighted images (Figs. 14-2, 15-6 and 15-7). In many cases, this abnormal tissue is more apparent on T1-weighted images. These findings can be seen at the hepatic hilum and within intrahepatic portal tracts, where they cause a collar surrounding portal vein branches. This high-signal collar is not seen surrounding branches of hepatic veins. There is some overlap, however, between the periportal inflammation seen with sclerosing cholangitis and other conditions, such as biliary obstruction, hepatitis, allograft rejection, and periportal malignancy.[323]

Sclerosing cholangitis is associated with occult-main or segmental-portal vein thrombus, presumably secondary to periportal inflammation (Fig. 15-6). This may be the cause of segmental atrophy (Fig. 15-8), a common finding in patients with sclerosing cholangitis.[183]

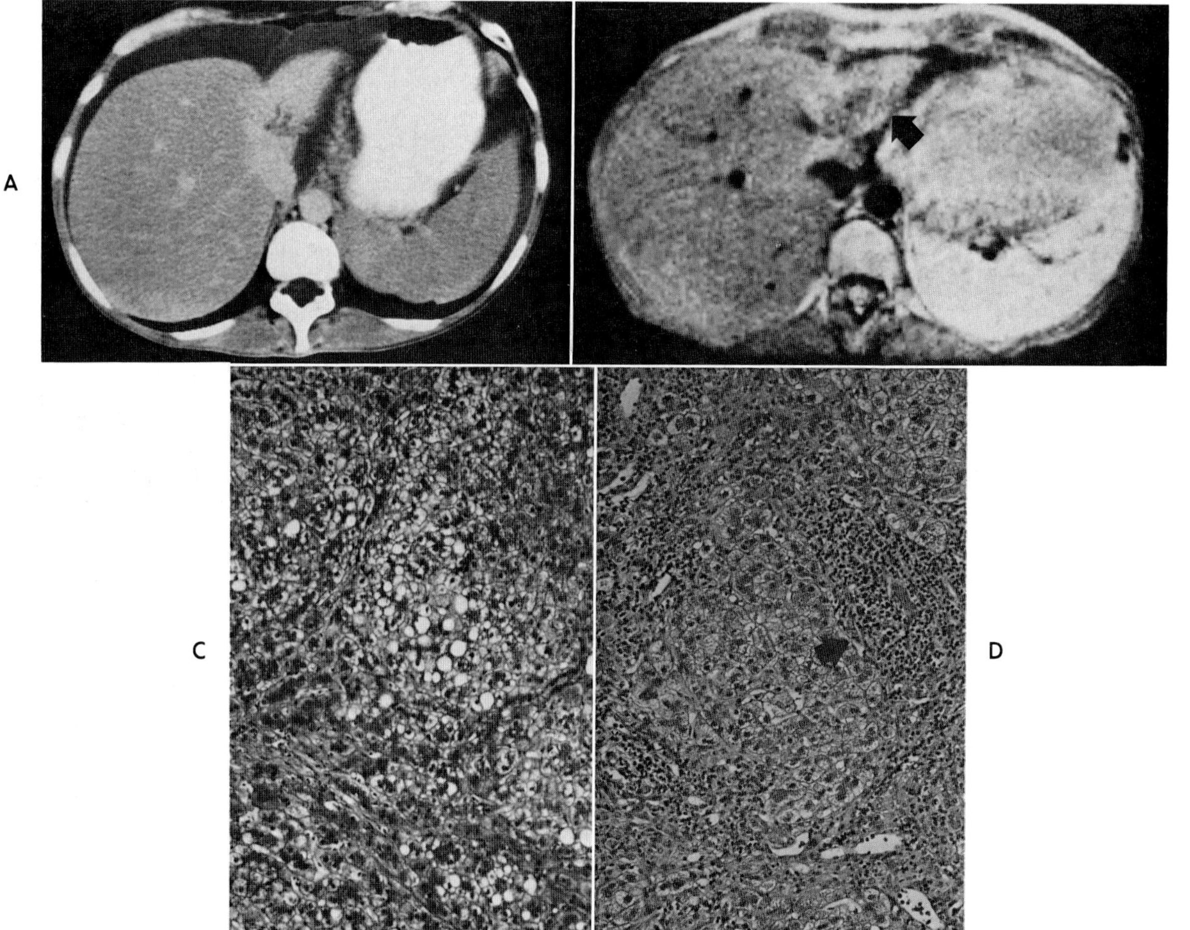

Fig. 15-1   Patient with alcoholic pancreatitis and hepatitis. **A,** CT scan after infusion of contrast material; low attenuation of the right lobe of the liver, relative to the spleen, suggests fatty infiltration. The left lobe of the liver is atretic but has normal attenuation. **B,** SE 2000/28 image at 0.6 T demonstrates normal intensity of the right lobe of the liver. The intensity of the left lobe of the liver *(arrow)* is increased. **C,** Biopsy of the right lobe of the liver *(trichrome stain)* reveals moderate cirrhosis and fatty infiltration without evidence of hepatitis. **D,** Biopsy of the left lobe reveals moderate cirrhosis and hepatitis *(arrow)* without evidence of fatty infiltration.

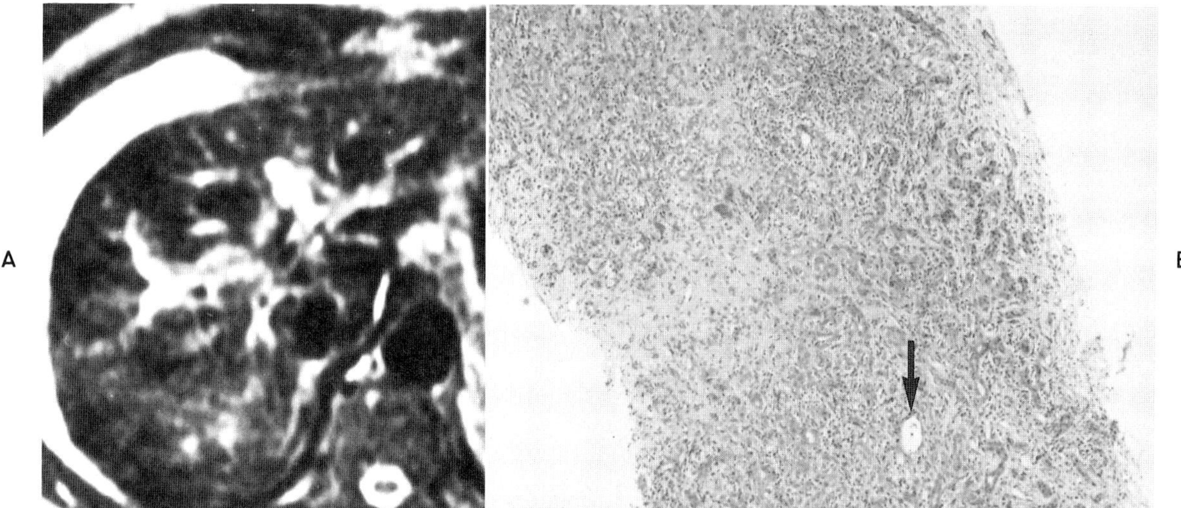

Fig. 15-2   Acute fulminant hepatitis. **A,** T2-weighted image at 1.5 T (SE 2500/100) reveals heterogeneous areas of increased intensity, most severe in the posterior segment of the right lobe. **B,** Histologic section (H & E) shows severe inflammation and virtual destruction of hepatic parenchyma. *Arrow* indicates central vein.

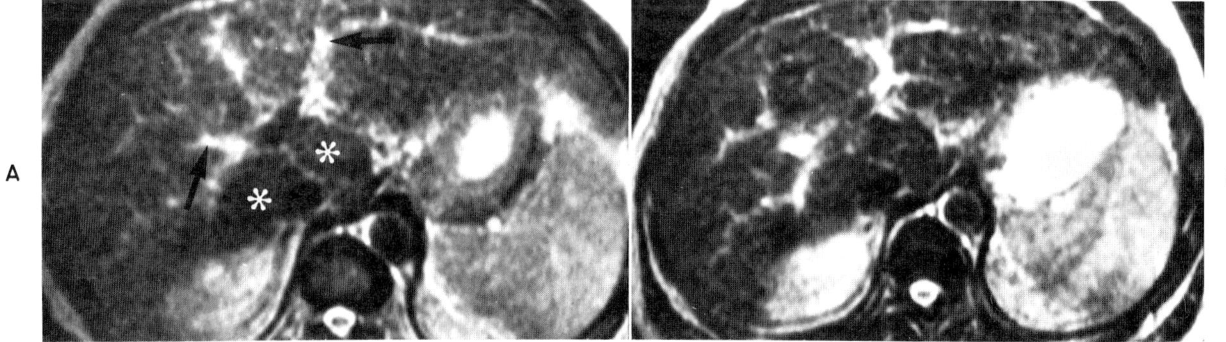

Fig. 15-3   Treatment of biopsy-proven chronic active hepatitis and cirrhosis with interferon, monitored by MRI at 1.5 T. **A,** Axial T2-weighted image (SE 2500/100) reveals heterogeneous areas of high signal, most marked between the right anterior segmental and left branches of the portal vein *(arrows)*. The tissue in the region of the inferior vena cava is relatively spared *(asterisks)*. **B,** About 9 months later, these areas of focal signal abnormality have resolved. The liver is slightly smaller, and the left portal vein is positioned more toward the right than in **A.** Nodular impressions on vessels, indicative of cirrhosis, are still present.

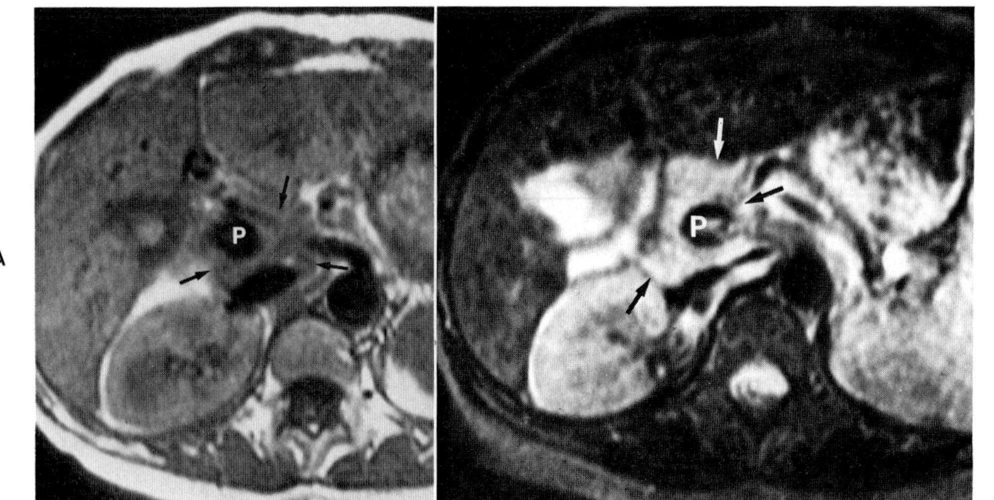

Fig. 15-4 Inflammatory lymph nodes *(arrows)* secondary to hepatitis B. **A,** SE 400/12 image at 1.5 T. There is abnormal soft tissue surrounding the portal vein *(P)*. **B,** SE 2500 image depicts the nodes as high signal intensity.

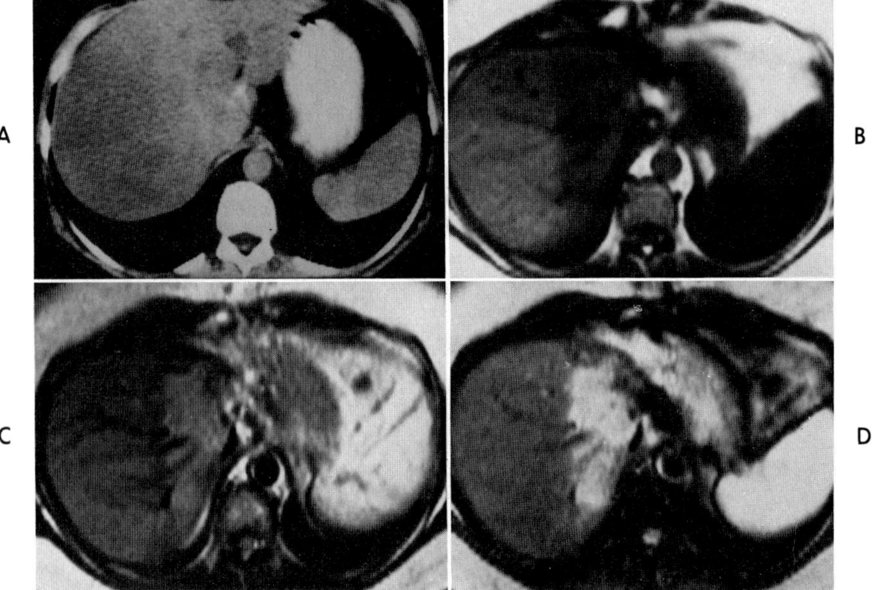

Fig. 15-5 Radiation hepatitis of the left side of the liver. Hepatic edema and noninvolvement by fatty infiltration. **A,** Increased attenuation on contrast-enhanced CT scan is due to nonfatty liver. **B,** Decreased intensity on T1-weighted MR image is due to edema and absence of fat. **C,** Note the increased intensity on SE 2000/60 image from edema. **D,** Opposed-phase 2000/60 image (compare with **C**) shows fatty infiltration of the right side of the liver, decreasing its intensity. The irradiated left side of the liver is not fatty.

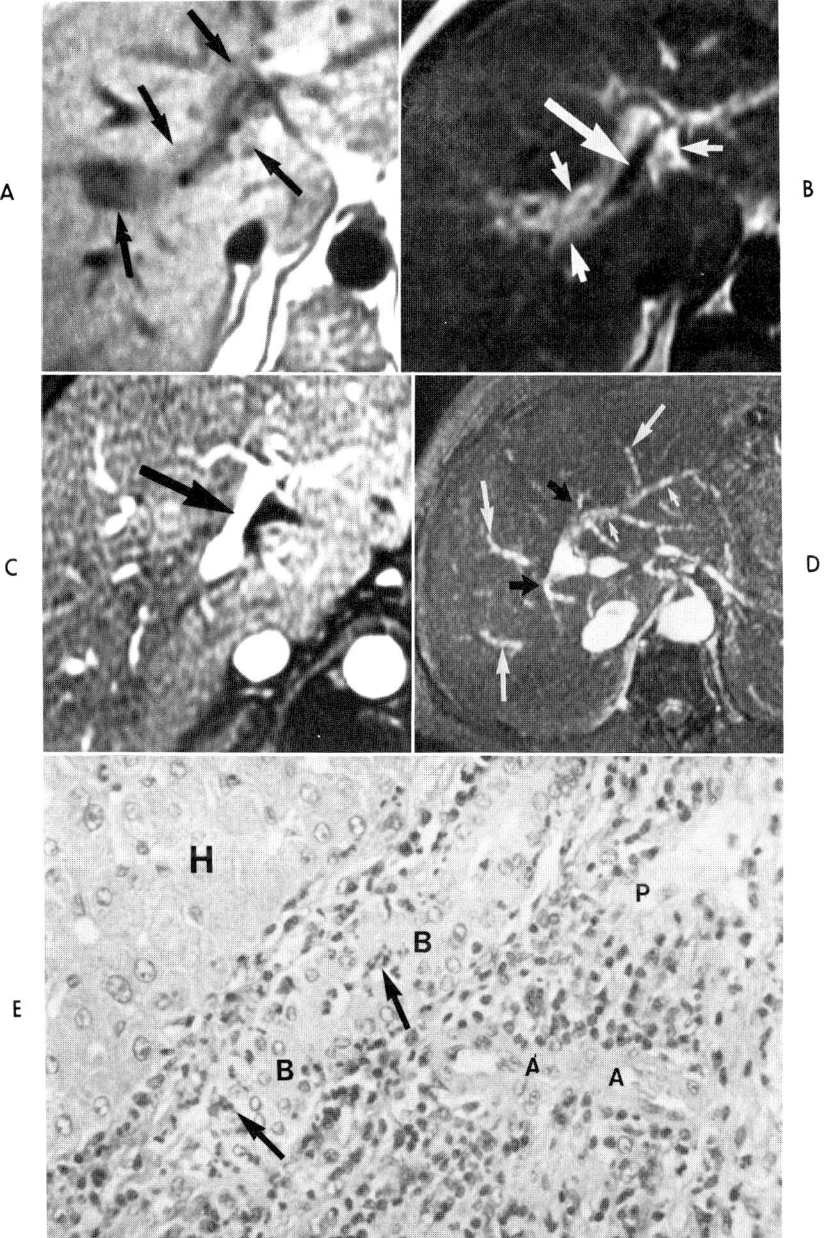

Fig. 15-6   Sclerosing cholangitis with periportal inflammation and thrombosis of the right and left medial branches of the portal vein. **A,** Axial T1-weighted image (SE 400/12) at the level of the portal vein bifurcation. Intermediate–signal-intensity tissue is noted along the course of the portal veins *(arrows)*. **B,** Corresponding T2-weighted image (SE 2500/100) depicts this periportal inflammation as high signal *(small arrows)*. A signal void is noted in the patent left portal branch *(large arrow)*, but there is no signal void in the thrombosed right branch. **C,** Gradient-echo image (GRASS; 25/13, flip angle 20 degrees) confirms flow in the left branch *(arrow)* and absence of flow in the right. **D,** Composite-MR angiographic slab approximately 4-cm thick, demonstrating the patient's left lateral segmental portal vein *(small arrows)* and abrupt termination of the right and medial left portal vein branches. *Thick arrows* = hepatic veins. **E,** Histologic section (H & E) shows marked expansion of a portal tract by inflammatory cells surrounding bile duct *(B)*, hepatic artery *(A)*, and portal vein *(P)* branches. Note inflammatory cells *(arrows)* within the lumen of the bile duct. Hepatocytes *(H)* are normal.

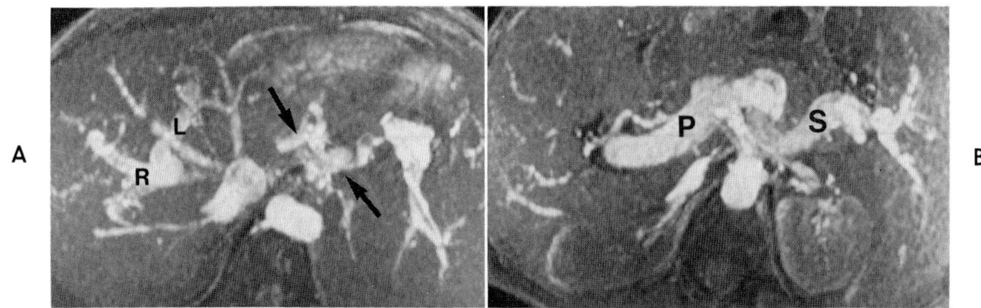

Fig. 16-12 Dilated intrahepatic and extrahepatic portal system in a patient with portal hypertension secondary to sclerosing cholangitis, depicted by MR angiography at 1.5 T. **A,** The left *(L)* and right *(R)* branches of the portal vein are dilated. *Arrows* = gastroesophageal varices. **B,** Inferiorly, the splenic *(S)* and main portal *(P)* veins are dilated.

sion causes or exacerbates complications of cirrhosis, such as variceal bleeding, ascites, and splenomegaly. During the early stages of portal hypertension, the portal system dilates, but flow is maintained (Fig. 16-12). Later, significant portosystemic shunting develops, reducing the volume of flow to the liver and decreasing the size of the portal vein (Fig. 16-13). With advanced portal hypertension, portal flow may actually become reversed.

Portal varices, caused by increased portal pressure, shunt portal blood into systemic veins, bypassing hepatic parenchyma and sinusoids. Nutrients absorbed from the gut are thus metabolized less effectively, and hepatic function decreases. Additionally, toxic metabolites such as ammonia accumulate in the blood, producing clinical manifestations such as hepatic encephalopathy. These physiologic alterations result regardless of the anatomic site of the shunting. Since diminished portal flow to the liver parenchyma is a significant factor in the production of liver atrophy and prevention of regeneration,[297] it is likely that portosystemic shunting plays a role in the development of hepatic atrophy in advanced cirrhosis.

Esophageal varices are especially significant because they may rupture through the esophageal mucosa and produce life-threatening hemorrhage. Esophageal varices arise from dilated left gastric (coronary) veins and drain into systemic veins of the thorax, such as azygous, hemiazygous, or intercostal veins.[600] Varices at other sites, such as splenorenal and paraumbilical, may thus benefit the cirrhotic individual by decompressing esophageal varices and forestalling hemorrhage, although they may exacerbate hepatic encephalopathy.[365,388] Esophageal varices may be treated by sclerotherapy or surgical decompression by creation of alternative portosystemic shunts.

Esophageal varices are difficult to demonstrate by sonography because of their high epigastric location and because they are often small.[511] Like other varices, they

are identified readily by T1-weighted or flow-sensitive gradient-echo images anterior to the aorta at the level of the diaphragmatic hiatus (Figs. 16-14 and 16-15).[40,585] Flow-sensitive gradient-echo images appear to be at least as sensitive as contrast angiography and endoscopy for detecting varices, whether single-slice tomographic or projection technique is used.[115]

Low flip angles should be used for gradient-echo images to decrease pulsatile artifact from the aorta and heart, since this may obscure small varices. If ghost artifact obscures esophageal varices, their presence can be inferred by demonstrating dilated left gastric veins in the gastrohepatic ligament.

Spontaneous splenorenal shunts, connecting splenic varices to the left renal vein, are difficult to visualize sonographically because of jejunal or colonic gas.[401] Collaterals to paravertebral veins, as well as to hemorrhoidal veins in the pelvis via the inferior mesenteric vein, are even harder to detect sonographically. Spontaneous retroperitoneal portosystemic shunts can be identified by MRI (Figs. 16-13, 16-14, 16-16). If enough blood is shunted through a splenorenal collateral, mesenteric blood is shunted away from the liver. This can be depicted by directional MR angiographic techniques as reversed flow in the central portion of the splenic vein (Fig. 16-17) (see also Color Plate VII).

Patent paraumbilical veins shunt blood from the left portal vein to superficial veins at the umbilicus. They can be found best by following the left portal vein, from which patent paraumbilical veins arise and course adjacent to the ligamentum teres (the obliterated umbilical vein) (Figs. 16-16, 16-18, and 16-19). Patent paraumbilical veins pass anteroinferiorly towards the abdominal wall, along which they course to a network of systemic veins at the umbilicus. When these superficial veins dilate, they produce a characteristic spider-web appearance at the umbilicus, referred to as a *caput medusa.*

In patients with isolated splenic vein occlusion, large

Text continues on p. 172.

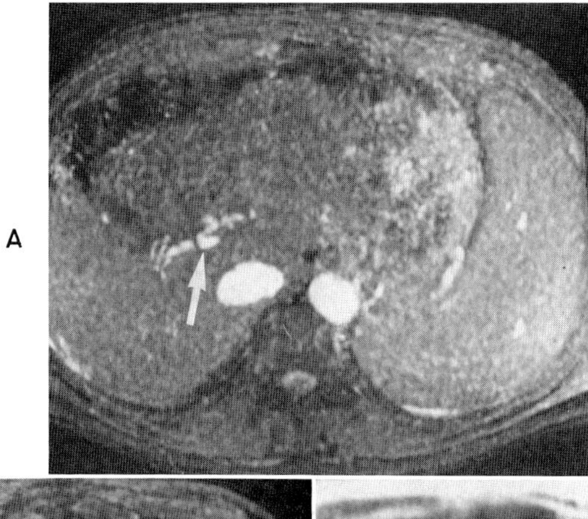

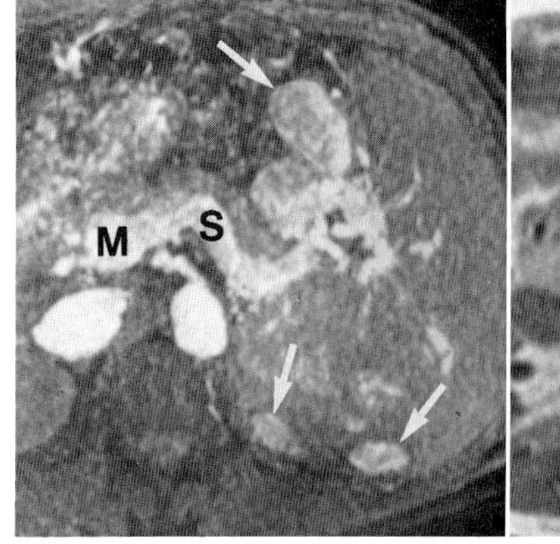

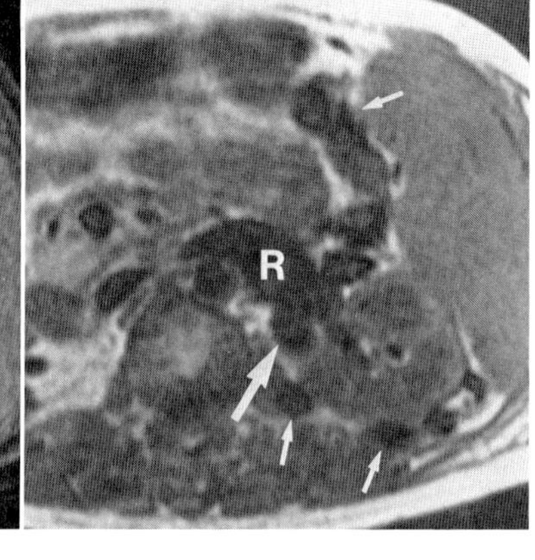

Fig. 16-13 Dilated extrahepatic portal system with small intraheptic portal veins resulting from massive portosystemic shunting. **A,** MR angiographic slab at 1.5 T at the level of the portal bifurcation *(arrow),* demonstrating its small size. **B,** Inferiorly, the splenic *(S)* and superior mesenteric *(M)* veins are dilated. Note dilated splenic and retroperitoneal varices *(arrows).* **C,** SE 400/12 image inferior to **A** and **B.** There is a large spontaneous splenorenal shunt *(large arrow)* draining into a dilated left renal vein *(R). Small arrows* = splenic and retroperitoneal varices.

Fig. 16-14 Large gastric, espophageal, and splenorenal varices secondary to portal hypertension, depicted at 1.5 T. **A,** Axial SE 2500/100 image. There are extensive varices depicted as flow voids *(arrows).* Note irregular intrahepatic vessels secondary to cirrhosis. **B,** Corresponding breath-hold gradient-echo image (TR/TE/flip angle = 25/13/20 degrees). *Long arrow* = dilated coronary vein adjacent to esophagus. The liver is at a different level relative to the varices than in the breathing-averaged spin-echo image in **A,** because of different position of the diaphragm. **C,** Composite-MR angiographic slab, approximately 4-cm thick. *Large arrows* = gastric varices, *small arrows* = esophageal varices, *P* = portal bifurcation. **D,** MR angiographic slab at an inferior level. *I* = inferior vena cava, *L* = dilated left renal vein, *P* = portal vein, *S* = splenic vein, *V* = retroperitoneal varices, *large arrow* = splenorenal collateral vein. **E** and **F,** Coronal-MR angiographic slabs. *Short arrows* = gastric varices, *long thin arrow* = dilated coronary vein and esophageal varices, *large arrow* = spenorenal collateral. *A* = aorta, *I* = inferior vena cava, *P* = portal vein, *S* = splenic vein.

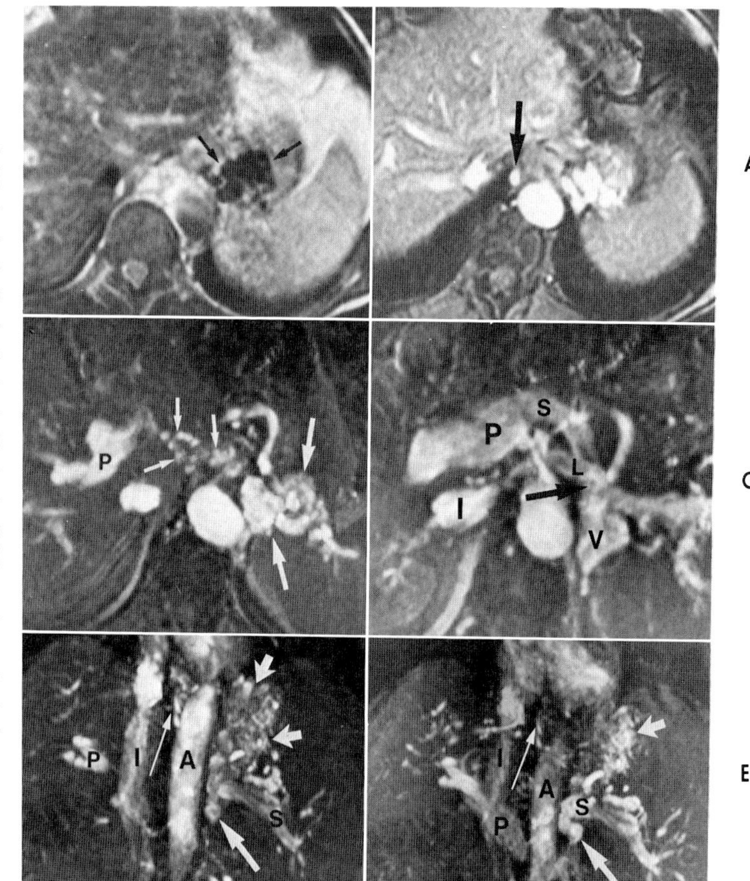

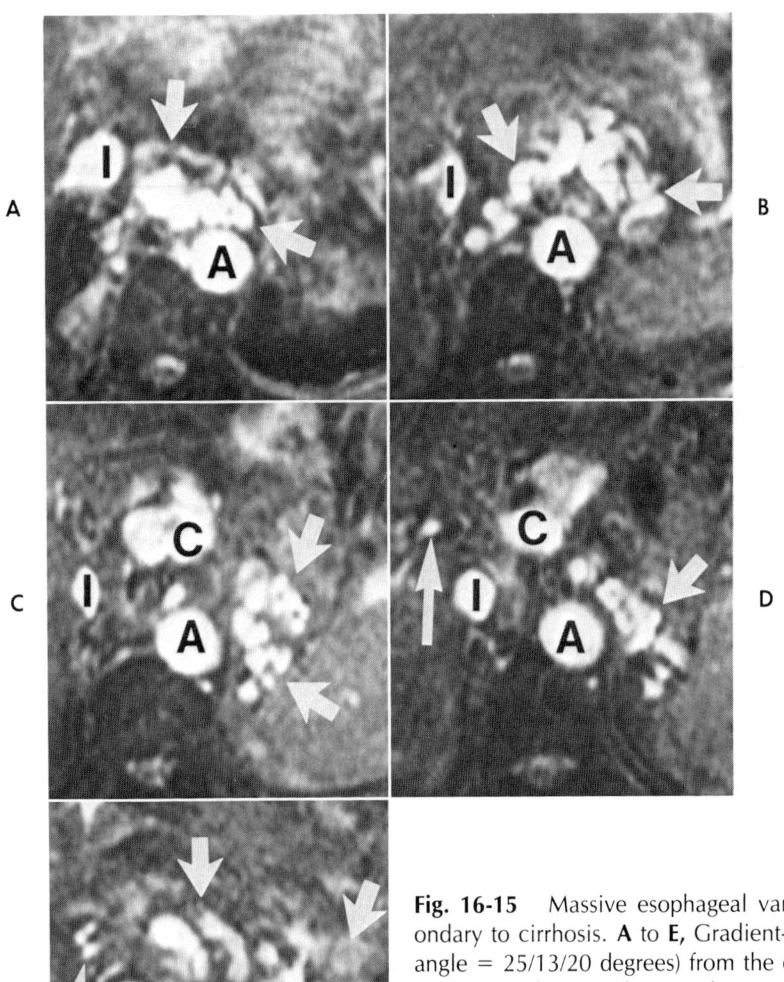

Fig. 16-15 Massive esophageal varices *(short arrows)* secondary to cirrhosis. **A** to **E,** Gradient-echo images (TR/TE/flip angle = 25/13/20 degres) from the esophageal hiatus down to the portal vein. The portal veins *(long arrows)* are small due to end-stage portal hypertension and massive shunting away from the liver. *A* = aorta, *C* = dilated coronary vein, *I* = inferior vena cava.

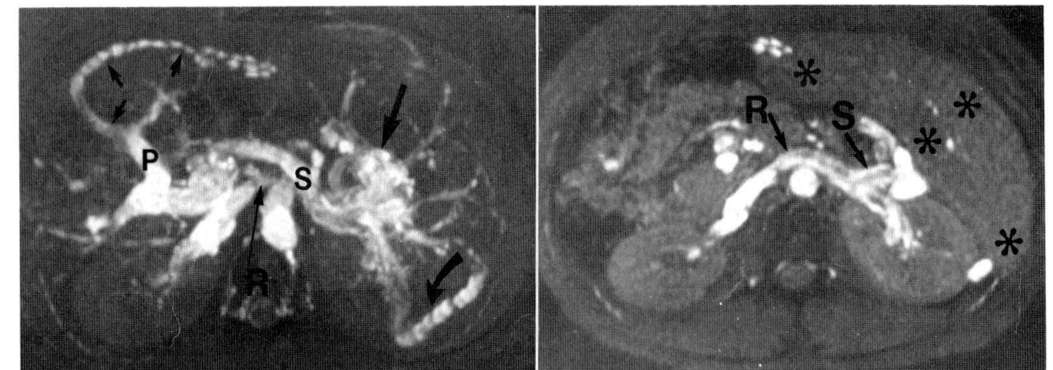

Fig. 16-16 Portosystemic shunting from splenorenal and retroperitoneal collaterals and a patent paraumbilical vein in a patient with portal hypertension. **A,** Axial MR angiogram (GRASS 25/13, flip angle 20 degres) shows the patent paraumbilical vein *(small arrows)* arising from the left portal vein *(P)*. Splenic collateral veins *(large arrow)* can be seen, but the splenorenal shunt, between the splenic vein *(S)* and left renal vein *(R)*, is obscured. Portosystemic collateral veins can be seen posterior to the spleen *(curved arrow)*. **B,** Limited MR angiogram with most of the liver excluded, demonstrating the spontaneous splenorenal collateral *(S)* joining a dilated left renal vein *(R)*. The spleen *(asterisks)* is enlarged.

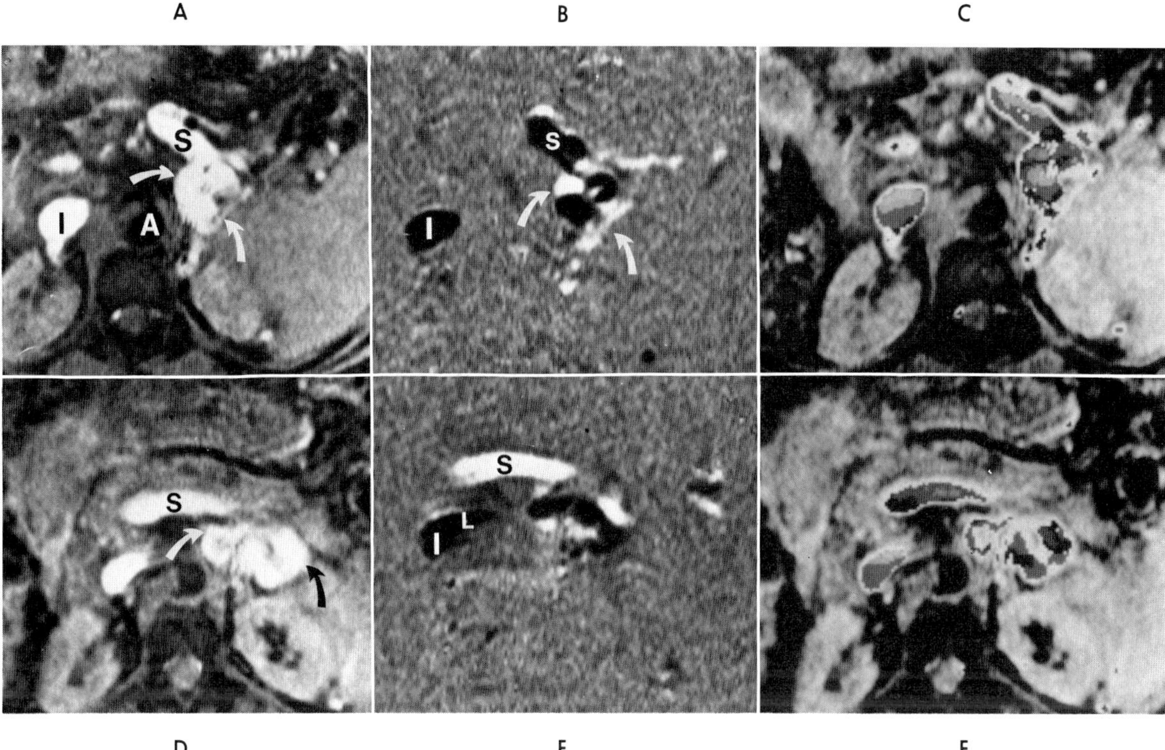

Fig. 16-17 Reversed flow in the splenic vein resulting from portosystemic shunting, depicted at 1.5 T by phase-sensitive color flow MR angiography. **A,** Magnitude image at the level of the proximal (peripheral) splenic vein *(S)*. *Curved arrows* indicate large tortuous perisplenic collataral veins. *I* = inferior vena cava. Vessels are bright because of inflow of unsaturated blood (time-of-flight phenomenon). Superior presaturation has produced a signal void in the aorta *(A)*. **B,** Corresponding phase-contrast image. Flow from left to right, as in the splenic vein *(S)*, is encoded as black, whereas flow from right to left is encoded as white. Background is grey. Perisplenic collaterals *(curved arrows)* are encoded as black and white because of their tortuosity. *I* = inferior vena cava. **C,** Color flow MR image produced by encoding phase changes in **B** as blue and red, rather than as black and white, respectively. This information was superimposed on the grey scale depiction of anatomy in **A.** (See Color Plate VII.) **D,** Magnitude image inferior to **A** through **C.** *S* = central splenic vein, *curved arrows* = perisplenic collaterals. **E,** Phase-contrast image corresponding to **D.** Flow in the splenic vein *(S)* is reversed, from right to left. This indicates that flow from the superior mesenteric vein is being shunted away from the liver. Lower images (not shown) revealed a large splenorenal shunt. *L* = left renal vein, with flow from left to right toward the inferior vena cava *(I)*. **F,** Color flow MR image corresponding to **D** and **E.** (See Color Plate VII.)

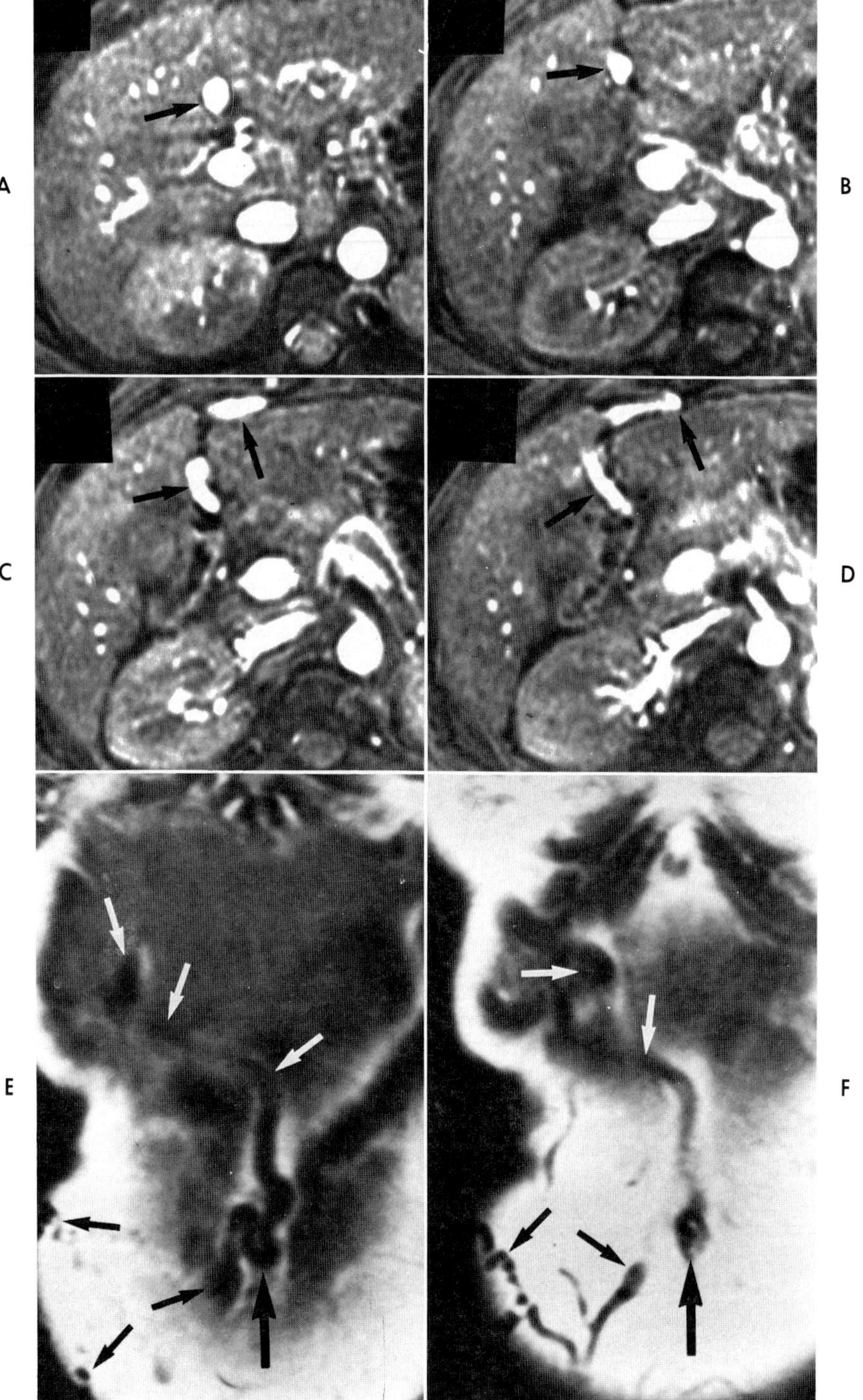

Fig. 16-18 Patent paraumbilical vein in a patient with portal hypertension. **A** to **D,** Axial GRASS images at 1.5 T (25/13, flip angle 20 degrees) from cephalad to caudad, depicting a patent paraumbilical vein *(arrows)* extending from the flaciform ligament towards the umbilicus. **E** and **F,** Coronal SE 600/20 images depict the patent paraumbilical vein *(white arrows)* anteriorly as it leaves the liver to supply a network of collateral veins at the umbilicus *(large black arrow).* Note the dilated superficial collaterals over the right lower quadrant *(small black arrows),* consitituting the systemic side of the portosystemic anastomosis.

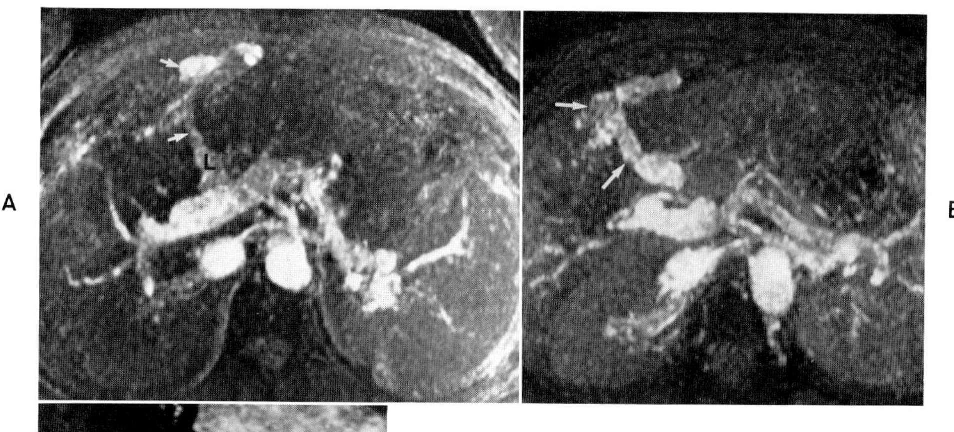

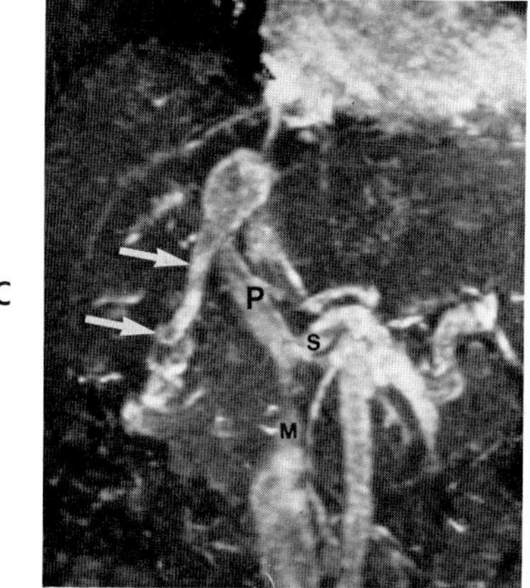

Fig. 16-19   Patent paraumbilical veins, depicted by MR angiography at 1.5 T. **A,** A large patent paraumbilical vein *(arrows)* extends from the left portal vein *(L)* toward the umbilicus. **B,** In a different patient, right lobe atrophy has cause the paraumbilical vein *(arrows)* to assume a more rightward direction. **C,** Coronal-MR angiographic slab depicts the paraumbilical vein *(arrows)* descending toward the abdominal wall, where it joins a network of collateral vessels. The umbilicus itself is anterior to the plane of this slab. *M* = superior mesenteric vein, *P* = main portal vein, *S* = splenic vein.

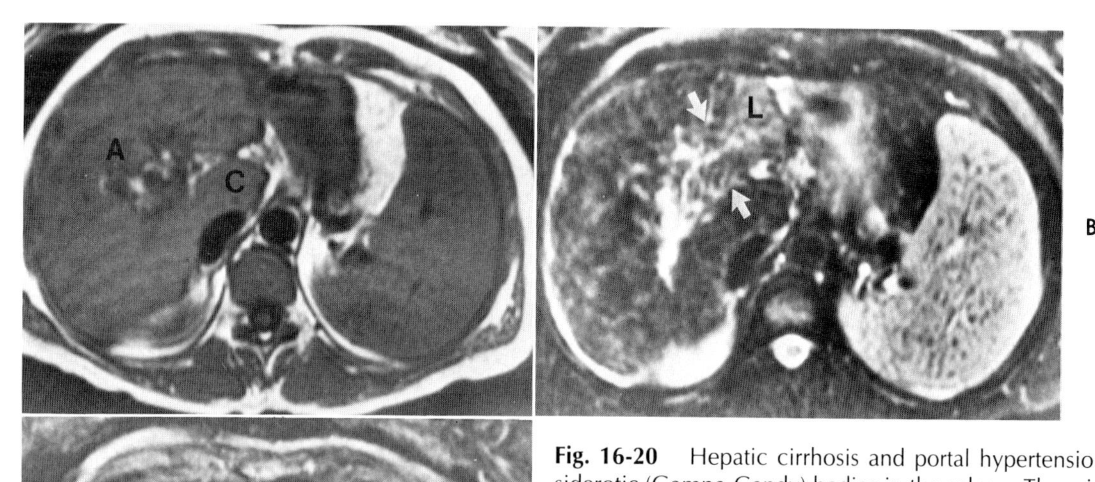

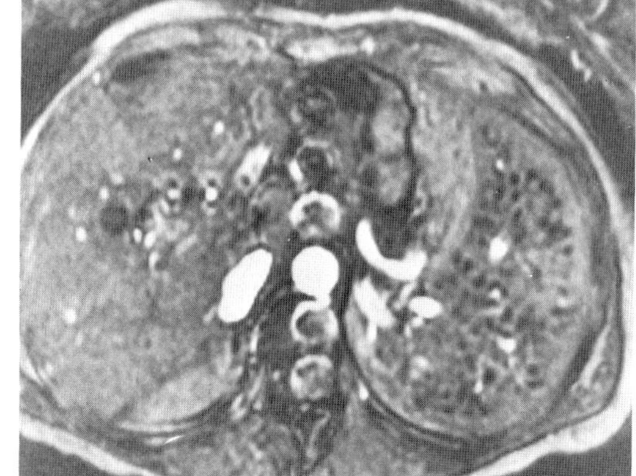

Fig. 16-20   Hepatic cirrhosis and portal hypertension, with siderotic (Gamna-Gandy) bodies in the spleen. There is recurrent hepatocellular carcinoma in the left lobe medial segment with invasion of portal veins after resection of a lateral segment tumor. **A,** Axial SE 500/20 image at 1.5 T reveals enlargement of the caudate lobe *(C)* and atrophy of the anterior segment *(A)* of the right lobe. The lateral segment of the left lobe has been resected. **B,** Corresponding T2-weighted image (SE 2500/100). Ascites provides a clear depiction of the nodular surface of the liver. Hepatic texture is markedly heterogeneous. The left lobe *(L)* has high signal extending into the porta hepatis *(arrows),* consistent with recurrent hepatocellular carcinoma. Note the enlarged spleen with numerous low-signal siderotic nodules. **C,** Corresponding GRASS image (25/13, flip angle 20 degrees) reveals absence of a normal portal vein, confirming invasion by tumor. The splenic nodules are even more evident.

gastroepiploic veins may develop along the greater curvature of the stomach, draining toward esophageal varices. Large gastroepiploic veins appear to be specific for splenic vein occlusion, since they are uncommon in patients with portal hypertension whose splenic veins are patent.[313] A patent paraumbilical vein, however, indicates portal hyperension, since it does not occur with isolated splenic vein occlusion.[313] Gastroesophageal and retroperitoneal collaterals may be seen with either condition.

Portal vein velocity can be measured by bolus tracking techniques (see Chapter 3, Short TR "Angiographic" Image).[115,527] By multiplying velocity by the area of the portal vein as measured on oblique short-axis images, portal vein flow can be estimated. Portal vein velocity[7] and flow volume[448] can also be measured by two-dimensional phase-contrast techniques. Increased portal flow has been noted by two-dimensional phase-contrast MRI in patients with well-compensated cirrhosis, whereas decreased or reversed flow is common in patients with clinically severe cirrhosis.[448]

Gallbladder walls are often thickened in patients with cirrhosis, whether or not there is any intrinsic gallbladder disease. Hypoalbuminemia may play a role,[551] although patients with ascites and low serum albumin are more likely to have thickened gallbladder walls if these findings accompany cirrhosis rather than renal failure.[248] Cystic veins may be dilated in patients with portal hypertension because of congestion and/or portosystemic shunting.[311] When these varices are large enough, they can be detected on gradient-echo images.[598] Conceivably, less-dilated cystic veins might contribute to gallbladder wall thickening in patients with cirrhosis and portal hypertension.

Other findings of portal hypertension include ascites and splenomegaly.[494] Siderotic nodules in the spleen (Gamna-Gandy bodies) can develop in patients with portal hypertension (Fig. 16-20). These nodules can be detected on T2-weighted images but are conspicuous on gradient-echo images with TE $\geq$ 10 msec.[339,456]

Iron Overload

Because of the liver's important functions as digestive and reticuloendothelial organs, iron is deposited in the liver via several mechanisms. Iron reaches the liver after intensinal absorption of dietary iron. Particulate iron, such as in damaged red blood cells, is also absorbed in part by Kupffer cells in the liver. In normal individuals, hepatic iron is cleared effectively and delivered to the bone marrow for production of red blood cells. In some pathologic conditions, however, excessive iron accumulates in the liver.

Iron overload within tissues reduces T2 and T2* relaxation times significantly, allowing MRI to be sensitive and specific for iron overload and for its regional distribution. Increased hepatic iron occurs in hemochromatosis, transfusional siderosis, hemolysis, and cirrhosis. In most cases the cause can be determined by MRI by noting the distribution of excessive iron outside the liver.

HEMOCHROMATOSIS

Hemochromatosis is a common but poorly understood disease that involves increased absorption and parenchymal accumulation of dietary iron. This increased iron is stored primarily as ferritin and hemosiderin.[214,329,413]

Most clinical manifestations of hemochromatosis involve malfunction and/or malignancy of the liver, pancreas, and heart.[243,329,382,413] The majority of patients with hemochromatosis have cirrhosis at the time of diagnosis. Cardiomyopathy and diabetes mellitus are also particularly common. Death is usually from disease in the previously mentioned organs, with HCC being particularly common.[329,382] Other clinical manifestations include dermal hyperpigmentation, decreased libido, and a slightly increased incidence of extrahepatic malignancies. Clinically significant hemochromatosis is rare in women, presumably because of menstruation.

In addition to abnormally increased absorption of dietary iron, patients with hemochromatosis may have decreased reticuloendothelial function. This theory is supported by slightly decreased levels of iron in the spleen and bone marrow of patients with hemochromatosis.[329] On the other hand, both parenchymal and reticuloendothial overload occur in patients without hereditary hemochomatosis who ingest massive quantities of iron (i.e., Bantu siderosis).

Hemochromatosis refers specifically to parenchymal, rather than reticuloendothelial, iron overload; *hemosiderosis* is a less specific term.[300,329] With iron overload from multiple transfusions, such as in patients with aplastic anemia or sickle cell disease, iron is primarily within reticuloendothelial cells; hepatocytes, pancreas, and other parenchymal organs are relatively spared. This distinction is significant, since reticuloendothelial iron overload is less toxic than parenchymal overload.[329,413,467] Parenchymal cells are only involved by transfusional siderosis when iron overload is especially massive.[219,300,413]

In most cases, hemochromatosis is a primary genetic disorder. The gene for primary hereditary hemochromatosis is present in approximately 2% of the population. Thus the homozygous form of this autosomal recessive disease should occur in one per 2500 individuals.[25,329,413] The gene can be located by HLA typing, allowing early screening of family members. If hemochromatosis is detected before severe cirrhosis or HCC have occurred, patients are treated by repeated phlebotomy until serum iron levels have returned to normal.

Serum iron and ferritin are usually elevated in patients with hemochromatosis, but these tests are nonspecific, limiting their diagnostic value.[25] CT has been used for the diagnosis of hepatic iron overload, but its sensitivity is only 60%.[178] Additionally, measurement of CT density is also confounded by other factors, such as fatty infiltration, increased density after hemodialysis,[223] or fluctuations in the concentration of hepatic glycogen.[104,105] Therefore elevated CT density is not sensitive or specific for iron overload. Additionally, CT is not effective for detecting extrahepatic iron overload. Definitive diagnosis is by biopsy, which reveals massive iron overload within hepatocytes.[413,492,497]

Hemochromatosis is manifested on MR images as low signal, especially on T2-weighted or T2*-weighted gradient-echo images (Figs. 17-1 to 17-3) (see also Color Plate VIII).[72,483] Transverse (T2 and T2*) relaxation time reduction accounts for this loss of signal intensity (Fig. 17-4). Decreased intensity of the pancreas and myocardium on MR images confirms systemic iron

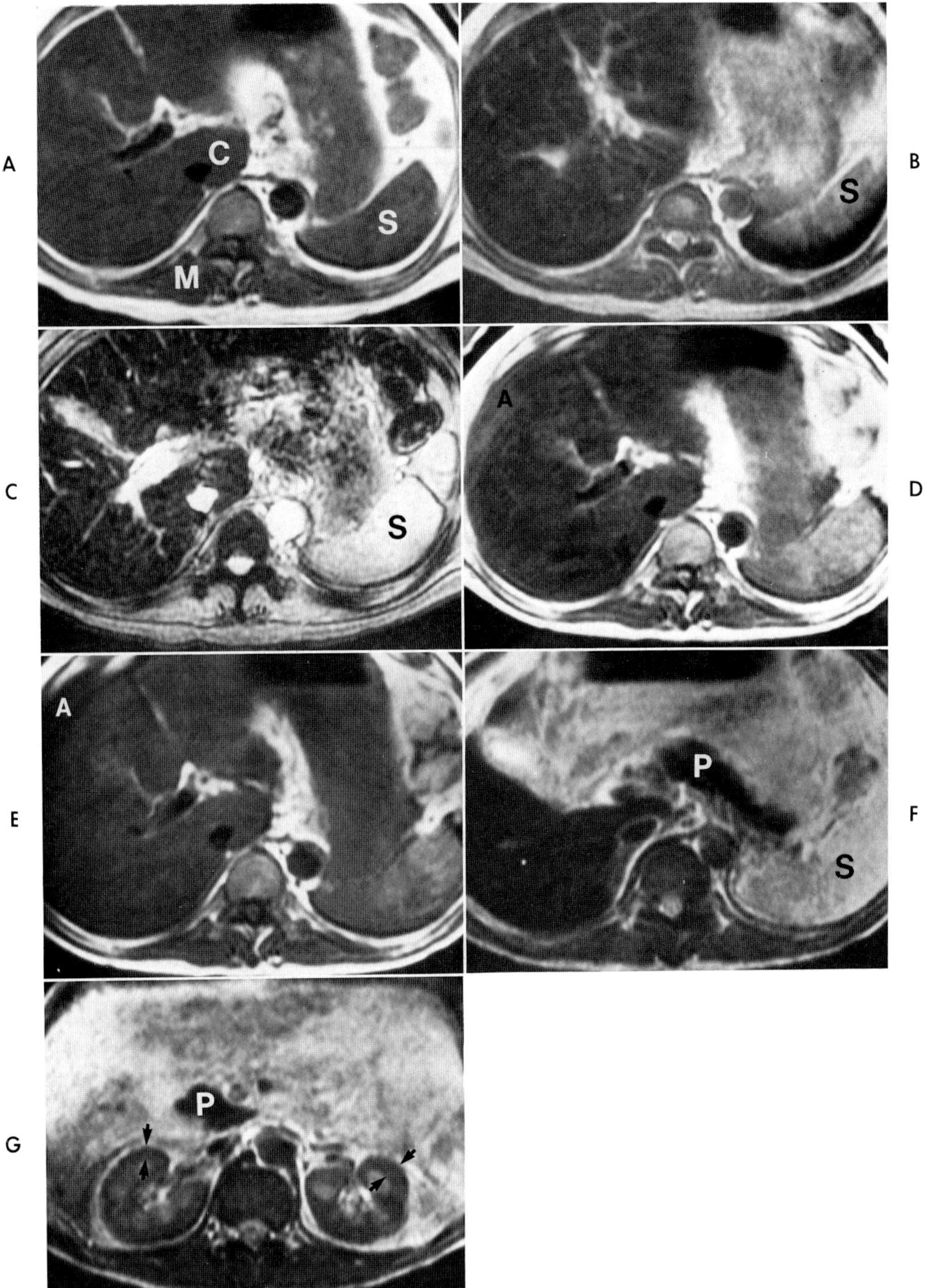

Fig. 17-1 Hemochromatosis progressing over 6 months, depicted by MRI at 1.5 T. Multi-system iron overload was confirmed at autopsy. **A,** Axial SE 400/20 image reveals decreased signal of liver, which is nearly isointense with muscle *(M)* and spleen *(S)*. Also note caudate hypertophy *(C)*, indicative of cirrhosis. **B,** Corresponding SE 2500/50 image. **C,** Corresponding GRASS image (25/13/20 degrees) The spleen *(S)* has normal intensity. **D,** SE 400/20 image 6 months later reveals heterogeneity and markedly decreased signal intensity of the liver, which is now less intense than muscle and spleen (compare with **A**). Note the development of moderate ascites *(A)*, which is slightly more intense than the liver. **E,** Corresponding T1-weighted image with TE = 12 msec. With reduced T2 "contamination" of the image, the liver now is more intense than ascites *(A)*. T2 relaxation can be evaluated by comparison with **D. F,** SE 2500/50 image at the level of the pancreatic body *(P)*. The pancreas and liver are signal voids, but the spleen *(S)* has normal intensity. **G,** SE 2500/50 image at the level of the pancreatic head *(P)*. Note that the intensity of renal cortex *(arrows)* is also reduced, unusual in hemochromatosis. *Figure continues.*

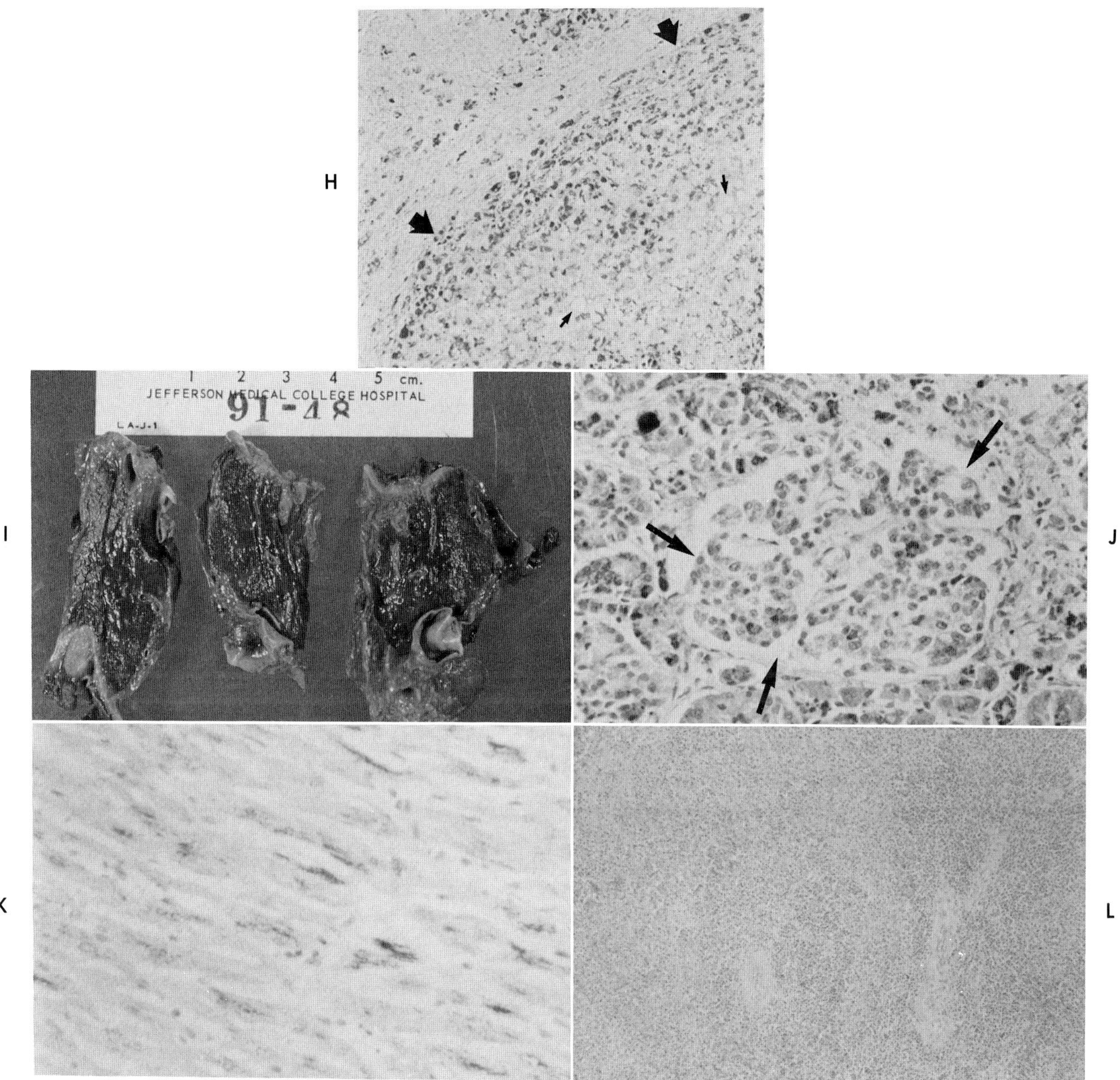

Fig. 17-1, cont'd   H, Histologic section of liver, prussian blue stain for iron. A regenerative nodule *(thick arrows)* with abundant iron and moderate fatty change *(small arrows)* is seen surrounded by fibrotic parenchyma, which also contains abundant iron. **I,** Gross sections of pancreas demonstrate an abnormal red color resulting from massive iron overload. **J,** Iron stain of pancreas depicts marked iron deposition (blue) within acinar cells. Pancreatic islets are relatively spared *(large arrows),* except for B cells . **K,** Iron stain of heart reveals marked myocardial iron deposition. **L,** Iron stain of spleen reveals no demonstrable iron. (See also Color Plate VIII.)

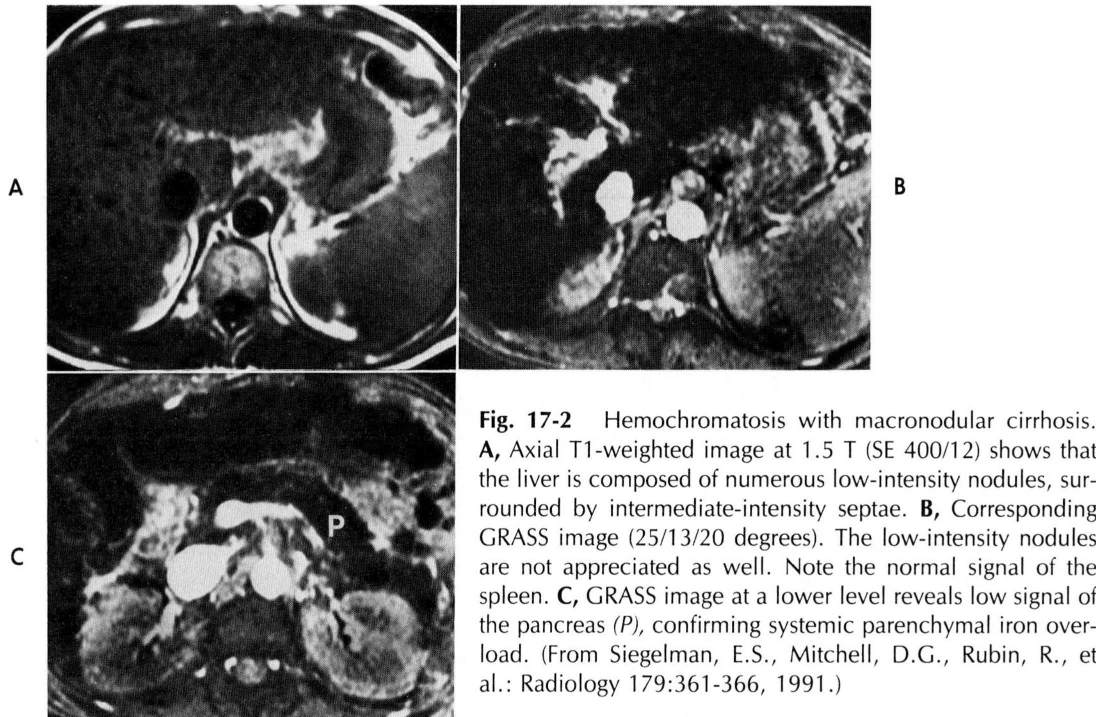

Fig. 17-2   Hemochromatosis with macronodular cirrhosis. **A,** Axial T1-weighted image at 1.5 T (SE 400/12) shows that the liver is composed of numerous low-intensity nodules, surrounded by intermediate-intensity septae. **B,** Corresponding GRASS image (25/13/20 degrees). The low-intensity nodules are not appreciated as well. Note the normal signal of the spleen. **C,** GRASS image at a lower level reveals low signal of the pancreas *(P)*, confirming systemic parenchymal iron overload. (From Siegelman, E.S., Mitchell, D.G., Rubin, R., et al.: Radiology 179:361-366, 1991.)

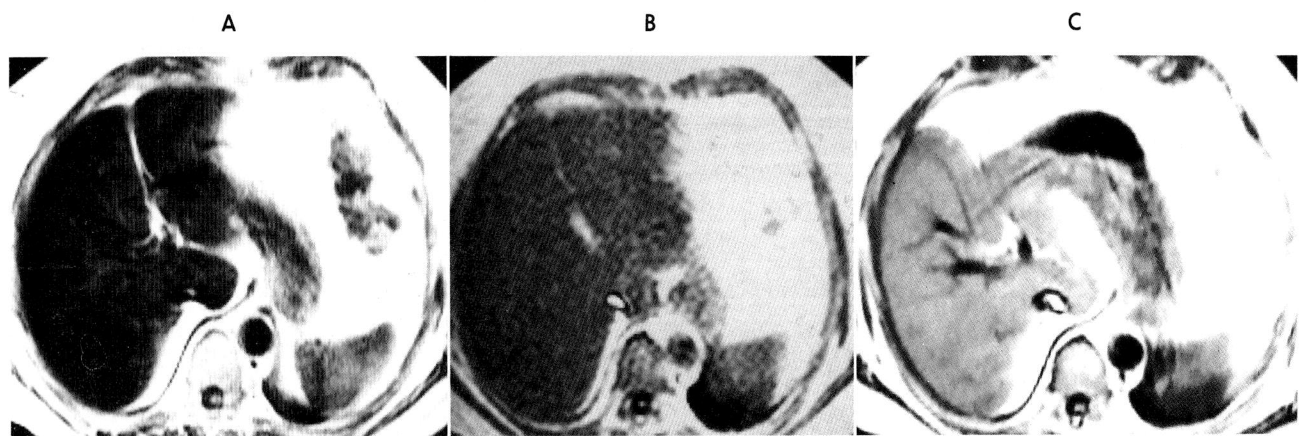

Fig. 17-3   Quantitation of hepatic iron overload and treatment monitoring by MRI at 0.6 T. **A,** SE 500/32 image before treatment. Liver signal intensity is reduced to the level of background noise. Liver biopsy showed an iron level of 4.6 mg/gm wet weight of liver tissue. **B,** SE 500/10 image. Short TE minimizes signal loss resulting from T2 relaxation. Increased liver SNR allows reproducible measurement of intensity, and by varying TE from 10 to 32 msec, a series of measurements allows calculation of T2 = 23 msec. **C,** SE 500/32 image after 1 year of phlebotomy therapy. Liver signal intensity has returned to normal (calculated T2 = 36 msec). Liver biopsy showed an iron level of 0.195 mg/gm wet weight, which is within normal limits.

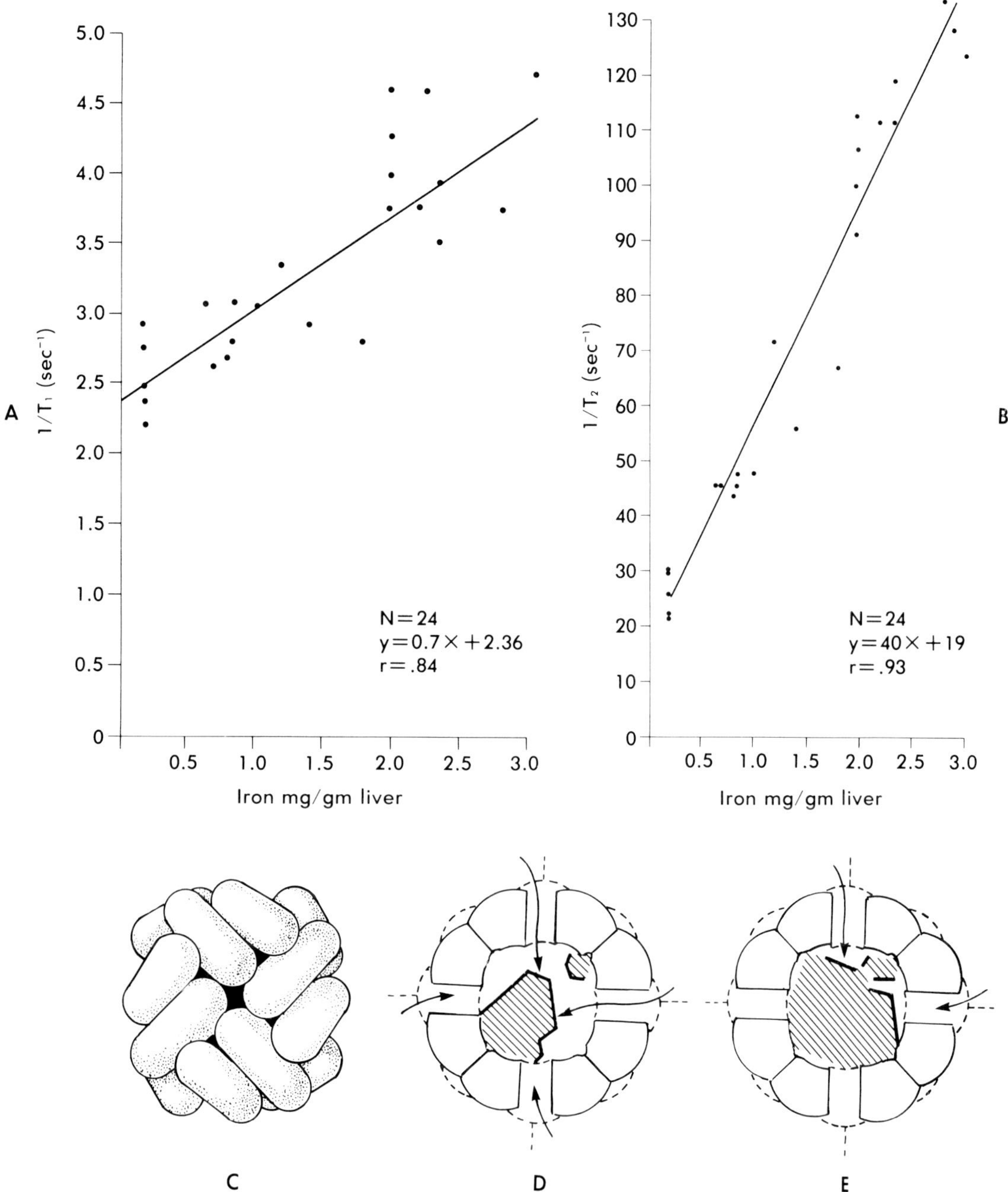

Fig. 17-4   Relaxometry of hepatic iron overload in vitro. **A,** Longitudinal (spin-lattice) relaxation rate 1/T1 shows a linear relationship to liver iron concentration. The slope 0.7 sec^{-1} mg^{-1} gm defines the T1 relaxivity (R1) of iron in liver iron overload. **B,** Transverse (spin-spin) relaxation rate (1/T2) shows a linear relationship to liver iron concentration. The slope 40 sec^{-1} mg^{-1} gm demonstrates much greater T2 relaxivity (R2) than T1 relaxivity (R1) of iron in liver iron overload. **C** to **E,** Ferritin structure. **C,** The three-dimensional protein shell of ferritin (apoferritin) has a molecular weight of 450,000 and consists of multiple protein subunits. **D,** A cross section of the ferritin molecule shows free access of cytosol water and low–molecular-weight solutes to the forming iron-oxyhydroxy crystal core. **E,** Ferritin may contain as many as 4500 iron atoms and have a molecular weight of 900,000 (i.e., 50% iron content by weight). Liver ferritin usually contains approximately 25% iron. (From Jacobs, A. and Worwood, M.: Iron in biochemistry and medicine, II, New York, 1980, Academic Press.)

overload. Patients with hemochromatosis usually have normal splenic signal, which excludes parenteral iron overload such as transfusional siderosis. Since normal liver is more intense than skeletal muscle on all sequences, and skeletal muscle is unaffected by hemochromatosis, skeletal muscle is a suitable reference tissue for detecting and quantifying decreased hepatic signal intensity.[72,207,291]

MRI is particularly sensitive to hepatic iron, which causes heterogeneous magnetic susceptibility. Susceptibility can be measured directly and accurately by SQUID (superconducting quantum interference detection), but this technology is not available at many centers.[46]

Normal liver iron levels are less than 250 μg/g, and patients with mild iron overload secondary to cirrhosis usually have hepatic iron levels in the range of 0.5 to 1.5 mg/gm.[497] At 0.6 Tesla and below, conventional spin-echo pulse sequences show little change in signal intensity of hepatic tissue until iron levels reach 1 mg/gm. These images are sensitive to hepatic iron overload in the range of greatest clinical significance, 1 to 10 mg iron/gm liver net weight (Fig. 17-5). Increased sensitivity can be achieved using T2* weighted gradient-echo technique. Sensitivity to iron also increases with magnetic field strength.

Early attempts to quantify hepatic iron levels using conventional spin-echo techniques failed because of the uniformly low-signal intensities of all livers with iron levels in excess of 2 mg/gm. Since these livers appear equally dark, no meaningful signal intensity ratios or relaxation time calculations were possible. Using short TE, however, it is possible to obtain sufficient signal from iron overloaded tissue with variable TR and TE to calculate T1 and T2 relaxation times (see Fig. 17-3).[171,497]

Satisfactory quantitative results can even be obtained at 1.5 T if short TE is used. In one study at 1.5 Tesla, intensity relative to muscle and estimated T2 were both highly correlated with hepatic iron content in rats (r = −0.89 and r = −0.66, respectively; p < .001 for both).[224] In patients with minimal iron deposition in preclinical hemochromatosis, even T2*-weighted gradient echo images at 1.5 T may be normal (Fig. 17-6) (see also Color Plate IX).[483] As hemochromatosis progresses, hepatic signal decreases.

Pancreatic signal remains normal early in the course of the disease, especially in menstruating women (Fig. 17-7). In patients with clinical symptoms of hemochromatosis, however, pancreatic signal is usually decreased. Spleen signal is normal in nearly all cases.

MR images obtained before and after treatment show a return of liver signal intensity to normal when the iron is removed by successful therapy (see Fig. 17-3). Similarly, MRI changes can document progression of iron overload (see Fig. 17-1). MRI may replace liver biopsy

for diagnosing and monitoring hemochromatosis once studies calibrating intensity with parenchymal iron levels at each field strength have been performed.

Cirrhosis can sometimes be detected in patients with hemochromatosis by depicting fibrous septa contrasted with low-signal parenchyma (see Fig. 17-2). These septa are seen best with short TE. With long TE, the heterogeneous magnetic field in these livers extends across the septa causing a "blooming" effect, whereby the entire liver loses signal. In many cases of hemochromatosis, the cirrhosis is micronodular. In these cases the thin, fibrous septa cannot be depicted by MRI.

Many patients with HCC have previously unsuspected hemochromatosis. Since tumor cells do not contain excess iron,[532] they have especially high contrast relative to iron overloaded liver on MR images (Figs. 11-13, 17-8, and 17-9). In patients with hemochromatosis, focal lesions have high signal on all sequences, and long TE is not necessary for their detection. In fact, the use of long TE may obscure small lesions because of the blooming effect from hepatic parenchymal iron.

Patients with end-stage liver disease resulting from hemochromatosis may be candidates for hepatic transplantation. Although the new liver does tend to reaccumulate iron (Fig. 17-10) (see also Color Plate IX), the hepatotoxic effects of iron overload are expected to take many years to develop. Interestingly, the livers of patients with hemochromatosis can be used as donor organs if death occurs before severe hepatic disease develops.[98] The iron in these livers is mobilized rapidly, since hemochromatosis appears not to involve a primary hepatic defect.

TRANSFUSIONAL SIDEROSIS

Among patients with decreased hepatic signal intensity, hemochromatosis can usually be distinguished from parenteral iron overload (e.g., transfusional siderosis) by noting the signal intensity of the spleen and pancreas (Figs. 17-11 to 17-14) (see also Color Plates XI, XII, and XIII). Splenic signal is decreased in patients with transfusional siderosis, whereas it is usually normal in patients with hemochromatosis. Pancreatic signal is usually normal with transfusional siderosis but decreased with hemochromatosis.[483]

The pancreas is typically involved in clinically significant hemochromatosis but is only effected by transfusional siderosis if overload is extreme, such as after transfusion of more than 100 units of red blood cells.[483] Similarly, gated images usually show normal intensity of the myocardium in patients with transfusional siderosis, whereas myocardial intensity is usually decreased in patients with hemochromatosis.[243]

Anemia in which bone marrow is hyperplastic, such as thalassemia major, is also accompanied by increased absorption and parenchymal accumulation of iron. Iron overload in these patients is compounded by multiple

Text continues on p. 186.

COLOR PLATES

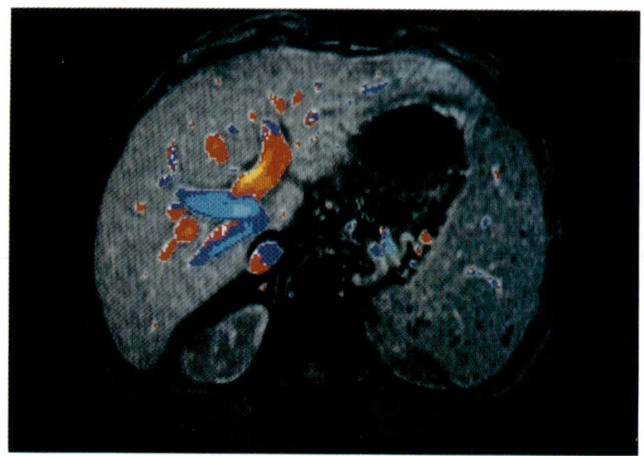

PLATE I/ Fig. 3-7, C/ Page 20

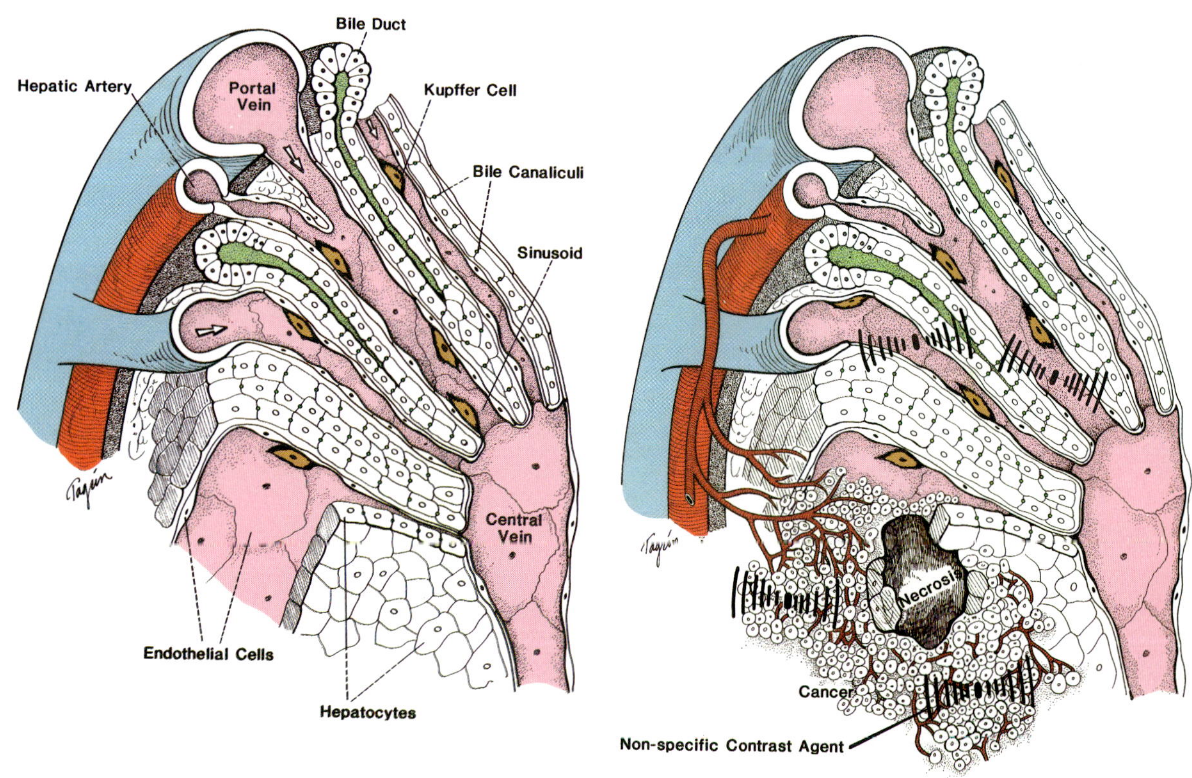

PLATE II/ Fig. 6-4, A-F/ Pages 38-39

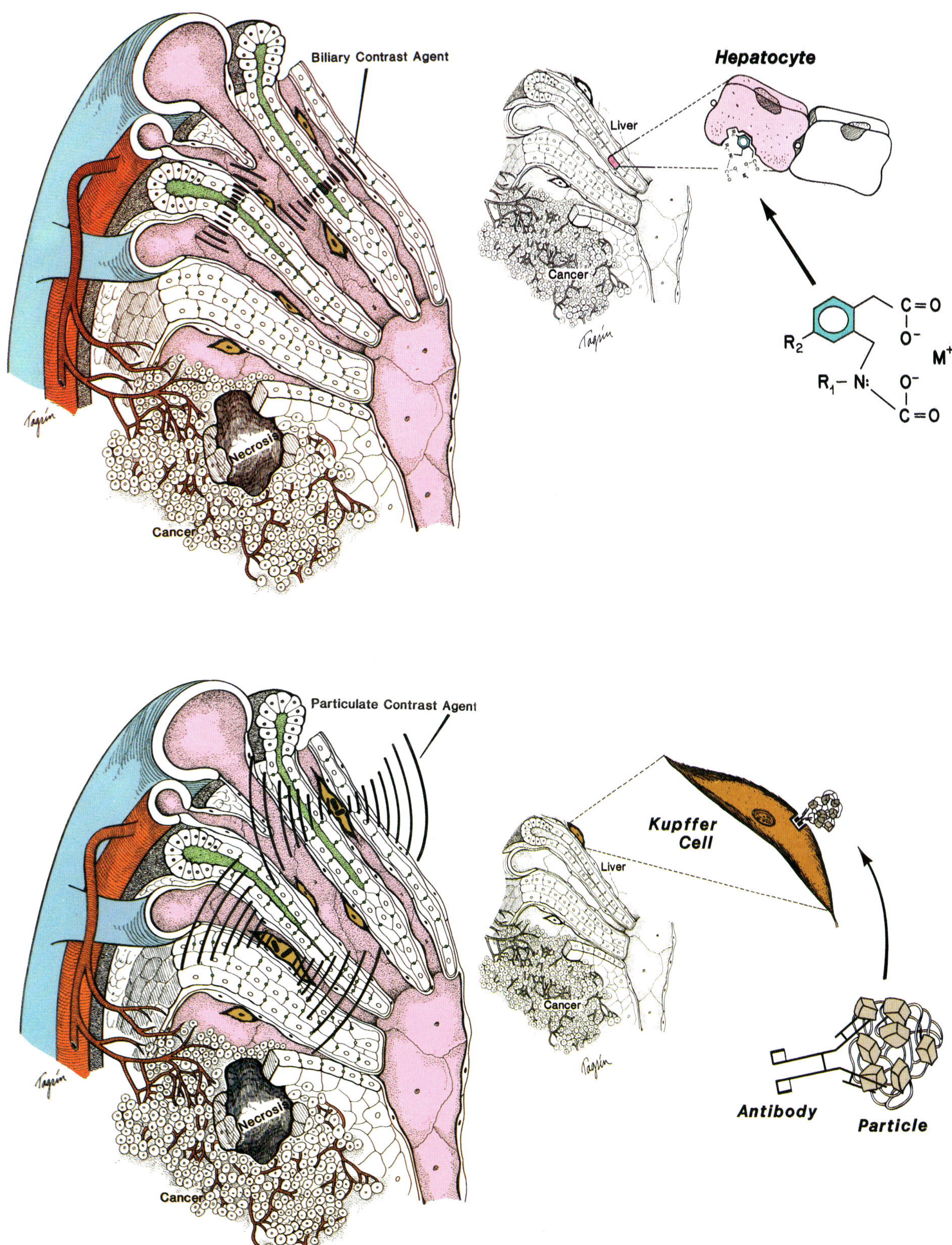

PLATE II, cont'd/ Fig. 6-4, A-F/ Pages 38-39

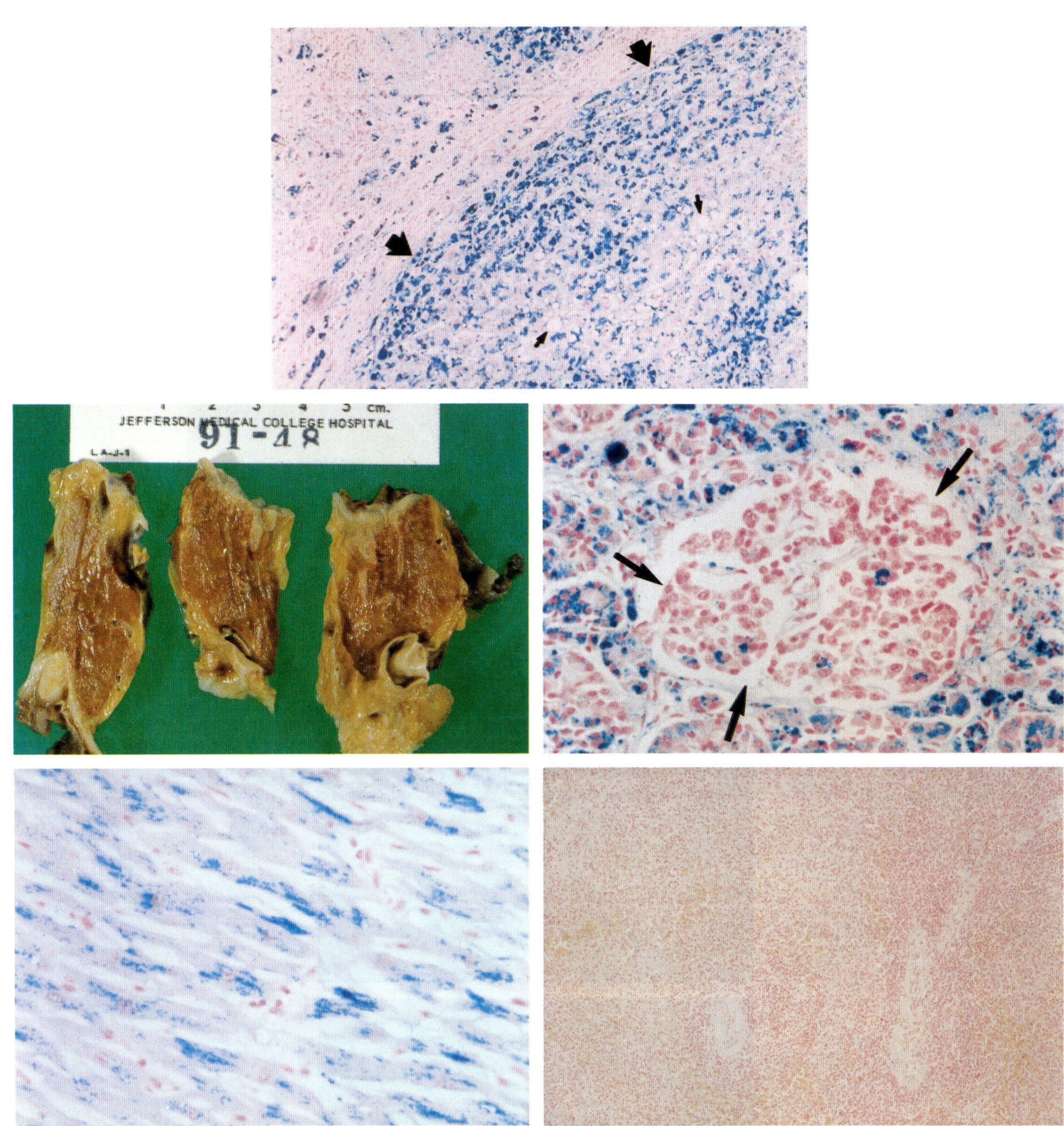

PLATE VIII/ Fig. 17-1, H-L/ Page 175

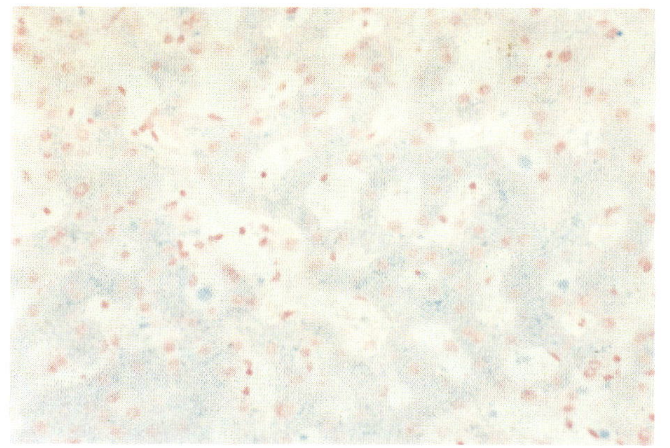

PLATE IX/ Fig. 17-6, D/ Page 180

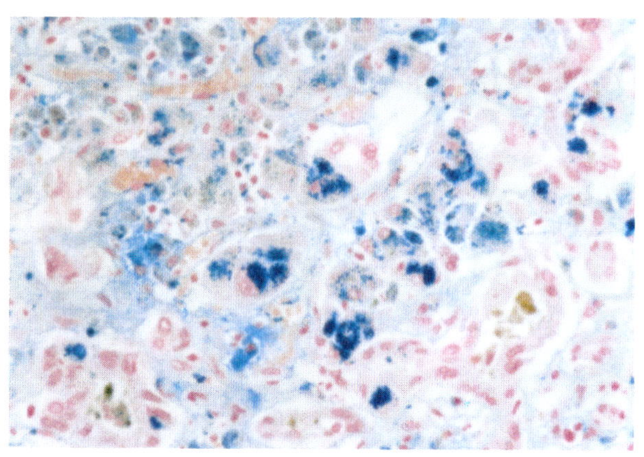

PLATE X/ Fig. 17-10, B/ Page 182

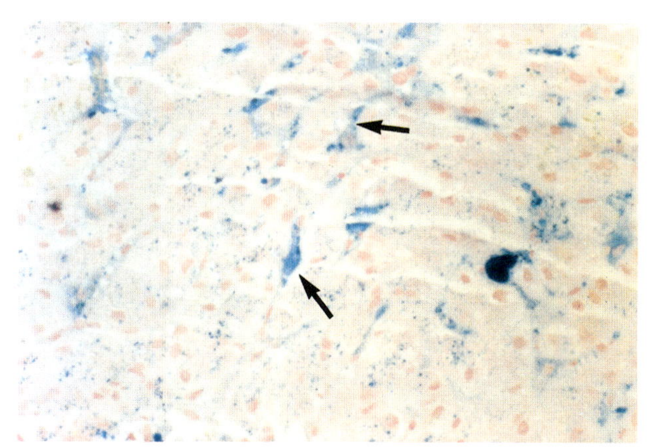

PLATE XI/ Fig. 17-11, C/ Page 182

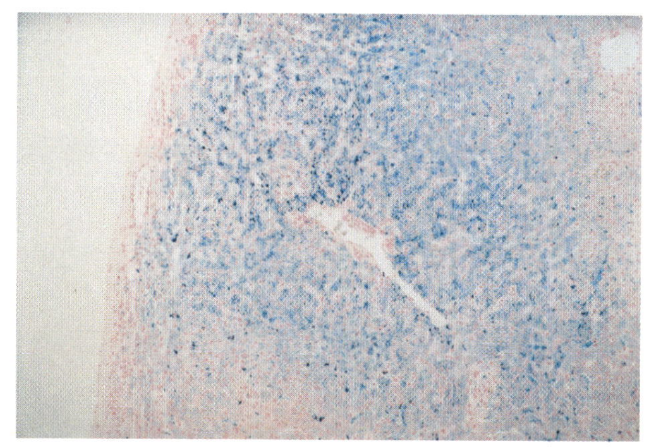

PLATE XII/ Fig. 17-12, A/ Page 183

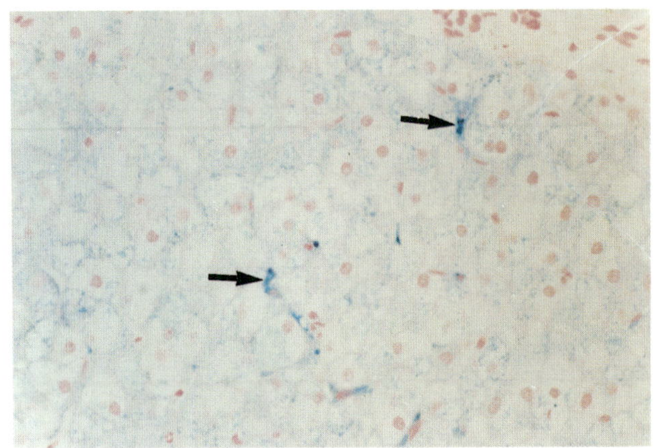

PLATE XIII/ Fig. 17-14, D/ Page 184

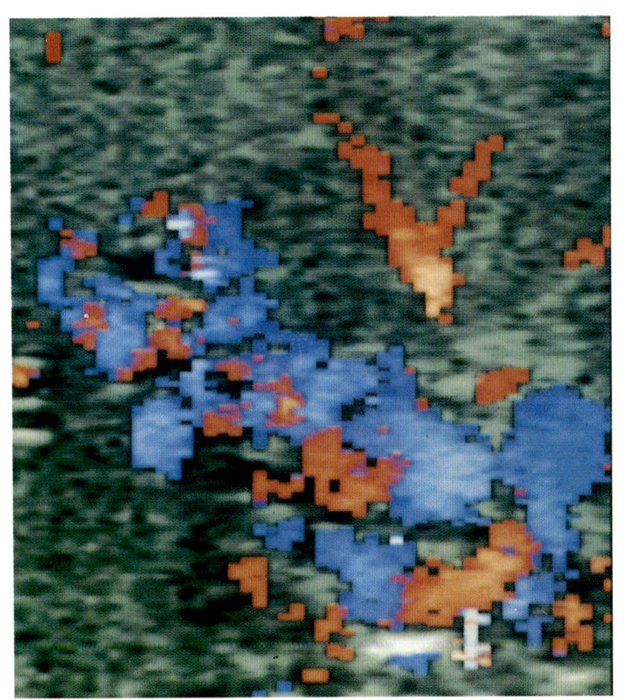

PLATE XIV/ Fig. 18-9, D/ Page 194

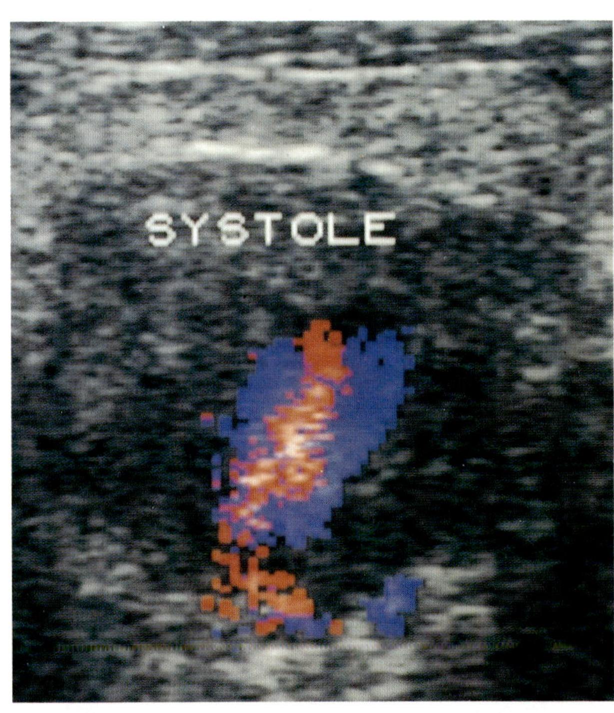

PLATE XV/ Fig. 22-24, C/ Page 263

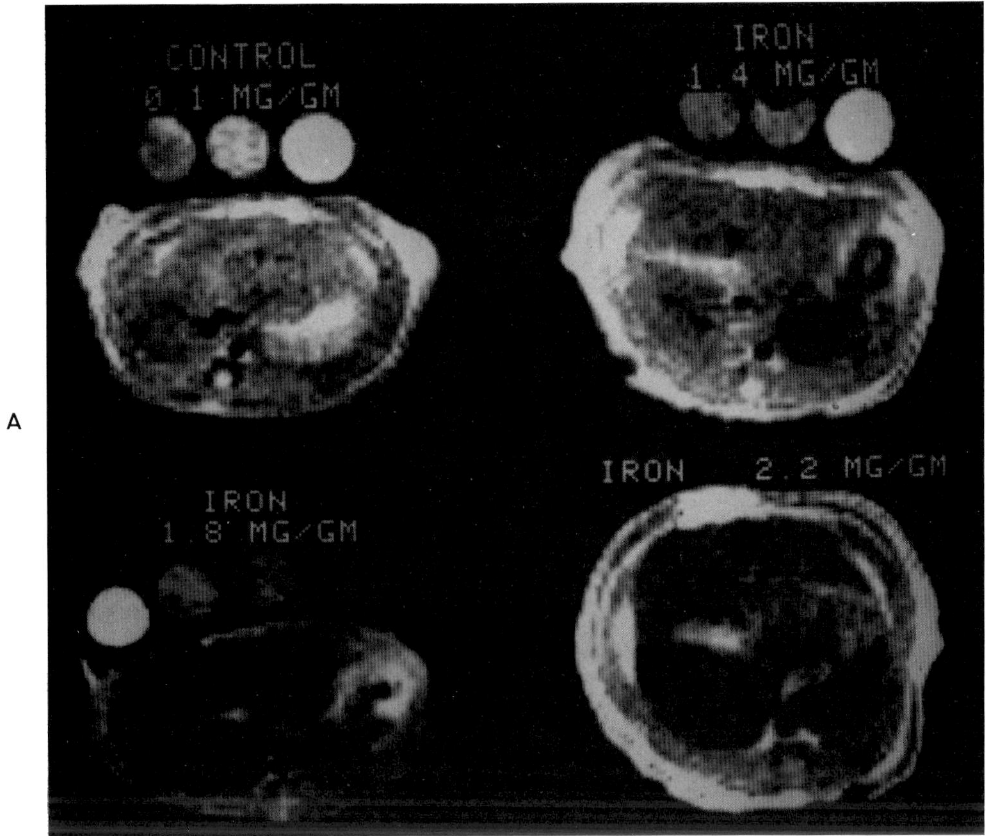

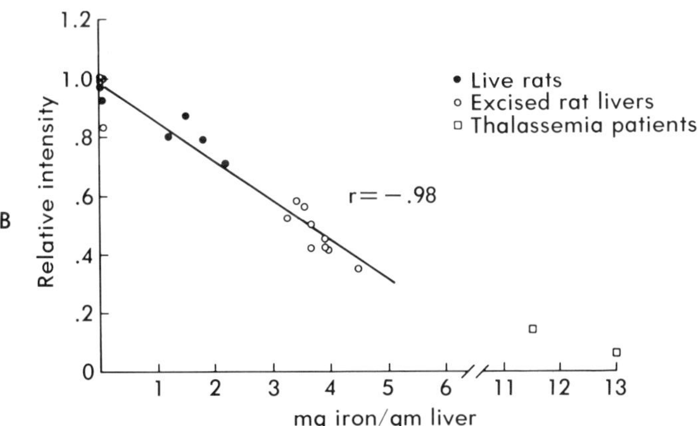

Fig. 17-5 Rat model of dietary-iron overload. **A,** SE 1000/28 images at 0.35 T through four different rat livers demonstrate progressive decreases in liver intensity as iron content increases. Round objects ventral to the animal are test-tube reference standards. **B,** Graph demonstrates linear relationship of MR signal intensity to liver iron content in live rats, excised rat livers, and two thalassemia patients who underwent liver biopsy (intensities standardized to control livers). (From Stark, D.D., Bass, N.M., Moss, A.A., et al.: Radiology 148:743-751, 1983.)

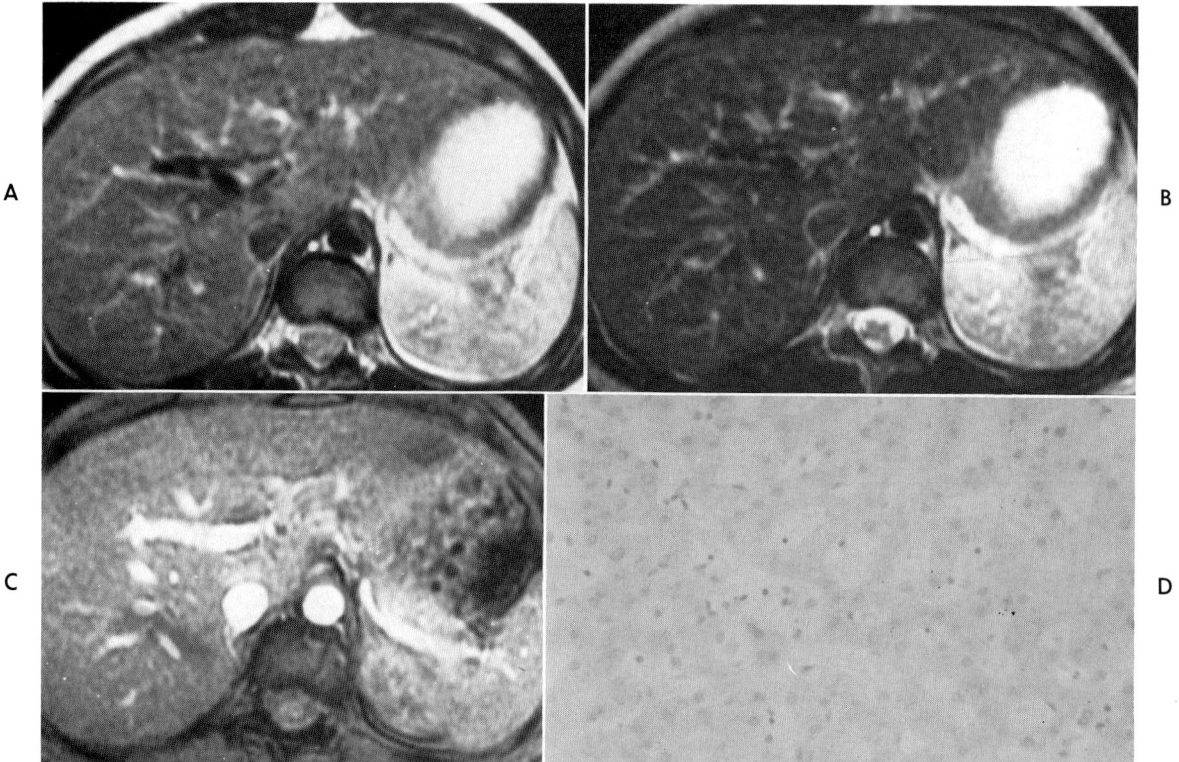

Fig. 17-6 Pathologically proven subclinical hemochromatosis in a 19-year-old woman, detected incidentally as a result of elevated serum iron and ferritin, which was followed by biopsy. **A,** SE 2500/50. Hepatic signal intensity is slightly increased. **B,** SE 2500/100. **C,** GRASS 25/13, flip angle 20 degrees. Hepatic signal intensity is normal. **D,** Iron stain reveals minimal iron within hepatocytes but none within Kupffer cells. (See also Color Plate IX.) (Siegelman, E.S., Mitchell, D.G., Rubin, R., et al.: Radiology 179:361-366, 1991.)

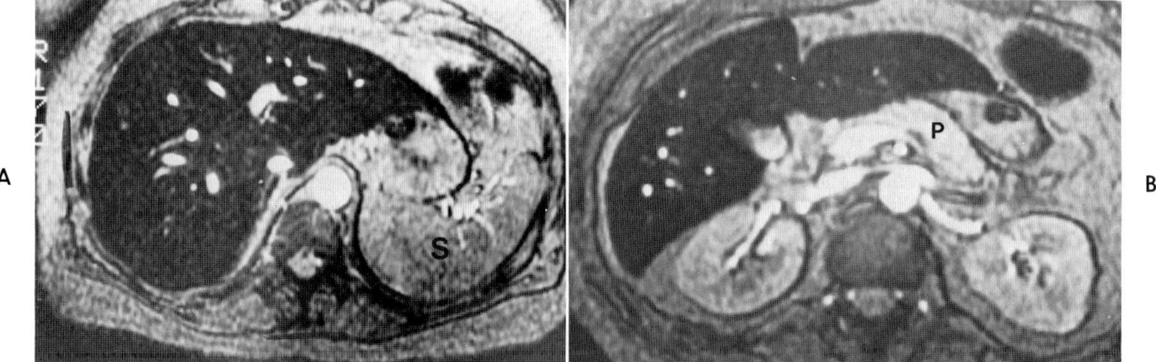

Fig. 17-7 Early hemochromatosis in a 45-year-old menstruating woman. **A** and **B,** Axial gradient-echo images (TR/TE/flip angle = 25/13/20 degrees) depict the liver as a signal void. The spleen (S) has normal signal intensity, which is consistent with hemochromatosis. Pancreatic (P) signal intensity is also normal, presumably because of the early stage of the disease. Iron stain from liver biopsy (not shown) demonstrated marked iron deposition within hepatocytes but no evidence of parenchymal damage.

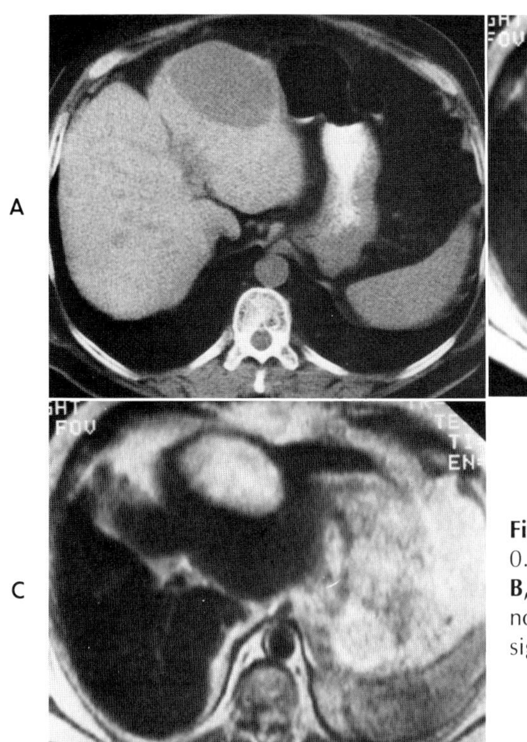

Fig. 17-8   Hepatocellular carcinoma in a patient with hemochromatosis at 0.6 T. **A,** Unenhanced CT scan shows a focal lesion in the left hepatic lobe. **B,** SE 275/14 image depicts the mass as slightly hyperintense because of abnormally low signal of the liver. **C,** SE 2350/60 image depicts the liver as a signal void resulting from iron overload, and the mass is obvious.

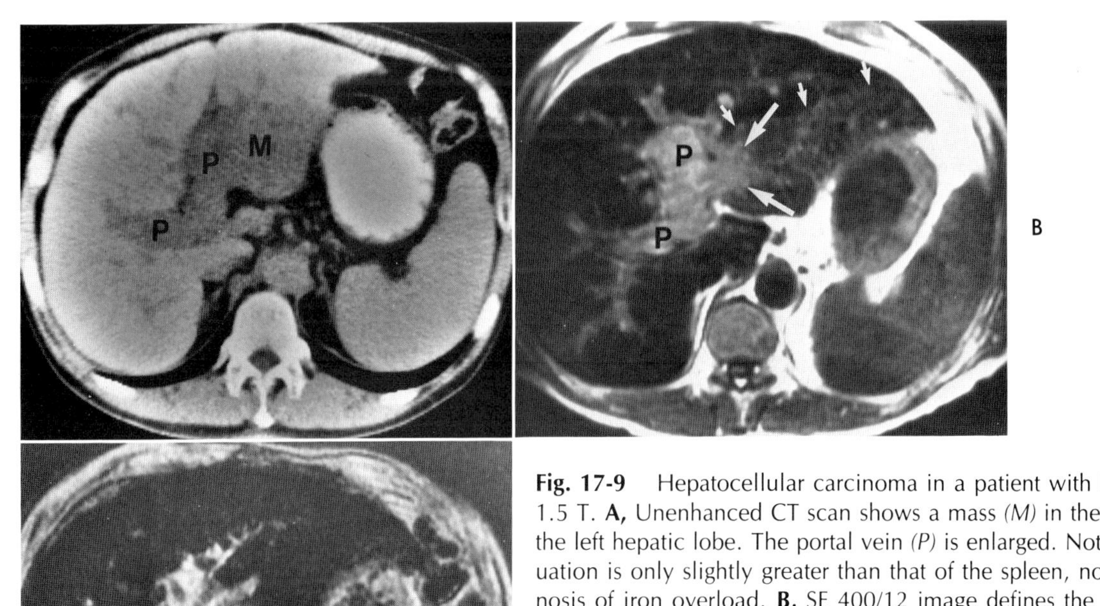

Fig. 17-9   Hepatocellular carcinoma in a patient with hemochromatosis at 1.5 T. **A,** Unenhanced CT scan shows a mass *(M)* in the posterior portion of the left hepatic lobe. The portal vein *(P)* is enlarged. Note that hepatic attenuation is only slightly greater than that of the spleen, not sufficient for diagnosis of iron overload. **B,** SE 400/12 image defines the primary mass *(large arrows)* as smaller than suggested in **A.** The portal vein *(P)* is filled with tumor. The posterior portion of the left lateral segment is filled with small nodules *(small arrows)*, presumably representing tumor emboli from portal vein invasion. The remainder of the liver is a signal void. This patient with hemochromatosis is unusual because the splenic signal is decreased as well. Lower sections (not shown) demonstrated a signal void in the pancreas. **C,** Gradient-echo image (TR/TE/flip angle = 25/13/20 degrees) confirms portal thrombus.

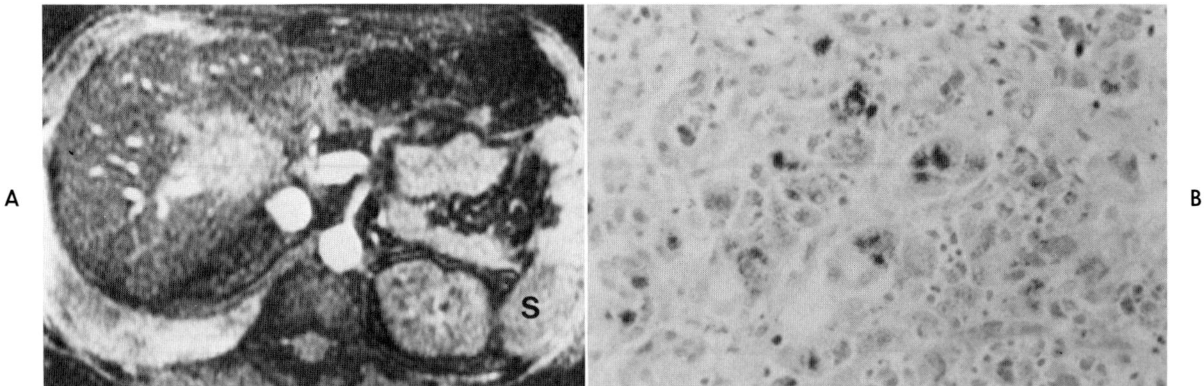

Fig. 17-10 Recurrent hemochromatosis 3 months after hepatic transplantation (same patient as Figs. 12-3 and 17-1). **A,** Gradient-echo image (TR/TE = 25/13/20 degrees). Hepatic signal is abnormally low, except for a periportal lymphoma mass. The spleen *(S)* has normal signal intensity, indicating that iron from transfusions during surgery has been cleared from it. **B,** Iron stain (Prussian blue) depicts marked iron deposition within hepatocytes. (See also Color Plate X.)

Fig. 17-11 Transfusional iron overload in a patient with chronic myelogenous leukemia. **A,** Axial SE 2500/50 image reveals decreased heptatic signal and absent splenic signal. Signal of the pancreatic tail *(P)* is normal. High-signal defects in the spleen may represent hemorrhage, but no histologic proof was available. **B,** Corresponding GRASS image (25/13, flip angle 20 degrees) shows similar findings. **C,** Iron stain (Prussian blue) reveals abundant iron within Kupffer cells *(arrows)* but only minimal iron within hepatocytes. (See also Color Plate XI.) (From Siegelman, E.S., Mitchell, D.G., Rubin, R., et al.: Radiology 179:361-366, 1991.)

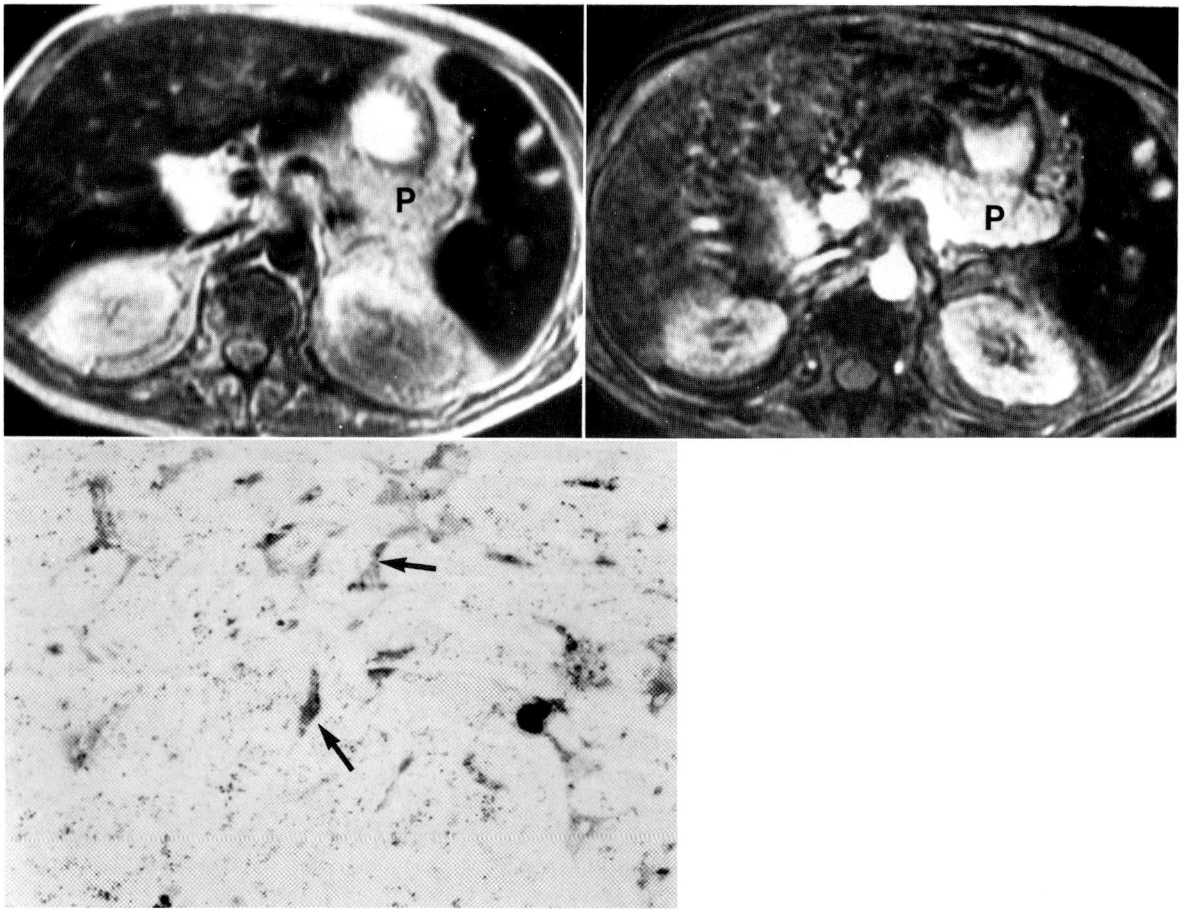

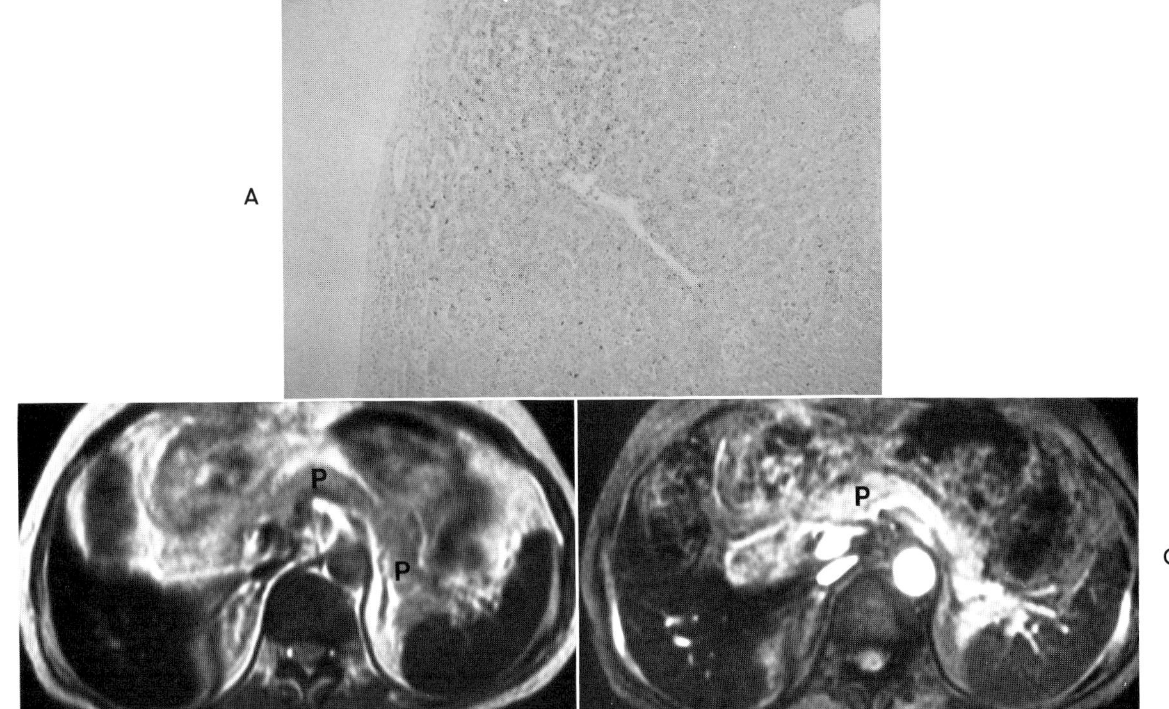

Fig. 17-12 Transfusional iron overload after surgery for renal transplantation. **A,** Prussian blue stain for iron. Iron overload is severe, involving hepatocytes and Kupffer cells. Systemic iron overload cannot be excluded, so MRI was recommended by the pathologist. (See also Color Plate XII.) **B,** Axial SE 2500/50 image at 1.5 T reveals decreased hepatic and splenic intensity but normal intensity of the pancreas *(P)*. The findings are thus consistent with transfusional siderosis. **C,** Corresponding GRASS image (25/13, flip angle 20 degrees).

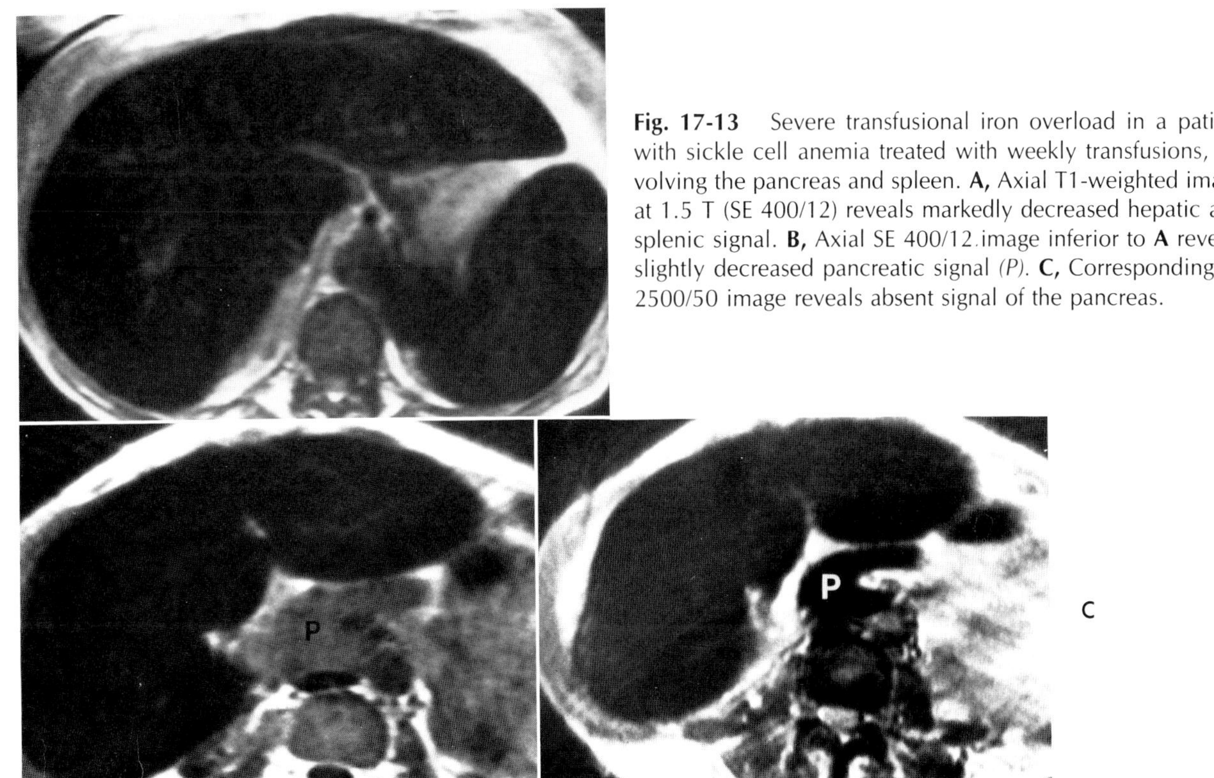

Fig. 17-13 Severe transfusional iron overload in a patient with sickle cell anemia treated with weekly transfusions, involving the pancreas and spleen. **A,** Axial T1-weighted image at 1.5 T (SE 400/12) reveals markedly decreased hepatic and splenic signal. **B,** Axial SE 400/12 image inferior to **A** reveals slightly decreased pancreatic signal *(P)*. **C,** Corresponding SE 2500/50 image reveals absent signal of the pancreas.

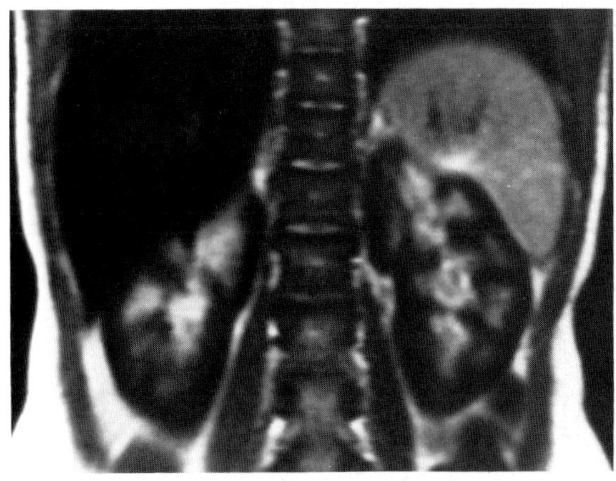

Fig. 17-18 Hepatic and renal parenchymal iron overload from intravascular hemolysis in a patient with paroxysmal nocturnal hemoglobinuria. Coronal SE 2500/40 image at 1.5 T reveals absent signal of the liver and renal cortex but normal signal of the spleen. Iron liberated from intravascular hemolysis is bound to haptoglobin and cleared by hepatocytes. If haptoglobin capacity is exceeded, hemoglobin is filtered through glomeruli and reabsorbed through the proximal tubules. (From Siegelman, E.S., Mitchell, D.G., Rubin, R., et al.: Radiology 179:361-366, 1991.)

transfusions. However, since the histologic result is similar to that of primary hemochromatosis, it is sometimes referred to as *erythropoietic hemochromatosis.*[413]

Parenteral overload can also be caused by rhabdomyolysis, since iron liberated from degraded myoglobin is taken up by reticuloendothelial cells (Fig. 17-15).[249] MRI findings are similar with parenteral iron overload because of rhabdomyolysis and transfusional siderosis.

CIRRHOSIS

Mild hepatocellular iron deposition is common in cirrhosis, especially in patients who abuse alcohol. The reasons for this are unclear. Hepatocellular iron decreases the signal intensity of cirrhotic livers slightly on T2-weighted and gradient-echo images (see Fig. 16-5). However, this should not be confused with the massive iron overload seen with hemochromatosis.[26,279,329,605] If signal is only mildly decreased (more intense than background noise) and if pancreatic signal is normal on T2- or T2*-weighted images, cirrhosis should not be attributed to hemochromatosis.

HEMOLYSIS

Hepatocellular iron overload can result from hemolysis. Extravascular (e.g., splenic) hemolysis causes RE deposition of iron (Fig. 17-16). Hemoglobin released by intravascular hemolysis, however, binds to plasma haptoglobin and is taken up by hepatocytes. If serum haptoglobin is saturated with hemoglobin, free hemoglobin is filtered through renal glomeruli, reabsorbed, and stored by proximal convoluted tubule epithelial cells.[606] Thus intravascular hemolysis can cause selective iron deposition in the liver and renal cortex, sparing the spleen (Figs. 17-17 and 17-18).

Intravascular hemolysis occurs in patients with paroxysmal nocturnal hemoglobinaria (see Fig. 17-18). These patients typically have decreased signal of the liver and renal cortex and normal signal of the spleen. Some patients with sickle cell disease also have sufficient intravascular hemolysis to decrease renal cortical signal (see Fig. 17-17). Some of these patients may have normal hepatic signal if they have not received many blood transfusions. The determinates of renal and hepatic iron deposition in sickle cell disease have not been elucidated fully. It is likely that MRI will provide new insights into iron metabolism and distribution in pathologic hematologic conditions.

CHAPTER
18

Vascular Thrombosis and Occlusion

PORTAL THROMBOSIS

Thrombosis of the portal vein can result from slow flow secondary to cirrhosis (Figs. 18-1 to 18-3); obstruction by porta hepatis lymphadenopathy; direct invasion by cancer; inflammatory changes secondary to pancreatitis; sclerosing cholangitis, or abdominal infections (Figs. 15-6, 18-4, and 18-5); polycythemia vera[572]; or even from benign masses.[6,379,402] Malignant portal vein thrombosis is more common with HCC but can occur with metastatic disease (Figs. 18-6).[10,13] Extrinsic obstruction from primary or secondary malignancies can also occur (Figs. 18-7 and 18-8).

Collateral periportal veins may maintain portal perfusion when the main portal vein is thrombosed. With time, this network of collateral venous channels dilates and the thrombosed portal vein retracts, producing "cavernous transformation" (Figs. 18-4 and 18-9) (see also Color Plate XIV).[374,595] When conventional B-mode ultrasound, rather than color Doppler, is used to set the range gate for duplex Doppler, flow in these periportal veins lying adjacent to a hypoechoic thrombosed portal vein may mimic patency. With MRI, there should be no confusion.

MRI can substitute for angiography and CT in evaluating suspected portal thrombosis. MRI is not restricted by body habitus or ascites, as is duplex Doppler ultrasound. With MRI, portal venous blood flow, intraluminal thrombus, and collateral circulation can all be identified noninvasively and without administration of contrast media.[134,283,548,604,627]

Examination of the portal vein for patency is important in planning shunt surgery or hepatic transplantation. Once shunt surgery is completed, MRI can confirm shunt patency.[31,495]

Spin-echo MR images can usually diagnose vascular patency by depicting a flow void. However, signal is often present in the center of the splenic-mesenteric venous confluence or with slow in-plane flow. Clot is usually isointense to liver on T1-weighted images and hyperintense on T2-weighted images,[283] and it should have the same shape and extent on all sequences. Flow-sensitive gradient-echo sequences can help confirm or exclude portal thrombosis.[485]

Lobar or segmental portal vein obstruction by tumor

can cause discrete wedge-shaped regions of increased intensity on T2-weighted images (see Figs. 9-2 and 18-7).[229] This phenomenon has also been noted with CT portography.[553] The apex of these abnormalities should be searched carefully for an obstructing tumor.[234] Obstruction of the portal vein can also cause segmental atrophy, with compensatory hypertrophy of other segments (Figs. 18-7 and 18-10).[60,297,523] In livers with fatty infiltration, segmental portal vein obstruction causes focal sparing, presumably because less fat is delivered to hepatocytes (see Fig. 18-8).[8]

BUDD-CHIARI SYNDROME

The Budd-Chiari syndrome involves obstruction of venous outflow from the sinusoidal bed of the liver, resulting in portal hypertension, ascites, and progressive hepatic failure.[491]

The optimum treatment or palliation depends on the cause of obstruction, which requires accurate assessment of the inferior vena cava (IVC) and right atrium.[316,495,571] Mebranous occlusion of the IVC, which is most prevalent in Asian patients, can be treated with membranectomy. In other occlusive conditions of the IVC sparing the hepatic veins, the IVC may be shunted to the right atrium. If hepatic veins alone are involved, a mesocaval shunt (superior mesenteric vein to IVC) may be inserted to decompress the portal system. If the hepatic veins and IVC are occluded, mesoatrial shunting must be performed. In many patients with tumors causing the Budd-Chiari syndrome, extensive surgery is contraindicated, and ascites is palliated via peritoneal shunting. Imaging is thus not only necessary for diagnosis but for choosing the most appropriate therapy.

Although sonography can be used to detect hepatic vein occlusion,[218] webs are difficult to visualize, and the IVC is not reliably evaluated. Ascites can also interfere with adequate visualization of the hepatic confluence. Therefore venography is required to complement sonography.[332] MRI alone appears to offer a complete noninvasive evaluation of the relevant intrahepatic and extrahepatic vascular anatomy.

Inferior vena cavography is often necessary to determine if there is a significant pressure gradient across the

Text continues on p. 196.

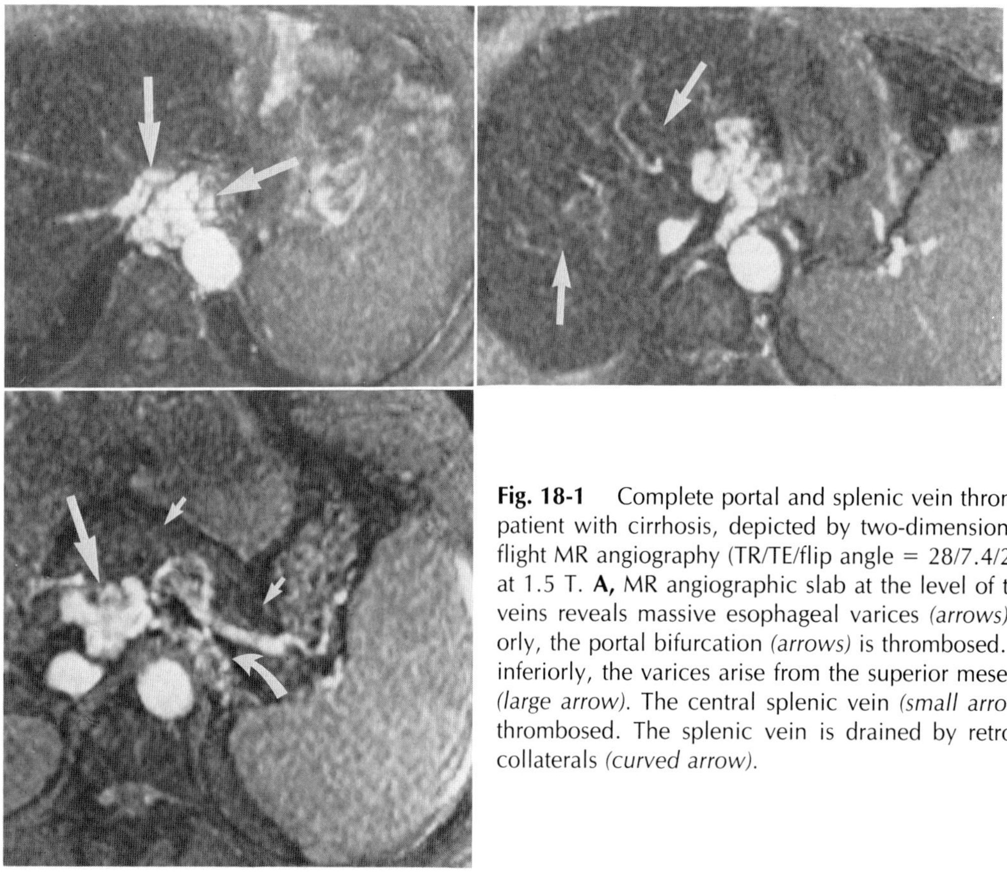

Fig. 18-1 Complete portal and splenic vein thrombosis in a patient with cirrhosis, depicted by two-dimensional time-of-flight MR angiography (TR/TE/flip angle = 28/7.4/20 degrees) at 1.5 T. **A,** MR angiographic slab at the level of the hepatic veins reveals massive esophageal varices *(arrows).* **B,** Inferiorly, the portal bifurcation *(arrows)* is thrombosed. **C,** Further inferiorly, the varices arise from the superior mesenteric vein *(large arrow).* The central splenic vein *(small arrows)* is also thrombosed. The splenic vein is drained by retroperitoneal collaterals *(curved arrow).*

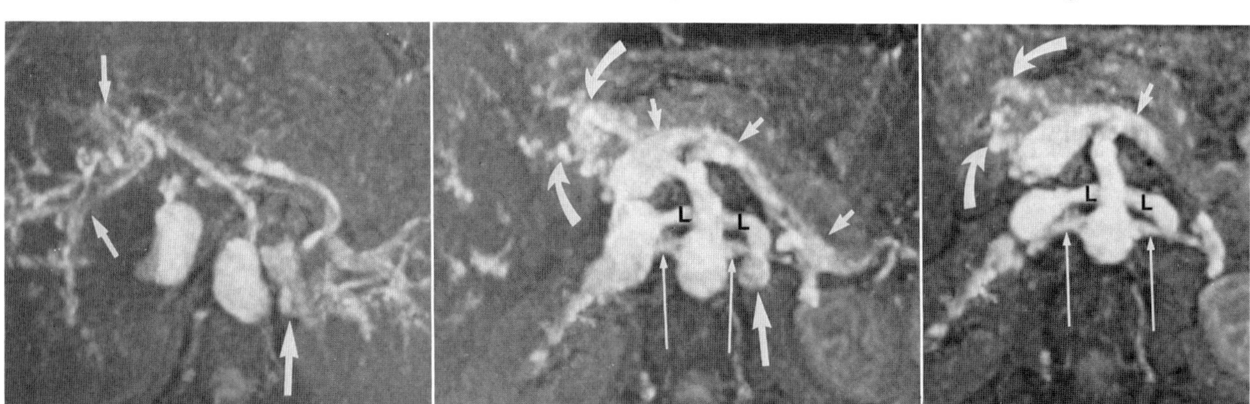

Fig. 18-2 Portal thrombosis in a patient with cirrhosis. Peripancreatic and splenorenal shunting demonstrated by MR angiography at 1.5 T. **A,** MR angiographic slab demonstrates a patent portal bifurcation *(small arrows). Large arrow* = splenorenal collateral veins. **B** and **C,** Inferiorly, the splenorenal collateral vein *(large arrow)* drains into the left renal vein *(L). Small arrows* = patent splenic vein, *curved arrows* = peripancreatic collaterals, *long thin arrows* = renal arteries.

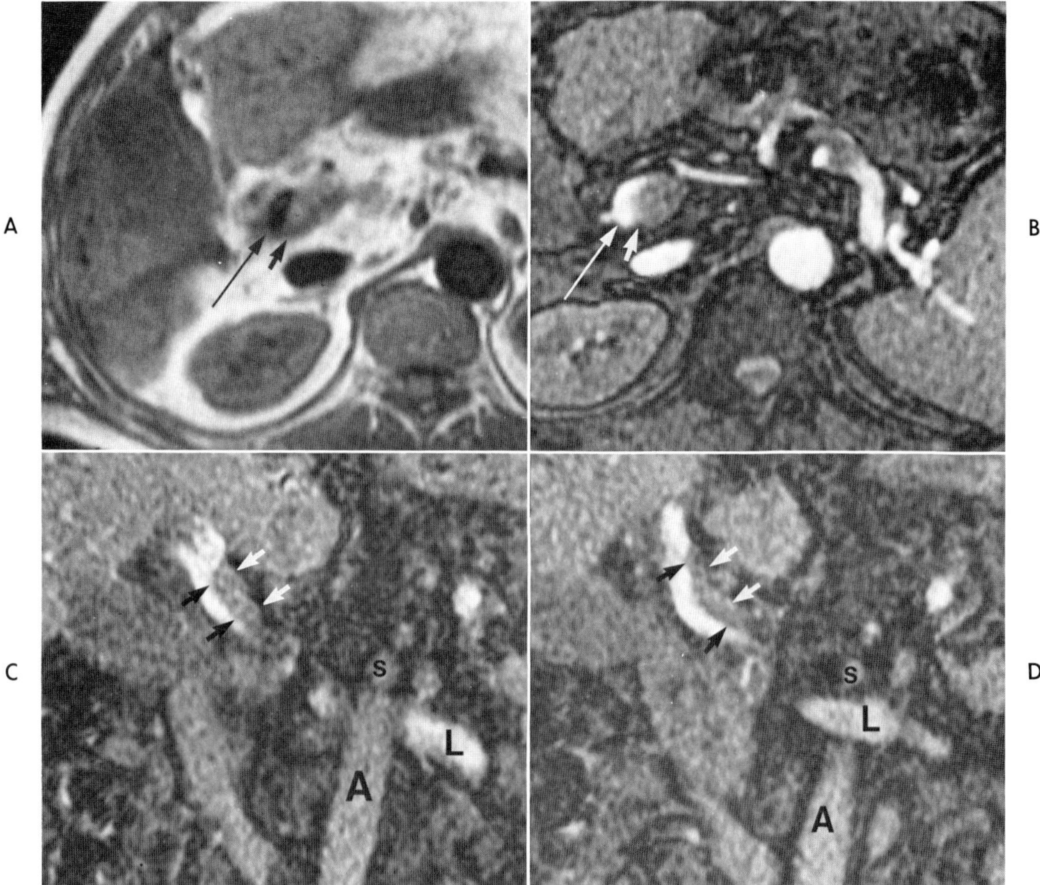

Fig. 18-3 Nonocclusive thrombosis depicted at 1.5 T in a patient with cirrhosis. The lateral portion of the portal vein is patent *(long arrow)* with thrombus present along the medial border *(short arrow)*. **A,** SE 400/12 image. **B,** Gradient-echo image (TR/TE/flip angle = 27/7.4/20 degrees). **C** and **D,** Coronal gradient-echo images (TR/TE/flip angle = 27/7.4/20 degrees). *Arrows* indicate portal thrombus. *A* = aorta, *L* = left renal vein, *S* = superior mesenteric artery origin.

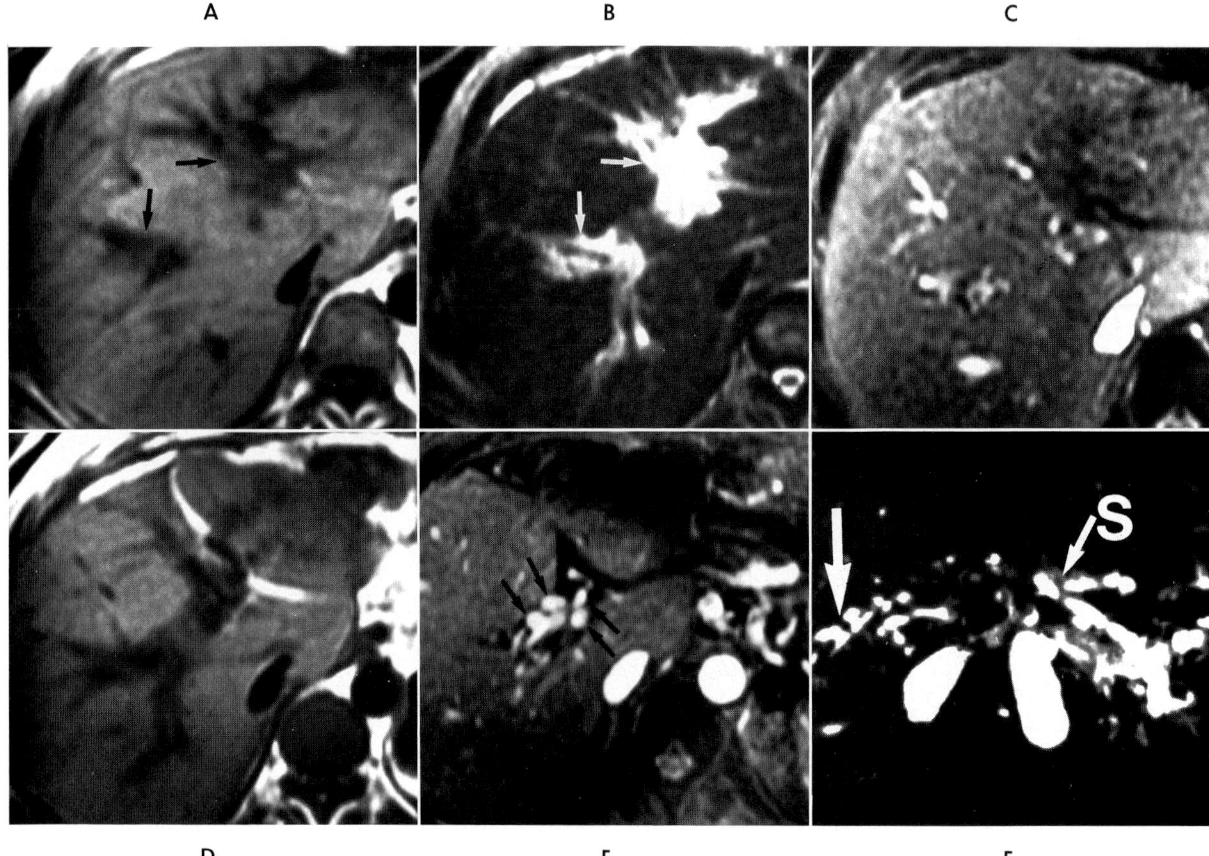

Fig. 18-4 Detection by MRI at 1.5 T of unsuspected portal vein obstruction with cavernous transformation in a patient with severe sclerosing cholangitis. Because of the portal vein obstruction, confirmed angiographically, hepatic transplantation could not be performed. **A,** Axial T1-weighted image (SE 400/12) cephalad to the portal bifurcation, showing extensive soft tissue *(arrows)* along the course of the left and right portal veins. **B,** T2-weighted image (2500/100) reveals diffuse high signal of this tissue *(arrows)*, consistent with inflammation. **C,** GRASS image (25/9, flip angle 20 degrees) shows that there is minimal flow in this region. **D,** T1-weighted image at the level of the porta hepatis. **E,** GRASS image (25/9, flip angle 20 degrees), depicting numerous collateral veins *(arrows)* in the expected location of the portal vein. **F,** MR angiogram depicts a patent splenic vein *(S)* ending proximal to its expected confluence with the superior mesenteric vein, which was thrombosed. *Arrow* indicates periportal collateral veins.

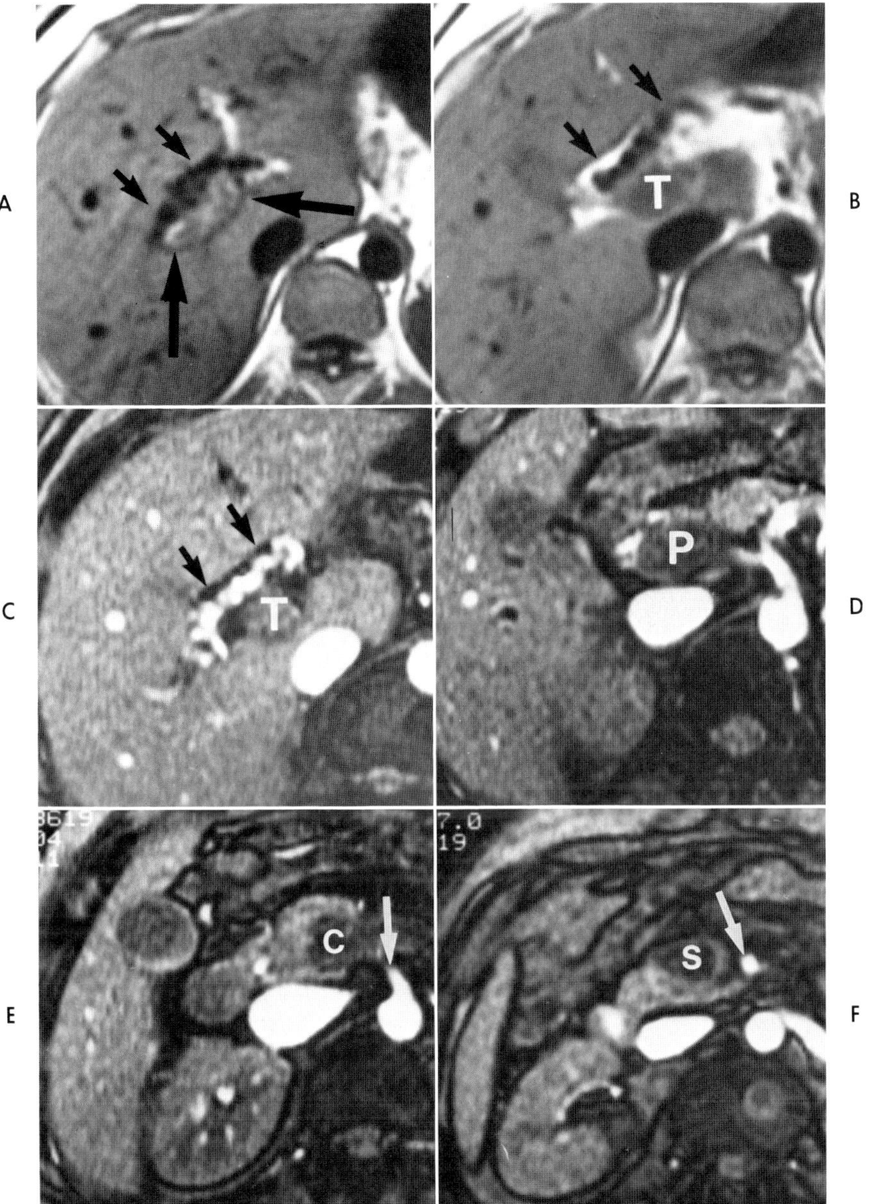

Fig. 18-5   Superior mesenteric and portal vein thrombus *(large arrows)* with cavernous transformation *(small arrows)* in a patient with ulcerative collitis. **A,** SE 400/12 image at 1.5 T. Thrombus in the portal bifurcation *(large arrows)* has high signal peripherally, indicative of methemoglobin. *Small arrows* = periportal collateral veins (cavernous transformation) anterior to the thrombus. **B,** SE 400/12 image shows intermediate signal intensity thrombus *(T)* within a dilated main portal vein. *Arrows* = periportal collateral veins (cavernous transformation). **C,** Gradient-echo image (TR/TE/flip angle = 25/13/20 degrees). **D** to **F,** Gradient-echo images further inferior demonstrate low-signal thrombus in the portal vein *(P)*, confluence of splenic and superior mesenteric veins *(C)*, and superior mesenteric vein *(S)*. *Arrow* = superior mesenteric artery.

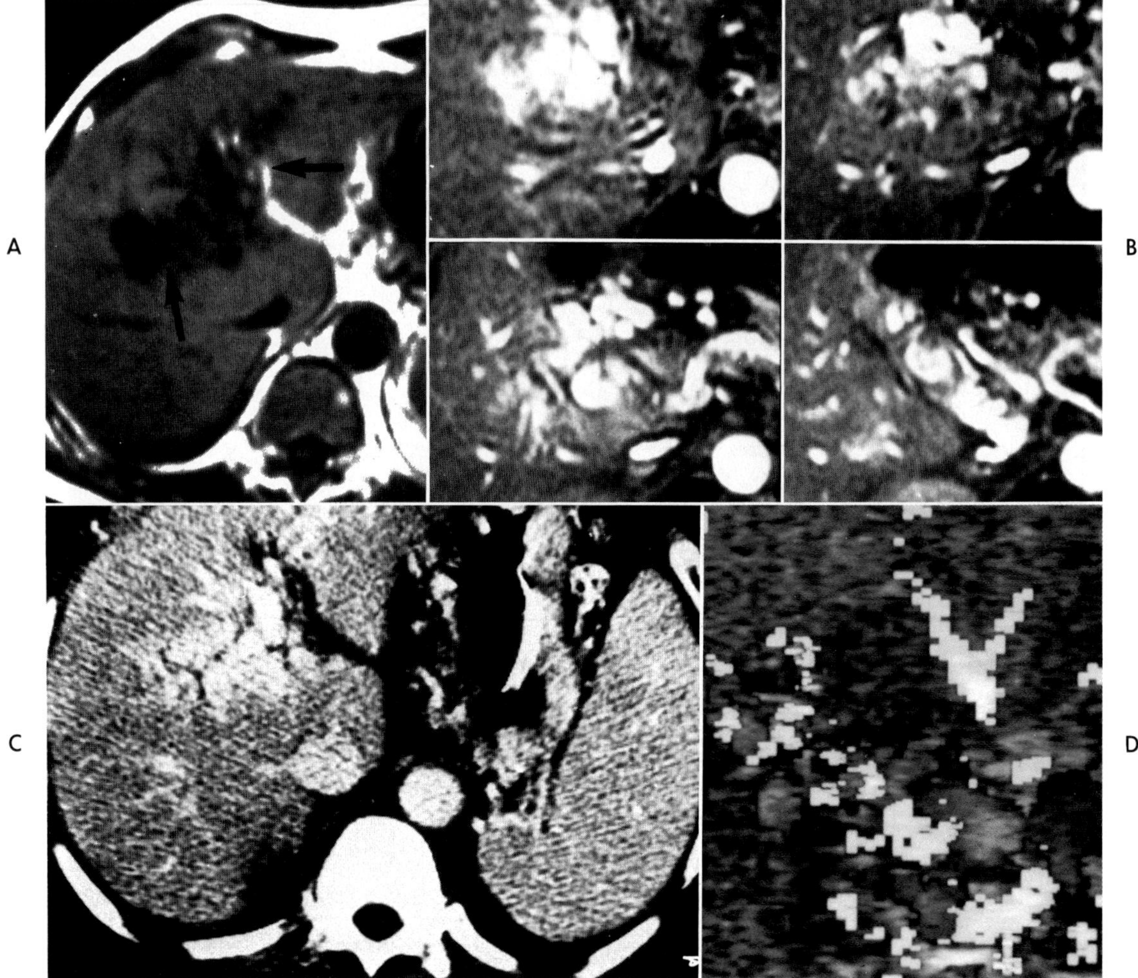

Fig. 18-9 Cavernous transformation of the portal vein. **A,** Axial T1-weighted image at 1.5 T (SE 350/12) shows numerous small channels in the expected location of the portal vein bifurcation *(arrows)*. **B,** GRASS images (25/13, flip angle 20 degrees), from cephalad to caudad, showing the cavernous transformation. **C,** Contrast-enhanced CT scan corresponding to **A. D,** Color Doppler image. (See also Color Plate XIV.)

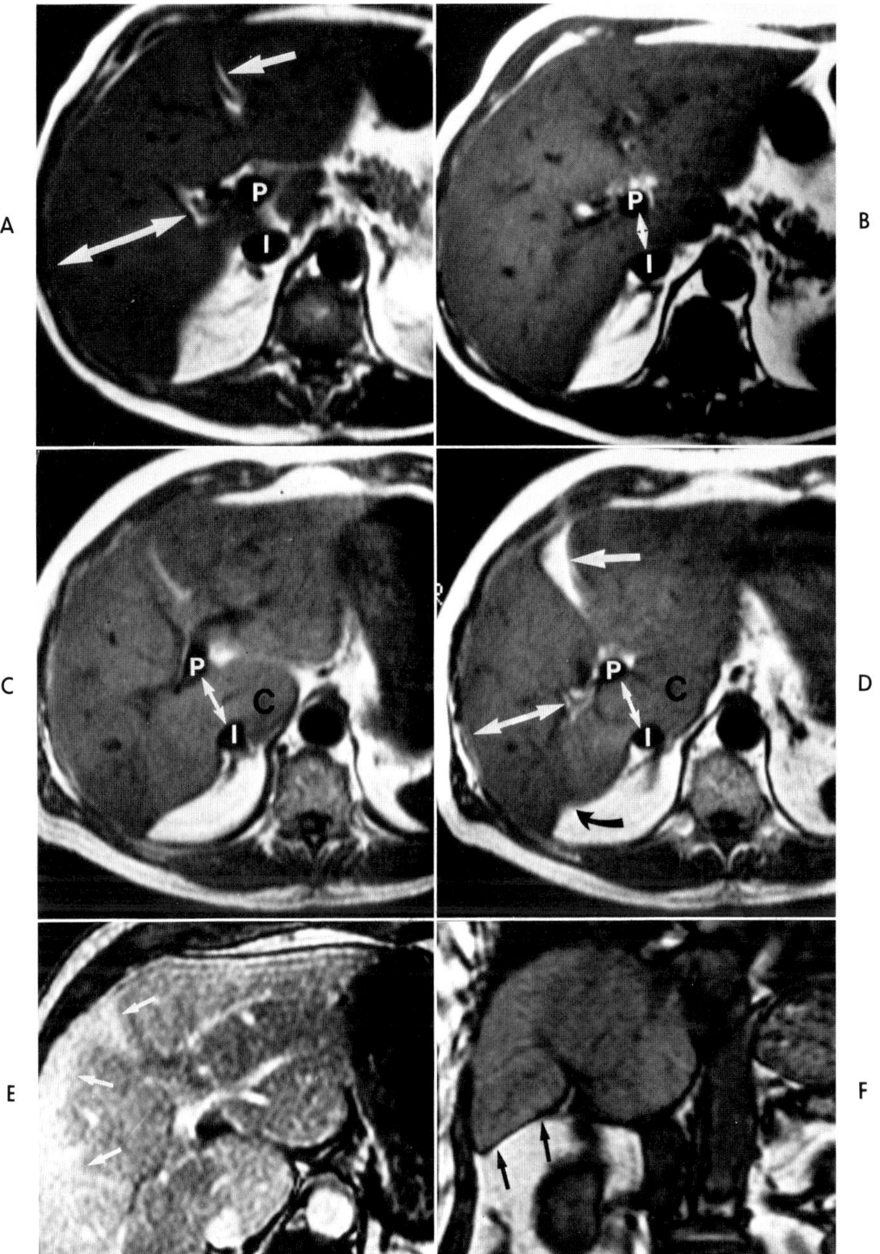

Fig. 18-10 Progressive right lobe and medial left segment atrophy secondary to right and medial left portal vein thrombosis in a patient with sclerosing cholangitis (same patient as in Fig. 15-6). **A** and **B,** SE 417/12 images at 1.5 T demonstrate mild caudate hypertrophy *(C)* but otherwise normal hepatic proportions. **C** and **D,** Corresponding SE 417/12 images 6 months later. Note rightward rotation of and increased fat in the falciform ligament *(arrow),* decreased distance between porta hepatis fat and the lateral liver surface *(large double-headed arrow),* and abnormal contour of the posterior hepatic surface *(curved arrow).* Caudate *(C)* hypertrophy has increased, increasing the distance *(small double-headed arrow)* between the inferior vena cava *(I)* and the portal vein *(P).* **E,** T1-weighted gradient-echo image (TR/TE/flip angle = 101/2.3/90 degrees) 1 minute after administration of gadopentetate dimeglumine demonstrates abnormally increased enhancement of the periphery of the right hepatic lobe *(arrows).* The mechanism of increased enhancement secondary to portal obstruction is unclear. **F,** Coronal T1-weighted gradient-echo image (TR/TE/flip angle = 101/2.3/90 degrees) demonstrates elevation of the inferior surface of the right lobe *(arrows)* resulting from atrophy.

IVC, even if other modalities demonstrate a patent IVC. If there is a pressure gradient across the inferior vena cava resulting from caudate lobe hypertrophy, a portacaval shunt is inappropriate; the portal venous system must be shunted into the right atrium or left inferior pulmonic vein in these cases.[31,495]

Vascular Features

MRI shows distinctive features that facilitate diagnosis and management of the Budd-Chiari syndrome. These features include striking reduction in caliber or complete absence of the hepatic veins, "comma-shaped" intrahepatic collateral vessels, and/or marked constriction of the intrahepatic IVC (Fig. 18-11 and 18-12). Occasionally, hepatic veins may be patent but not connected to the IVC (Fig. 18-13). Other times, hepatic venous occlusion may be one or more centimeters away from the IVC (Fig. 18-14).

MR findings allow a specific etiologic diagnosis in most patients with the Budd-Chiari syndrome. Obstruction of the IVC or right atrium by primary sarcomas or tumors of the liver, kidney, or adrenal gland can be readily demonstrated. Hepatic veins are obliterated in Budd-Chiari syndrome because of hypercoagulable states (e.g., polycythemia vera, paroxysmal nocturnal hemoglobinuria, oral contraceptive use, or the postpartum state). In patients with polycythemia vera, diffusely decreased marrow intensity and splenomegaly may be seen as incidental findings. Patients with paroxysmal nocturnal hemoglobinuria have an unusual combination of decreased hepatic and renal cortical signal intensity with normal splenic intensity (see Chapter 17, Hemolysis). Congenital webs can also be diagnosed by MRI.

Morphologic Features

Examination of patients with Budd-Chiari syndrome is often complicated by markedly altered hepatic morphology secondary to regional differences in hepatic venous outflow and portal venous inflow.[320,332,561] Awareness of the expected alterations may therefore be necessary for proper examination and interpretation. These alterations can be understood best by considering the pathophysiology of hepatic venous obstruction.

In most cases, hepatic venous outflow is not completely eliminated, since a variety of accessory hepatic veins may drain above or below the principal site of obstruction.[520] The most common of such sites include the inferior (accessory) right hepatic vein and caudate vein, which drain into the inferior portion of the IVC. Connections also exist to other systemic veins, such as the azygous, vertebral, and/or intercostal veins, and these may enlarge and provide hepatic venous drainage in patients with Budd-Chiari syndrome. Shunting is also common between hepatic and portal veins, producing reversed flow in at least some portal vein branches,[320,561] although main portal vein flow may remain antegrade.[218]

Some hepatic veinous drainage is usually preserved for the caudate lobe, and central regions of the left and right lobes may also be spared via drainage into caudate veins or other collaterals.[75,320,561] Compensatory hypertrophy is typical, especially in the caudate lobe, which may become massive and produce secondary obstruction of the IVC (see Figs. 18-12 to 18-14). Some venous drainage is also preserved in the periphery through capsular veins,[75,309] although this is usually not sufficient to prevent peripheral hepatic atrophy in patients with Budd-Chiari syndrome.

Text continues on p. 203.

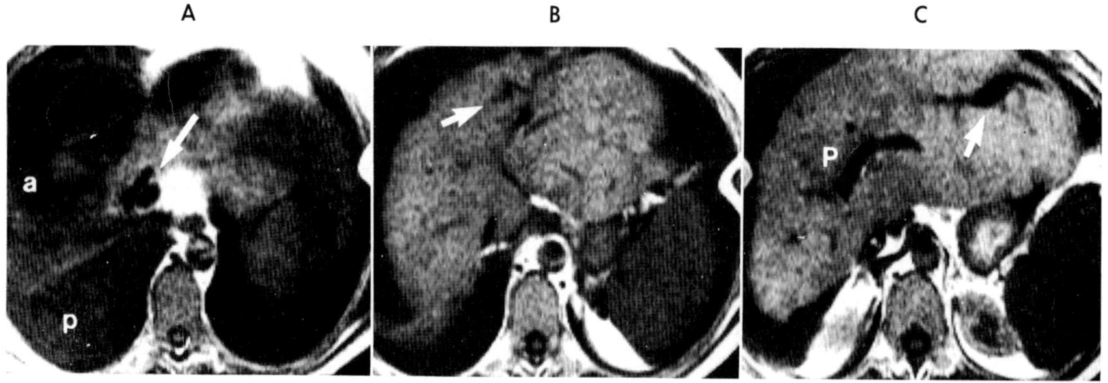

Fig. 18-11 Chronic, untreated Budd-Chiari syndrome secondary to membranous venous webs. **A,** SE 260/20 image at 0.6 T near the IVC-right atrial junction shows a vascular web *(arrow)* separating two channels of flowing blood. Note ascites *(a)* and a right pleural effusion *(p)*. **B,** Approximately 3 centimeters caudal, the IVC has a slitlike configuration and hepatic veins are absent. The liver is shrunken and irregular as a result of cirrhosis secondary to this patient's long-standing, untreated venous obstruction. Note prominent intrahepatic collateral venous drainage *(arrow)*. **C,** Further caudal, a patent portal vein *(P)* is seen. A large peripheral comma-shaped, collateral vein is seen in the left hepatic lobe *(arrow)*.

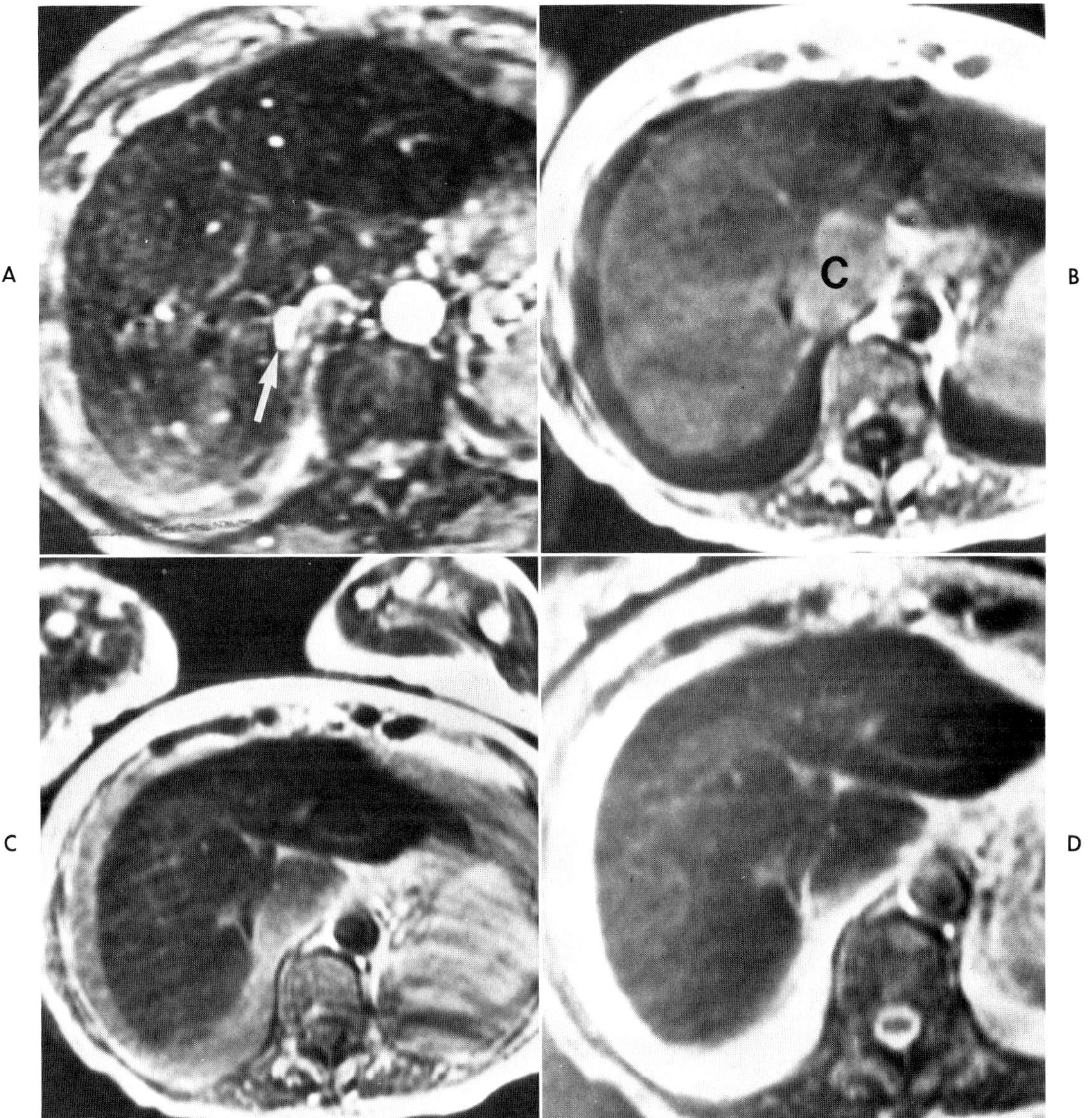

Fig. 18-12   Budd-Chiari syndrome: signal differences of caudate lobe. **A,** Axial GRASS image at 1.5 T (25/13, flip angle 30 degrees) reveals a patent IVC *(arrow)* but no flow in hepatic veins. A dilated caudate vein drains into the IVC. **B,** Corresponding SE 600/20 image reveals low signal of the liver, except for the caudate lobe *(C),* which is usually less severely affected in Budd-Chiari syndrome. **C,** SE 2500/30 image. **D,** On the T2-weighted image (SE 2500/80), the entire liver has decreased signal. Note ascites.

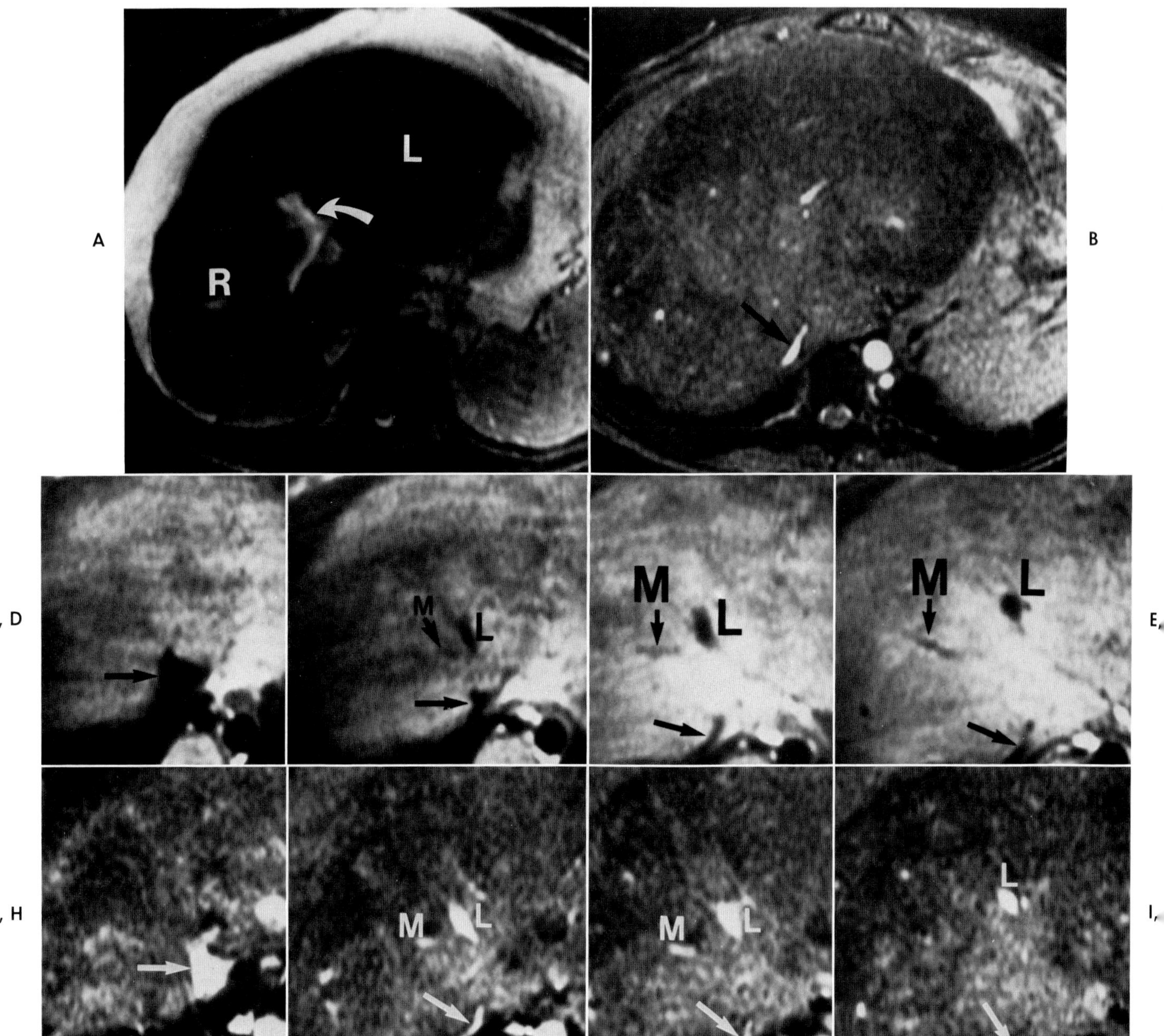

Fig. 18-13 Budd-Chiari syndrome with patent hepatic veins that do not drain into the IVC. **A,** Axial T2-weighted image at 1.5 T (SE 2500/100) reveals diffusely decreased hepatic signal intensity, marked hypertrophy of the left lobe *(L)* and atrophy of the right lobe *(R)*. The portal bifurcation *(arrow)* is rotated towards the right. **B,** GRASS image (25/13, flip angle 20 degrees) slightly higher reveals a compressed but patent IVC *(arrow)*. Hepatic parenchyma has normal intensity centrally but decreased intensity peripherally. **C** to **F,** T1-weighted (SE 400/12) images from cephalad to caudad show abnormally decreased signal intensity peripherally but normal intensity centrally, a common finding in Budd-Chiari syndrome. The IVC *(arrow)* is patent. The left hepatic vein *(L)* is large, and is rotated towards the usual location of the middle hepatic vein *(M)* by the enlarged left lobe. The middle and left hepatic veins join together but do not connect with the IVC. **G** to **J,** Corresponding GRASS images (25/13, flip angle 20 degrees) again show decreased hepatic signal intensity peripherally and similar vascular anatomy. *Figure continues.*

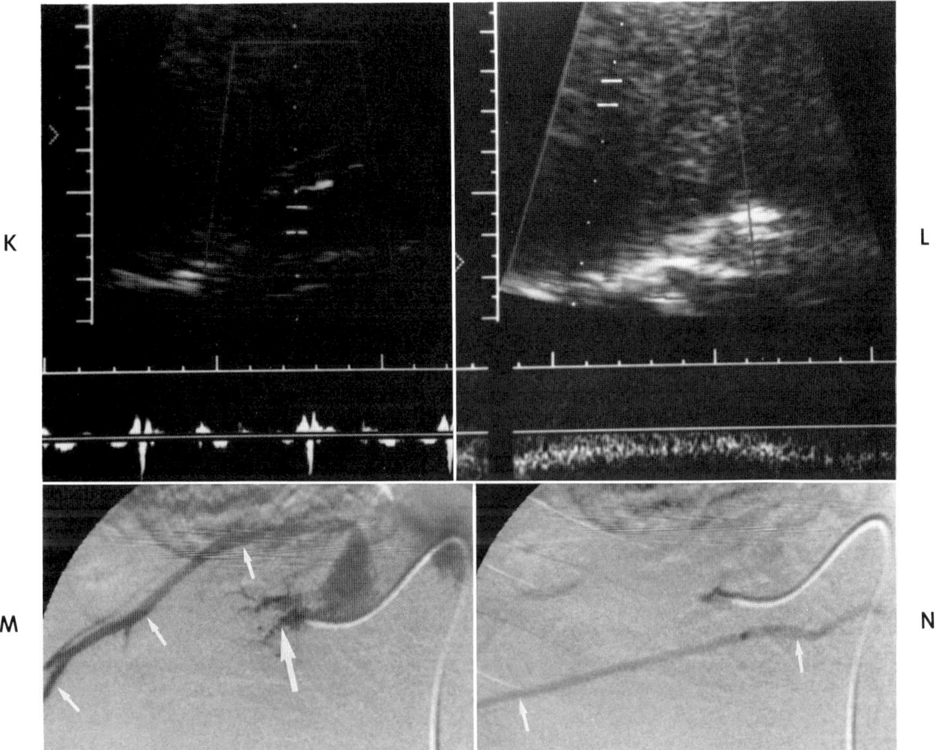

Fig. 18-13, cont'd   K, Duplex Doppler examination shows normal pulsatile flow in the IVC. **L,** Duplex Doppler examination of the left hepatic vein shows patency and normal direction of flow, but cardiac pulsations are absent. This results from discontinuity between the hepatic veins and the IVC. **M,** Digital subtraction hepatic venogram shows "spider-web" appearance of obstructed hepatic venous confluence *(large arrow).* An accessory hepatic vein is patent superiorly *(small arrows).* **N,** Delayed image reveals drainage via an intercostal vein *(arrows),* which emptied into the azygous vein on a later image (not shown).

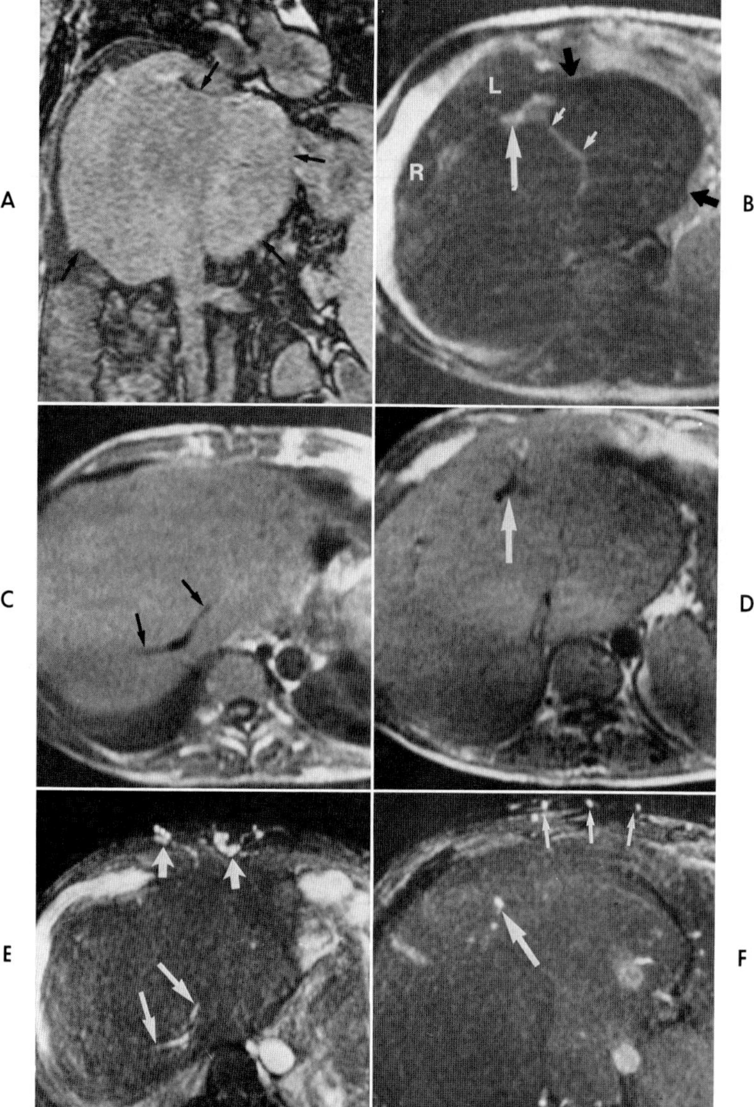

Fig. 18-14   Budd-Chiari syndrome with patent central hepatic veins and massive caudate hypertrophy. **A,** Coronal spoiled gradient-echo image (TR/TE/slip angle = 101/2.3/90 degrees) at 1.5 T reveals massive hypertrophy of the caudate lobe *(arrows)*. **B,** Axial SE 2500/50 image reveals decreased signal of the liver. The caudate lobe *(black arrows)* is markedly enlarged, and the left *(L)* and right *(R)* lobes are atrophied. *Large white arrow* = porta hepatus, *small white arrows* = portal branch to caudate. **C,** SE 400/12 image at the level of the central hepatic veins *(arrows)*, two of which are patent. The hepatic veins could not be imaged peripheral to this. **D,** SE 400/12 image corresponding to **B.** Hepatic signal is heterogeneous and decreased. *Arrow* = porta hepatus. **E,** MR angiographic slab approximately 2-cm thick, corresponding to **C.** *Long arrows* = hepatic veins, *short arrows* = abdominal wall collateral veins. **F,** MR angiographic slab corresponding to **B** and **D.** *Large arrow* = small portal vein, *small arrows* = body walls collateral veins.

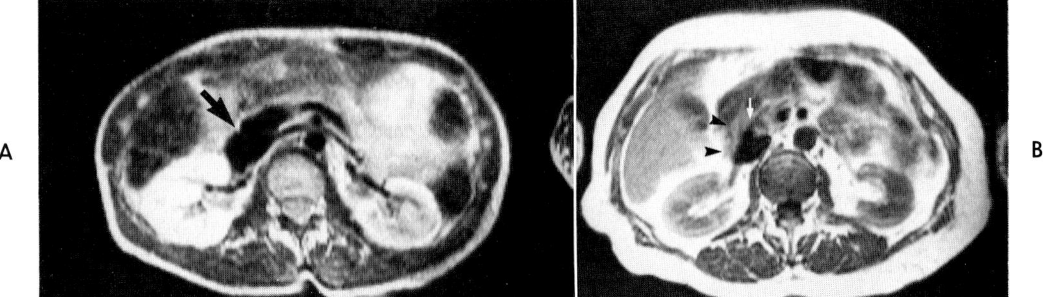

Fig. 18-15 Portacaval side-to-side shunts. **A,** T1-weighted MR image at 0.6 T demonstrates a widely patent shunt *(arrow)*. **B,** Another patient shows scar tissue *(arrowheads)* of intermediate signal intensity surrounding a small but patent shunt orifice *(arrow)*. The portal vein side of this shunt anastomosis was seen on a higher section.

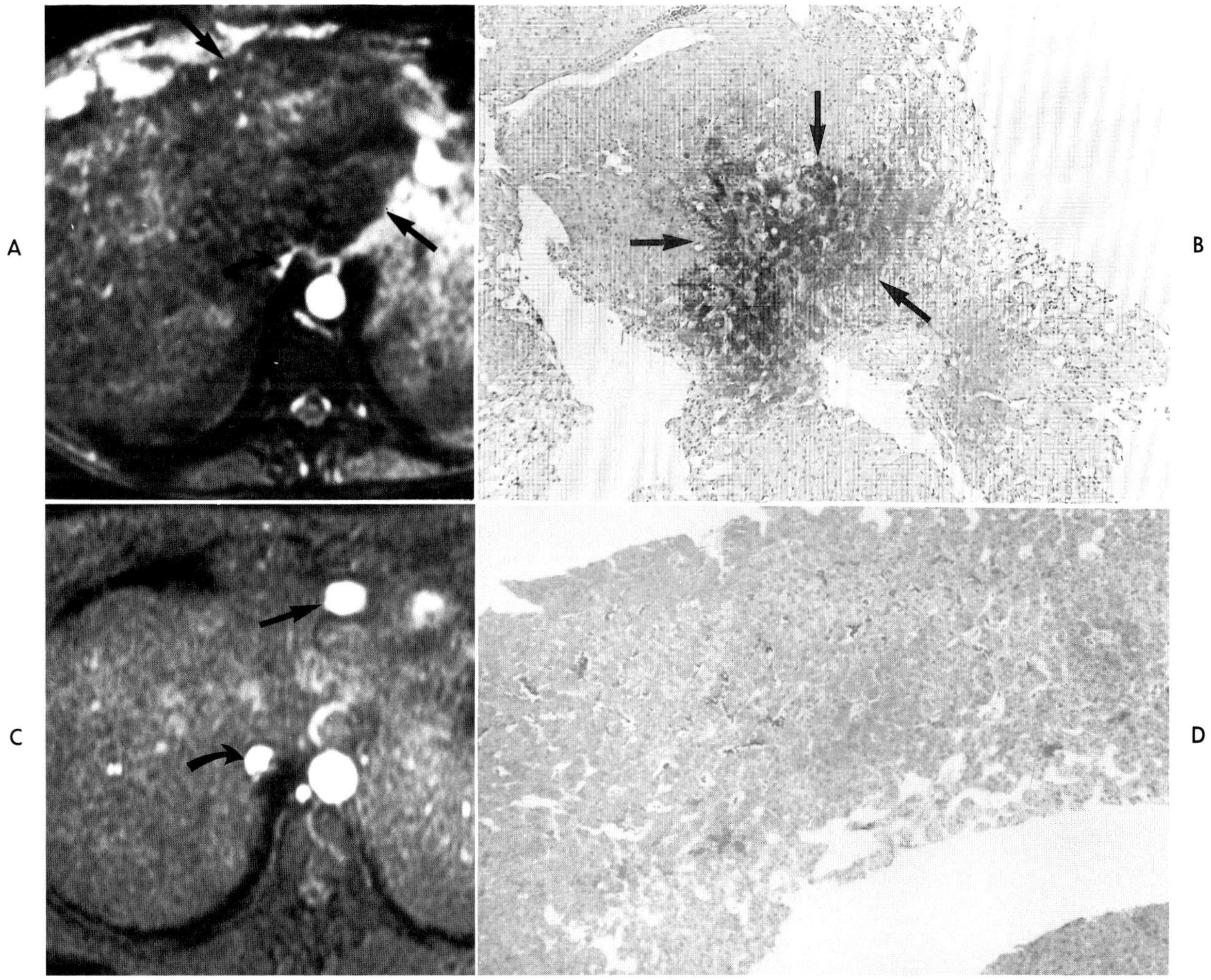

Fig. 18-16 Budd-Chiari syndrome treated by mesoatrial shunt. **A,** Axial GRASS image at 1.5 T (25/13, flip angle 20 degrees) at the dome of the liver reveals absent hepatic venous flow and marked compression of the IVC *(curved arrow)*. Note the swollen appearance of the left hepatic lobe *(straight arrows)*. **B,** Histologic section shows centrilobar venous congestion *(arrows)* consistent with Budd-Chiari syndrome. **C,** Corresponding GRASS image (25/13, flip angle 20 degrees) 2 years after surgical creation of a shunt between the superior mesenteric vein and right atrium. The shunt is patent *(arrow)*, just deep to the anterior abdominal wall. The IVC *(curved arrow)* is not compressed, but hepatic veins remain ocluded. Note that the liver now has normal shape. **D,** Repeat biopsy shows only mild congestion, significantly less than in **B.**

Figure continues.

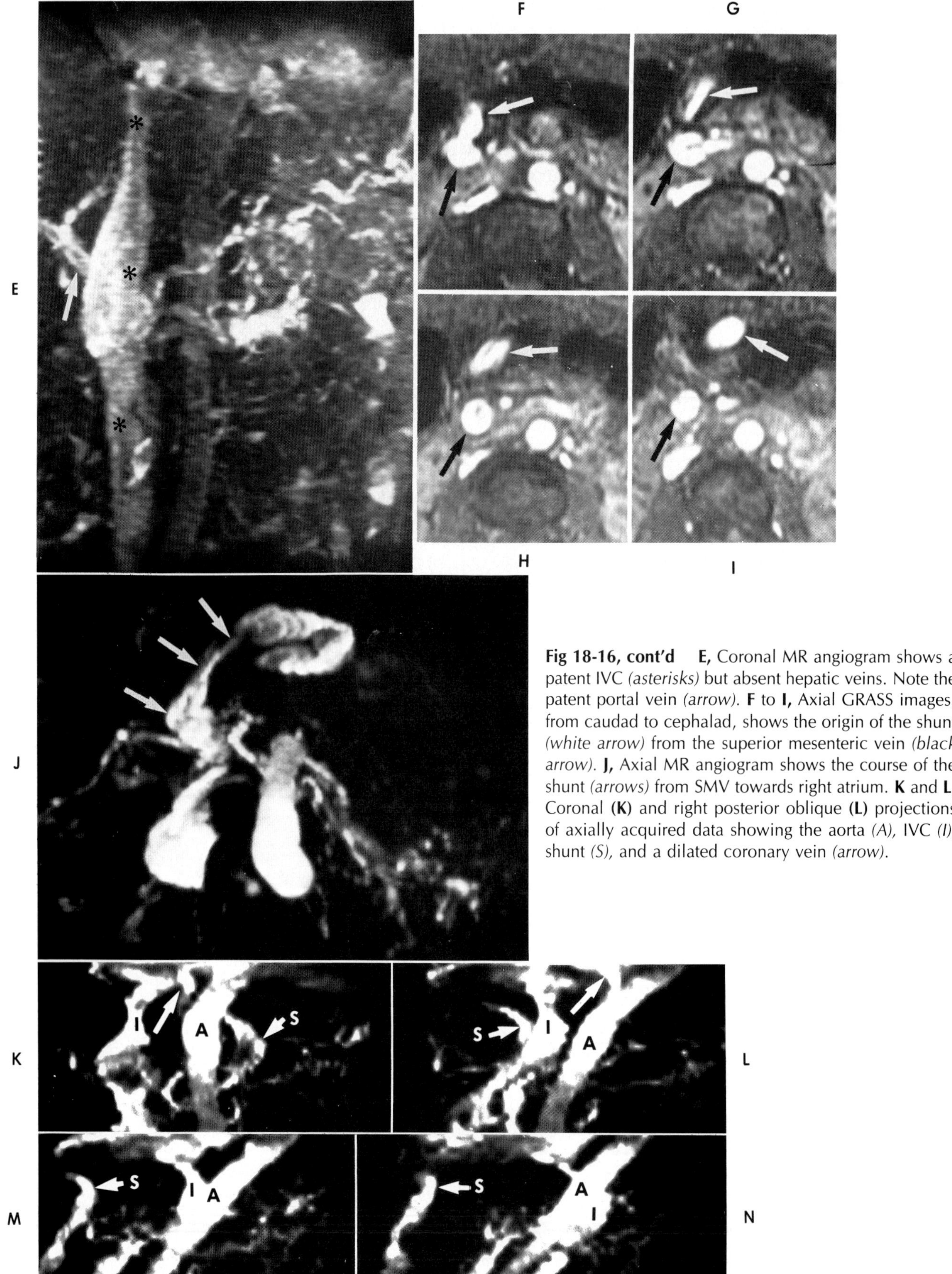

Fig 18-16, cont'd **E,** Coronal MR angiogram shows a patent IVC *(asterisks)* but absent hepatic veins. Note the patent portal vein *(arrow).* **F** to **I,** Axial GRASS images, from caudad to cephalad, shows the origin of the shunt *(white arrow)* from the superior mesenteric vein *(black arrow).* **J,** Axial MR angiogram shows the course of the shunt *(arrows)* from SMV towards right atrium. **K** and **L,** Coronal **(K)** and right posterior oblique **(L)** projections of axially acquired data showing the aorta *(A),* IVC *(I),* shunt *(S),* and a dilated coronary vein *(arrow).*

Regions with completely obstructed hepatic venous outflow tend to drain via shunting of hepatic veins and arteries to portal veins, producing reversed portal venous flow.[410] These regions of the liver will thus be deprived of portal vein supply. Since hepatic regeneration, hypertrophy, and atrophy depend in part on the degree of portal perfusion,[135,503,504] Budd-Chiari syndrome is typically associated with peripheral hepatic atrophy and caudate and central hypertrophy. The porta-hepatus may thus be displaced toward the anterior portion of the liver (see Fig. 18-14).

MR images may demonstrate regional differences in signal intensity because of hepatic vascular congestion, central lobular necrosis, and/or differences in hepatocellular fat or iron. Relative to the less severely involved caudate lobe, peripheral liver may have decreased signal on T1-weighted images and/or increased signal on T2-weighted images (see Figs. 18-12 and 18-13).

Patients with primary Budd-Chiari syndrome must be separated from patients who have cirrhosis as the primary pathologic process. Patients with Budd-Chiari syndrome usually have acute clinical symptoms and a large, tender liver without the nodular changes of cirrhosis. Patients with end-stage cirrhosis often have compressed, distorted hepatic veins, but flow can usually be noted on T1-weighted and flow-sensitive gradient-echo images. In addition, severely cirrhotic livers are distinguished by their small size, nodular surface, heterogeneous texture, and extrahepatic collateral varices. MRI may demonstrate ascites in patients with cirrhosis and Budd-Chiari syndrome, so it is not a valuable differential feature.

In patients who are treated by surgical shunts, patency can be monitored effectively by MRI (Figs. 18-15 and 18-16).[71,495]

Hepatic venoocclusive disease, another cause of hepatic venous obstruction, can be caused by chemotherapy, especially after bone marrow transplantation.[48] This disease involves diffuse obliteration of postsinusoidal venules, and the IVC and major hepatic veins remain patent. Definitive diagnosis is by biopsy. In one such patient, MRI was falsely normal and the true diagnosis was established only by wedged hepatic venography.[495]

BILIARY SYSTEM AND ACCESSORY ORGANS

The clinical impact of MRI on imaging the biliary system, pancreas, and spleen has been far less than for imaging the liver. Ultrasound and CT are superior for depicting intrahepatic biliary ducts. CT's superior spatial resolution and relative insensitivity to motion artifact and the availability of suitable oral contrast have enabled CT to retain superiority for most extrahepatic indications in the upper abdomen.

Recently, improved pulse-sequence design and motion-suppression techniques have enabled effective imaging of the pancreas, biliary tract, and spleen, allowing the superior tissue contrast characteristic of MRI to become available for diagnosis. We anticipate that further development of rapid-imaging techniques and contrast agents will enable MRI to reach parity with CT, if not surpass it, for extrahepatic diagnosis in the upper abdomen in the near future.

Biliary System

For most indications, ultrasound is the preferred modality for biliary diagnosis because of its sensitivity for calculi and bile duct dilatation. Patients who are referred for MRI to detect or characterize masses may also have biliary pathology. Proper MRI interpretation therefore requires familiarity with the appearance of the normal and pathologic biliary system.

BILIARY DILATATION

Bile ducts dilate proximal to intrahepatic or extrahepatic obstruction. Segmental or multifocal bile duct dilatation is common with sclerosing cholangitis (see Chapter 15).

At 0.6 T, T1-weighted images are best for delineating the relationship of dilated intrahepatic ducts to adjacent portal stuctures.[102,507] However, since hepatic bile has a long T1 and low signal intensity on heavily T1-weighted images, it can be difficult to distinguish bile ducts from the flow void of portal vessels (Figs. 20-1 and 20-2).

At 1.5 T, T2-weighted images are better for depicting bile ducts[490] (Figs. 20-3 and 20-4). This is because T1-weighted images at high field have less contrast than T1-weighted images at mid field. Additionally, T2-weighted images have a higher signal-to-noise ratio (SNR) at high field. Like most other fluids, hepatic bile has a long T2 relaxation time and extremely high signal on images acquired with echo delays of 100 msec or longer.

Congenital anomalies resulting in biliary dilatation include Caroli's disease and choledochal cysts. Choledochal cysts produce dilatation of the common duct (Fig. 20-5). Because continuity of the cyst with the biliary tree may be difficult to establish by cross-sectional imaging, cholangiography is usually performed to confirm the diagnosis.

CHOLELITHIASIS

Gallstones are encountered frequently in routine MR imaging as a signal void surrounded by high-intensity bile on T2-weighted images (Figs. 20-6 and 20-7). It is worthwhile to recognize gallstones when they are discovered incidentally, but ultrasound is the preferred technique for detecting cholelithiasis.

Recent success of nonoperative therapies for choleli-thiasis has renewed interest in characterizing gallstone composition. These therapies include extracorporeal shock wave lithotripsy, treatment with oral bile acids, and percutaneous catheter chemodissolution with methyl *tert*-butyl ether (MTBE). Although most gallstones appear as a signal void in vivo, calculi can be categorized based on in vitro T1-weighted imaging as dark (35%), rimmed (40%), laminated (14%), homogeneously bright (5%), or homogeneously faint (7%).[24] In an earlier report at 0.35 T using longer TE,[361] only 17% of dehydrated gallstones had discernible signal when imaged in vivo after rehydration. Signal within calculi is more likely to be recognized when TE is minimized (Figs. 20-7 and 20-8).

Since successful stone lysis may depend on the fraction and distribution of cholesterol and calcium bilirubinate within the stone, it was hoped that positive signal might relate to the stone lipid component. However, lipid content does not correlate with signal intensity, and signal intensity does not predict in vitro dissolution with MTBE.[23] Positive signal requires a sufficient proton density, and T1 shortening probably arises from diminished mobility of water molecules when bound to large molecules such as proteins and cholesterol. When this T1 shortening is extreme, the T2 shortening is also extreme and predominates, causing signal void.

Intrahepatic stones are more likely than gallbladder calculi to exhibit detectable signal on a clinical MR image. Calculi with short T1 have been demonstrated within saccular ductal dilatations in Caroli's disease.[318] The high lipid content of these calculi was supported by low x-ray attenuation observed on CT. A case of a short T1 intrahepatic biliary calculus rich in fatty acids has been reported.[359] Less commonly, gallbladder calculi can also have high signal (see Fig. 20-7). Common duct stones can occasionally be depicted by MRI (see Fig. 20-8), but ultrasound and x-ray cholangiography remain superior for their demonstration.

CHOLECYSTITIS

Acute cholecystitis is a common cause of fever and acute right upper quadrant pain, mandating urgent treatment. Chronic cholecystitis is a common cause of pain

Text continues on page 219.

bladders usually has increased water content, protein content also tends to be increased. The increased T1 or T2 relaxation times caused by increased water are therefore offset by the higher protein content, which decreases T1 and T2 relaxation times (Fig. 20-9). Thus T1 and T2 values cannot distinguish reliably between normal gallbladder bile and bile in patients with acute or chronic cholecystitis.[294]

Although MRI is not indicated as the initial modality for detection of acute cholecystitis, unsuspected cholecystitis might be detected when the patient's presenting symptoms are nonspecific. As with ultrasound, ancillary morphologic features may be useful in the MRI diagnosis of cholecystitis. Thickening of the gallbladder wall, fluid in the gallbladder fossa, or fluid within the gallbladder wall itself can occasionally be detected on T2-weighted MR images (Fig. 20-10). When present, these signs are more indicative of gallbladder disease than is analysis of the relaxation times of bile.[593] An inflamed gallbladder wall may have increased enhancement with intravenous gadopentetate dimeglumine. At present, neither the sensitivity nor specificity of this finding is known.

Thickening of the gallbladder wall, by itself, is nonspecific. In particular, it is a common finding in patients with acute hepatitis or portal hypertension, probably because of intrinsic liver disease. Although extremely low albumen may also be a causative factor for increasing gallbladder wall thickening, patients with low albumen and ascites resulting from renal failure and peritoneal dialysis are less likely to have thick gallbladder walls than are patients with liver disease.[248]

Decrease in bile T1 associated either with physiologic concentration or with elevation of biliary protein content should not be confused with the dramatic fall in bile T1 in hemobilia (Fig. 20-11). In hemobilia, production of paramagnetic methemoglobin from oxydation of extravasated hemoglobin presumably accounts for the T1 shortening. The heavier components rich in methemoglobin layer dependently, producing fluid-fluid levels.

GALLBLADDER CARCINOMA

Gallbladder carcinoma, the fifth most common malignancy of the GI tract, usually occurs in the setting of chronic cholecystitis with cholelithiasis.[447] It is discovered incidentally in about 1% of cholecystectomies. When the presentation suggests neoplasm, the tumor is usually advanced, with extensive involvement of the gallbladder, liver, and head of pancreas.[142] Prognosis with advanced gallbladder carcinoma is poor.

Gallbladder carcinoma is seen on T2-weighted images as focal thickening of the gallbladder wall, more intense than liver and less intense than bile (Fig. 20-12).[457] Although uncommon, a very desmoplastic short T2 gallbladder carcinoma has been reported.[603] Gallbladder carcinoma tumor tends to invade liver and spreads to lymph nodes along the common bile duct in the hepatoduodenal ligament. Duodenal invasion is also common. Prospective differentiation of gallbladder carcinoma from inflammatory thickening of the gallbladder wall or from tumors of the liver crossing the interlobar fissure may be difficult because the signal characteristics are similar.

BILE DUCT CARCINOMA

Bile duct carcinoma is depicted as low signal on T1-weighted images and high signal on T2-weighted images (Figs. 20-13 to 20-15). One preliminary report suggested that the scirrhous subtype of cholangiocarcinoma could be distinguished by a short T2 relaxation time,[103] but more experience is needed. Segmental biliary and portal vein obstruction are common, leading to segmental atrophy and compensatory hypertrophy of uninvolved segments.[60,297,523] There is a high rate of recurrence after resection of cholangiocarcinoma, so patients may present at a later date with widespread hepatic metastases (Fig. 20-16).

Central (hilar) cholangiocarcinomas are associated with biliary dilatation, which has higher signal intensity than the obstructing tumor on T2-weighted images (Fig. 20-17). The tumor may infiltrate along portal tracts (see Figs. 20-13 and 20-14). This infiltration may be difficult to detect because of partial volume averaging with nearby portal vessels and dilated bile ducts,[91] but it can be depicted as high signal on both sides of the portal vein. This appearance is different from that of dilated bile ducts, which appear on only one side of the portal vein. Other conditions can mimic this appearance of cholangiocarcinoma, including hepatic transplantation, metastases to porta hepatis lymph nodes, surgical exploration of the porta hepatis, hepatitis, cholangitis, obstruction of hepatic lymphatics, and recent biliary obstruction.[323]

Peripheral (intrahepatic) cholangiocarcinomas may present as large masses without biliary dilation (Fig. 20-15). The MRI characteristics of peripheral cholangiocarcinomas are similar to those of other tumors, but features characteristic of hepatocellular carcinoma, such as capsules and high intensity on T1-weighted images, should not occur.

Biliary cystic neoplasms are rare tumors that occur primarily in middle-aged women.[259] These tumors may be benign (cystadenoma) or malignant (cystadenocarcinoma). Even when malignant, these tumors are far more indolent than cholangiocarcinomas. Biliary cystic neoplasms are composed of large multiloculated cysts with mural nodules.

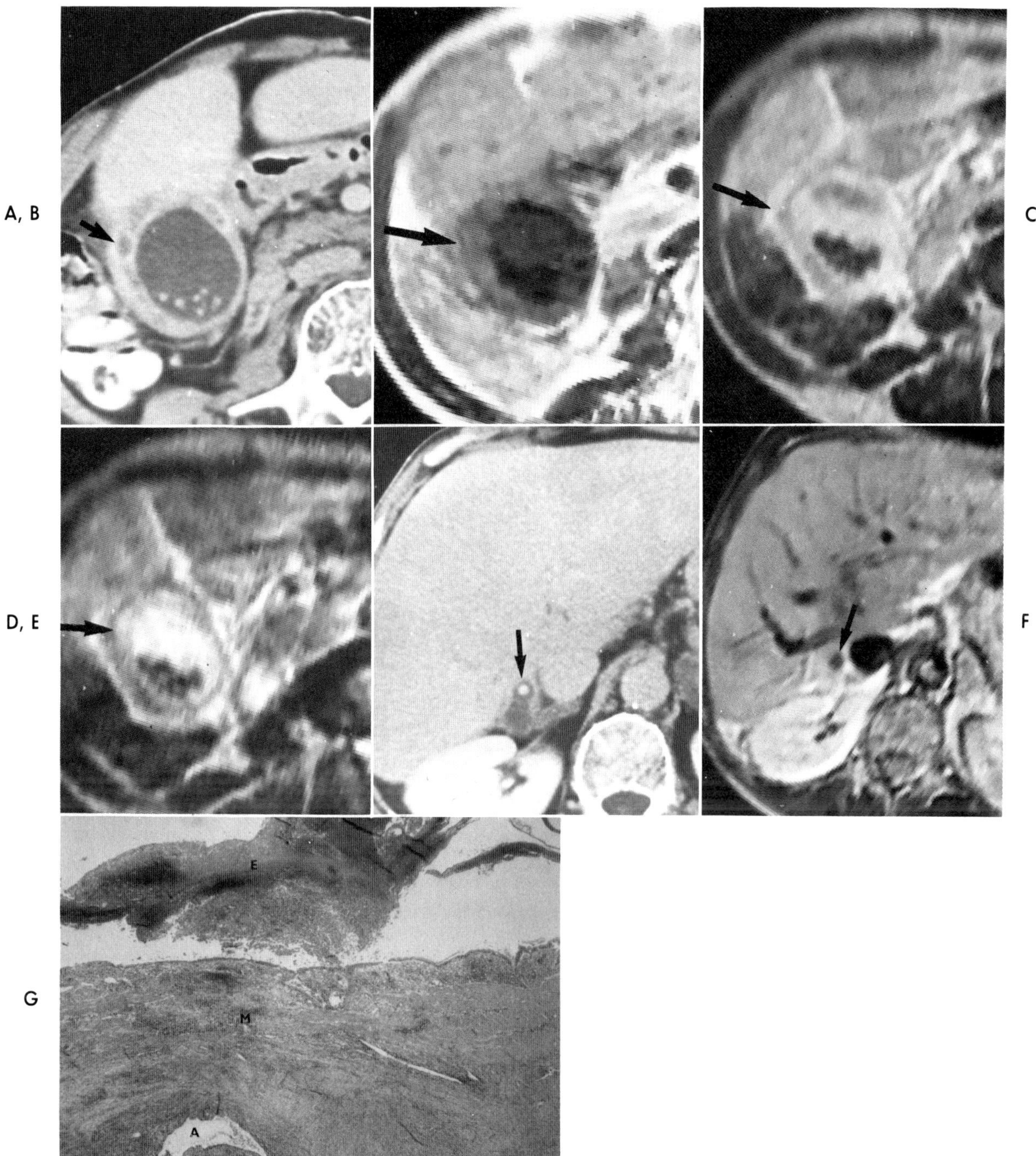

Fig. 20-10 Acute cholecystitis (**A** to **D**) with a gallstone impacted in the gallbladder neck (**E** to **G**). **A,** CT scan shows gallstones and fluid within thickened gallbladder wall *(arrow).* **B,** SE 300/14 image shows wall thickening *(arrow).* Bile in acute cholecystitis has increased water content and long T1 and therefore has a low signal intensity. Gallstones have an even lower signal intensity and can be seen in the most dependent part of the gallbladder. **C,** SE 2400/60 sequence shows multiple gallstones as low-intensity structures, layering beneath two distinct fractions of bile. The more anterior fraction has a lower signal intensity consistent with its lower specific gravity and longer T1 relaxation time. **D,** SE 2400/120. Fluid in the gallbladder wall *(arrow)* is clearly delineated. **E,** CT scan shows the calcified center and low-density periphery of impacted stone *(arrow).* **F,** SE 2400/60 sequence displays bile as the same intensity as liver parenchyma. Stone is a conspicuous signal void. **G,** Photomicrograph of hematoxylin- and eosin-stained histology of resected specimen, showing thickened, inflamed mucosa *(M),* mural microabscess *(A),* and exudate *(E)* in lumen. (From Weissleder, R., Stark, D.D., Compton, C., et al.: Magn. Reson. Imaging 6:345-348, 1988.)

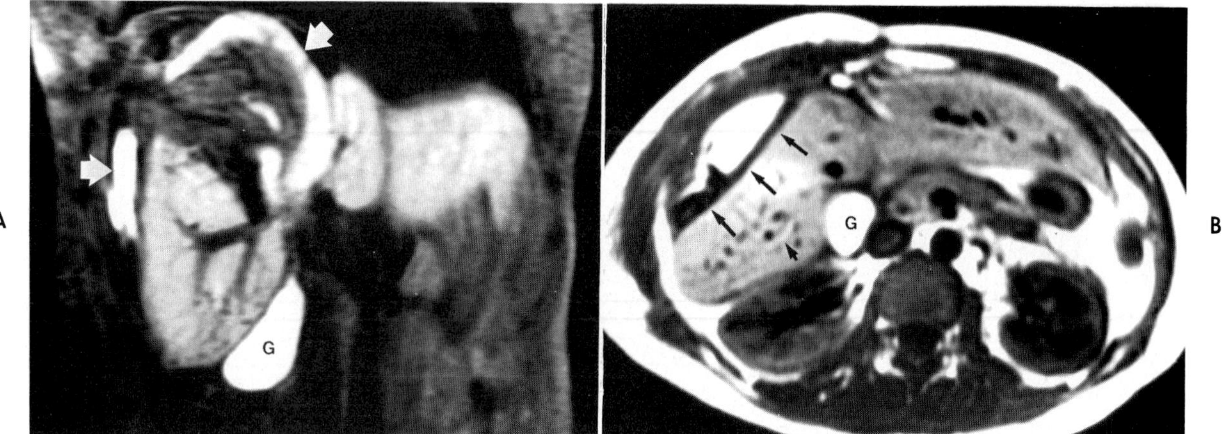

Fig. 20-11 Traumatic hemobilia. **A,** T1-weighted coronal image at 1.5 T shows acute and subacute subcapsular hematoma with short T1 methemoglobin forming at the periphery *(arrows)*. Methemoglobin-rich blood fills the gallbladder *(G)*. **B,** Axial T1-weighted image shows mixed signal intensities from peripheral subcapsular hematoma *(long arrows)* and blood in the bile ducts *(short arrow)* and gallbladder *(G)*. Surgical exploration revealed the hemobilia to be the result of a fistula from the hepatic artery to the bile duct.

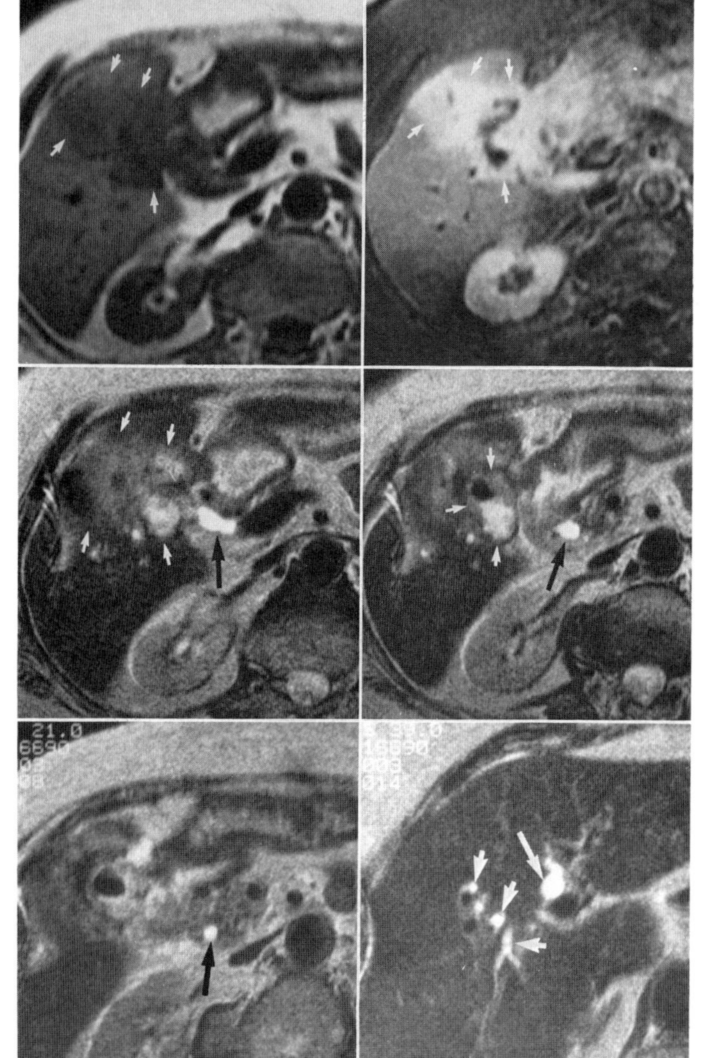

Fig. 20-12 Invasive gallbladder carcinoma depicted at 1.5 T. **A,** SE 400/12 image depicts a low-signal mass in the gallbladder fossa *(arrows)*. **B,** SE 400/12 image with fat suppression, approximately 5 minutes after administration of gadopentatate dimeglumine. The mass and adjacent tissues *(arrows)* enhance more than normal tissues. **C,** Corresponding multiple spin-echo conjugate (fast spin echo) image (TR/TE = 6000/102, 16 echoes per excitation), acquired using a 512 × 512 matrix and two signal averages in approximately 6 minutes. The mass *(short arrows)* has high signal. *Long black arrow* = dilated proximal common bile duct. **D,** Inferiorly, the abnormal gallbladder *(short arrows)* is indicated. *Long black arrow* = dilated common bile duct. **E,** Further inferiorly, the common bile duct *(arrow)* is not dilated. **F,** Superiorly, intrahepatic ducts *(arrows)* are dilated.

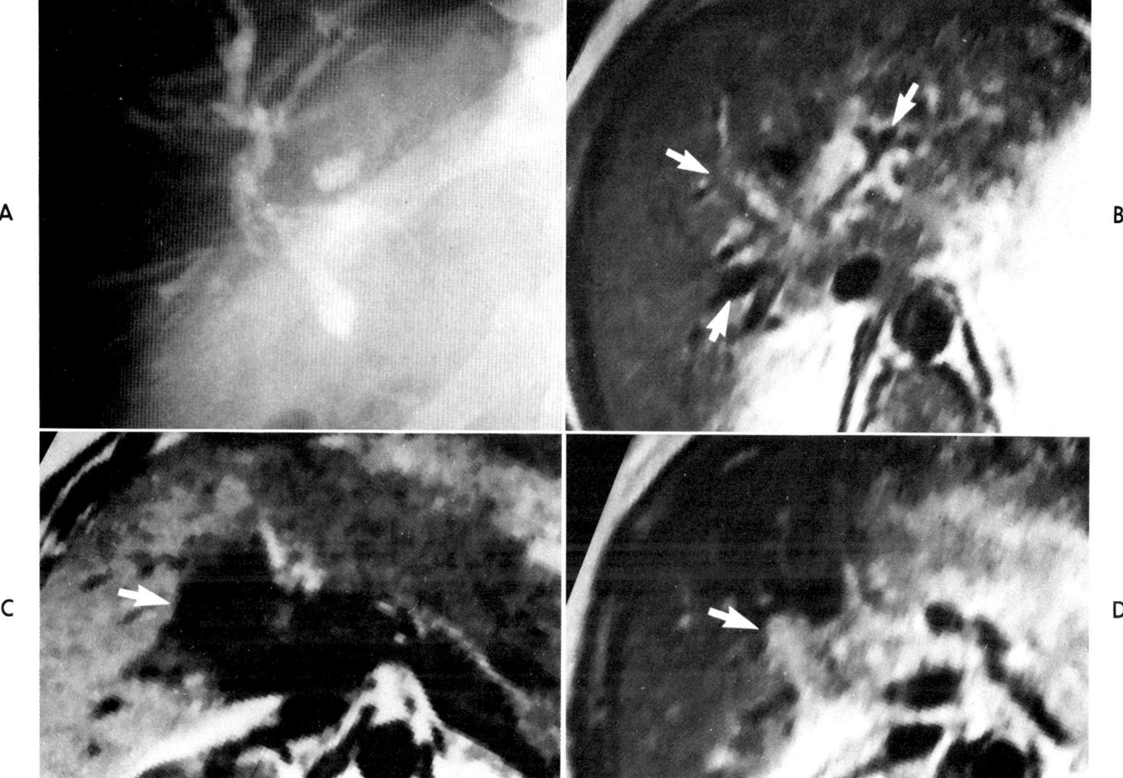

Fig. 20-13 Cholangiocarcinoma. **A,** Percutaneous transhepatic cholangiogram shows encasement of bile ducts in the porta hepatis with minimally dilated intrahepatic ducts. **B,** SE 2400/60 sequence separates low-signal portal veins *(arrow)* from surrounding high-signal—intensity tumor. This pulse sequence is particularly useful for distinguishing cholangiocarcinoma from dilated bile ducts. Bile ducts would not encircle the portal veins and are isointense to liver at this TR and TE. **C,** SE 300/14 image at the level of the porta hepatis. An abnormal soft tissue mass is seen *(arrow)*. **D,** SE 2400/60. T2-weighted sequence shows the tumor mass to be nearly isointense to the pancreatic head, fat, duodenum, and other structures adjacent to the porta hepatis. (Images at 0.6 T.)

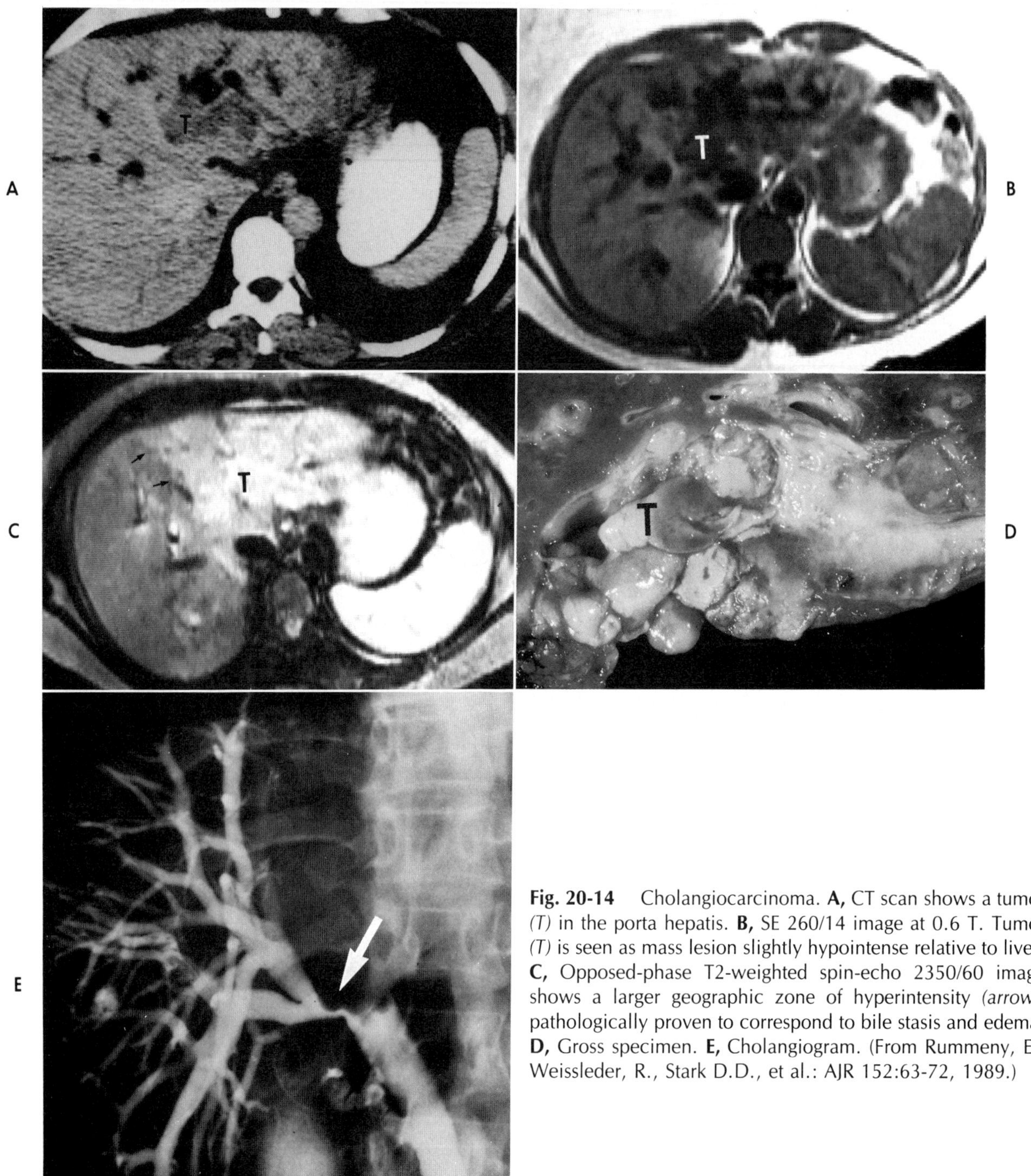

Fig. 20-14 Cholangiocarcinoma. **A,** CT scan shows a tumor *(T)* in the porta hepatis. **B,** SE 260/14 image at 0.6 T. Tumor *(T)* is seen as mass lesion slightly hypointense relative to liver. **C,** Opposed-phase T2-weighted spin-echo 2350/60 image shows a larger geographic zone of hyperintensity *(arrow)*, pathologically proven to correspond to bile stasis and edema. **D,** Gross specimen. **E,** Cholangiogram. (From Rummeny, E., Weissleder, R., Stark D.D., et al.: AJR 152:63-72, 1989.)

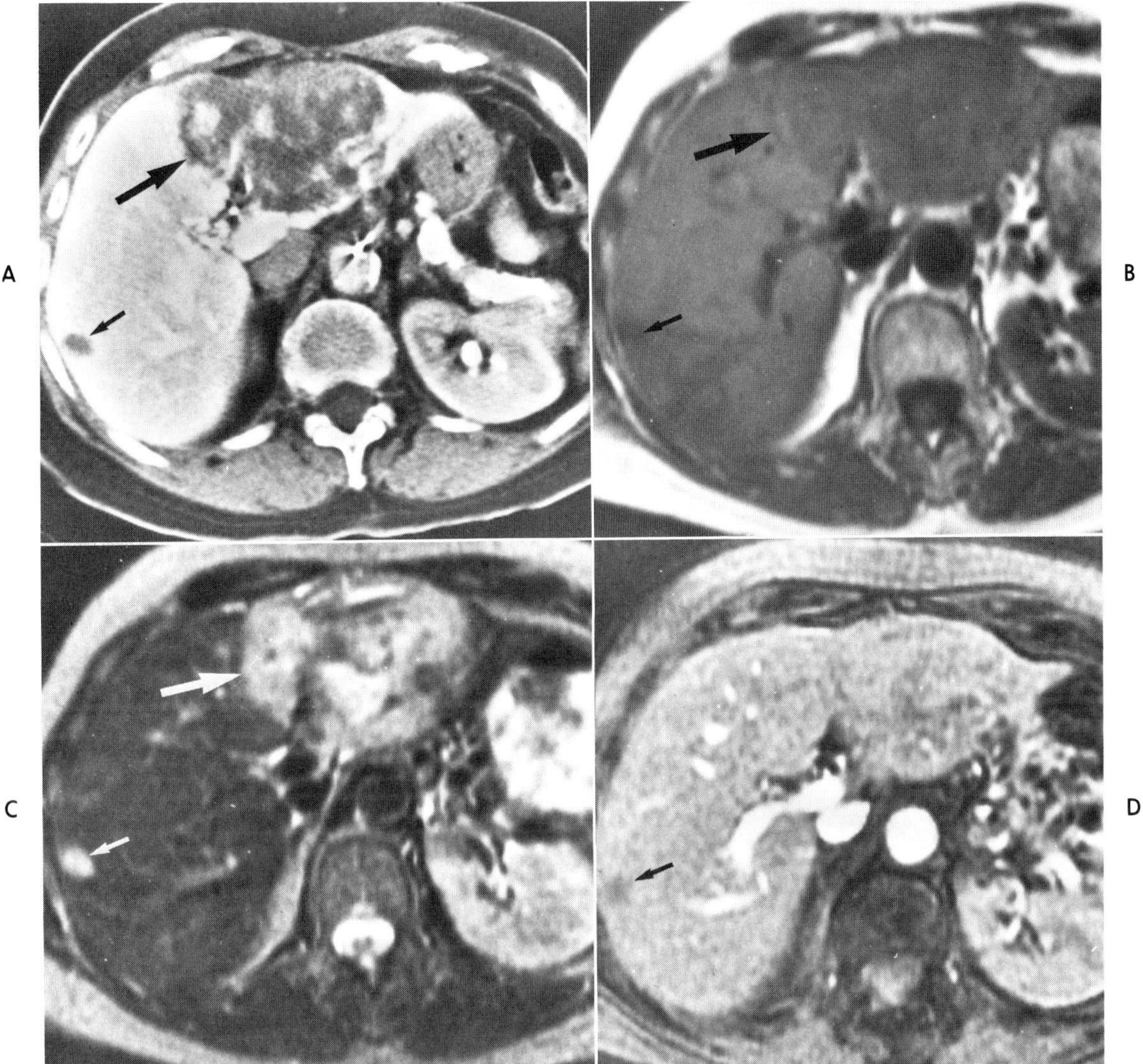

Fig. 20-15 Peripheral cholangiocarcinoma and benign cyst. **A,** CT during arterial portography reveals a large heterogeneous mass in the left lobe *(large arrow)* and a small lesion *(small arrow)* in the right lobe. **B,** On the SE 400/20 image at 1.5 T the mass in the left lobe *(large arrow)* is slightly hypointense, whereas the smaller mass in the right lobe *(small arrow)* is less intense. **C,** T2-weighted image (SE 2500/100). The mass in the left lobe is hyperintense and heterogeneous. The peripheral lesion, a surgically proven benign cyst with clear fluid, has higher signal intensity and distinct borders. **D,** On the corresponding GRASS image (25/13, flip angle 20 degrees), the cholangiocarcinoma is isointense and heterogeneous, whereas the cyst *(arrow)* is hypointense.

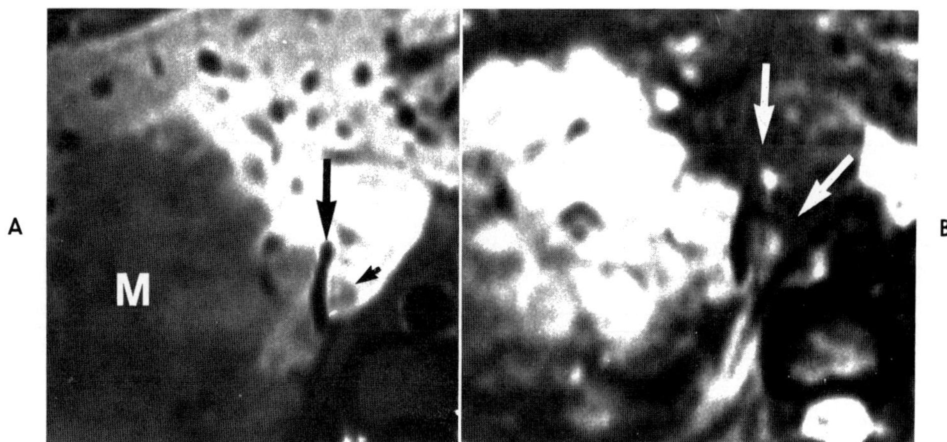

Fig. 20-16 Metastatic cholangiocarcinoma after resection of a central primary tumor, with compression of the inferior vena cava detected by duplex Doppler ultrasound. Patency could not be confirmed. **A,** Axial SE 600/20 image at 1.5 T. A lobulated low-signal mass *(M)* is noted, compressing a patent inferior vena cava *(large arrow)*. Note a small satellite nodule to the left of the inferior vena cava *(small arrow)*, **B,** Individual lesions are seen better on the corresponding T2-weighted image (SE 2500/80).

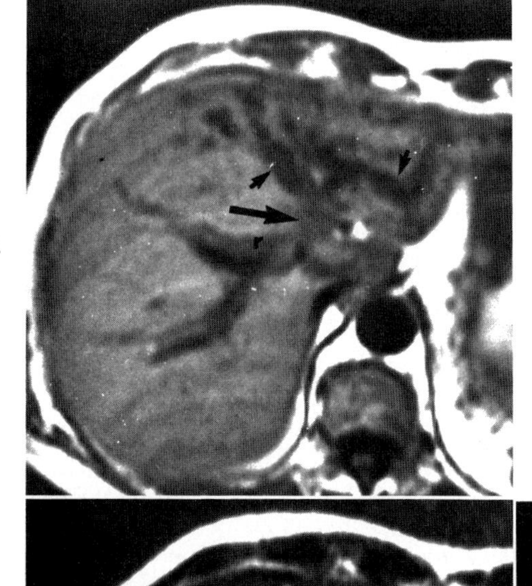

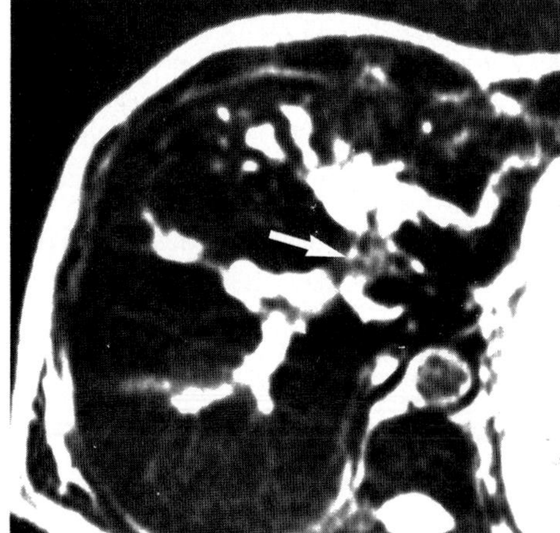

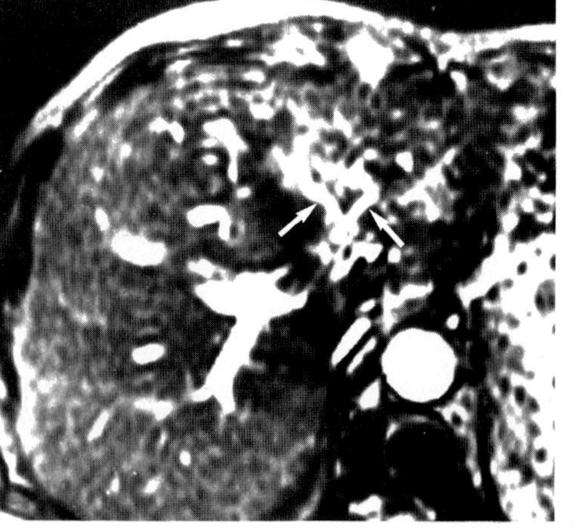

Fig. 20-17 Central cholangiocarcinoma with biliary and portal vein obstruction. **A,** Axial SE 400/20 image at 1.5 T reveals a low-signal mass *(large arrow)* associated with biliary dilatation *(small arrows)* in the left lobe. The right bile duct *(r)* is mildly dilated as well. **B,** On the corresponding T2-weighted image (SE 2500/100), the mass *(arrow)* is intermediate in intensity between liver and dilated bile ducts. Because of gradient moment nulling, hepatic vessels have high intensity, rendering them difficult to distinguish from bile ducts. **C,** Corresponding GRASS image (25/13, flip angle 20 degrees) depicts irregular collateral vessels in the left lobe *(arrows)*, indicating obstruction of the left portal vein.

Pancreatic Adenocarcinoma

Improved artifact suppression has made effective MR imaging of the pancreas possible. In general, T1-weighted images are more useful for imaging the pancreas, even at high field. This is because the T1 relaxation time of the pancreas is even shorter than that of the liver (see Table 7-1, p 56). At 1.5 T, T1-weighted images with fat suppression depict the pancreas as higher signal than other solid nonfatty tissues, even liver (Fig. 21-1). On these images, lower signal of pancreas than liver should be considered abnormal but non-specific. Morphologic signs should be examined for differential diagnosis of pancreatic disease. Improved resolution and signal-to-noise ratio (SNR) resulting from the combined use of breath-hold sequences and optimized surface coils may extend the use of MRI for pancreatic diagnosis (Fig. 21-2).

CLINICAL BACKGROUND

Most patients with pancreatic adenocarcinoma present with biliary or gastrointestinal obstruction or pain resulting from invasion of retroperitoneal nerves. By this time, the tumor is usually unresectable. The pancreas does not have a true capsule, and there is no barrier to spread beyond the confines of the gland. The only hope for cure is if the tumor can be detected when it is less than 2 cm in diameter and if it is confined entirely within the gland.[225,239] Since there is no effective method for screening the general population, few tumors are detected at this stage.[93]

In spite of the dismal prognosis in most cases, there is a role for effective noninvasive diagnosis and staging of pancreatic carcinoma. If the tumor can be identified, the diagnosis can be made by guided biopsy. Cross-sectional imaging is important for presurgical staging. Signs of unresectability include invasion of bowel or major vessels, such as the portal vein, superior mesenteric artery or vein, or common hepatic artery.[101,239,409] In patients with unresectable tumors who undergo palliative surgery, imaging can be useful for operative planning and/or intraoperative irradiation.

LOW- AND MID-FIELD MRI

Until recently, the image quality of MRI was inadequate for diagnosis of most pancreatic disease.[498] In a blinded retrospective study of 101 examinations performed for liver metastases, three times as many pancreatic masses were detected by CT as by MRI.[500] In a series of 29 patients with cancer of the pancreas, CT detected 27 and MRI only 20.[125] In another series, MRI was consistently unable to demonstrate pancreatic carcinomas smaller than 3 cm.[550] All of these studies were published in 1987 and used MRI technqiues with minimal or absent motion artifact suppression and without fat suppression or oral contrast.

At low and mid field, the MR tissue characteristics of normal pancreas are similar to those of normal liver. Like liver tumors, pancreatic tumors tend to have a longer T1 and longer T2 than either normal liver tissue or normal pancreatic tissue (Fig. 21-3). However, Steiner et al found that a difference in signal intensity was discernible in only 63% of cases on T1-weighted images and in only 40% of T2-weighted images.[507] In many of these cases the entire gland might have had abnormal signal resulting from pancreatic duct obstruction, preventing delineation of cancer as a low-signal mass. Even when signal intensity differences are visible, motion-induced artifact may cause the tumor to present only as a region of heterogeneity, not as segmentation of the pancreas into discrete zones of clearly differing signal intensity.

MRI reliably detects metastatic deposits of pancreatic carcinoma in the liver, therefore the limited success of MRI in detecting pancreatic adenocarcinoma by signal intensity differences alone may be due to increased noise over the pancreas. When motion-artifact suppression is suboptimal and when fat signal is not suppressed, detection of pancreatic adenocarcinoma depends largely on demonstration of a space-occupying mass deforming the pancreatic contour.[125] Experience with fat suppression at mid and low field is limited at the present time.

HIGH-FIELD MRI

At 1.5 T with fat suppression, cancer is depicted as a low-signal mass, with intensity similar to that of the spleen. The normal pancreas, on the other hand, is even brighter than the liver. When tumors are located in the body or tail of the pancreas, or when the tumor is small and has not obstructed the pancreatic duct, the cancer

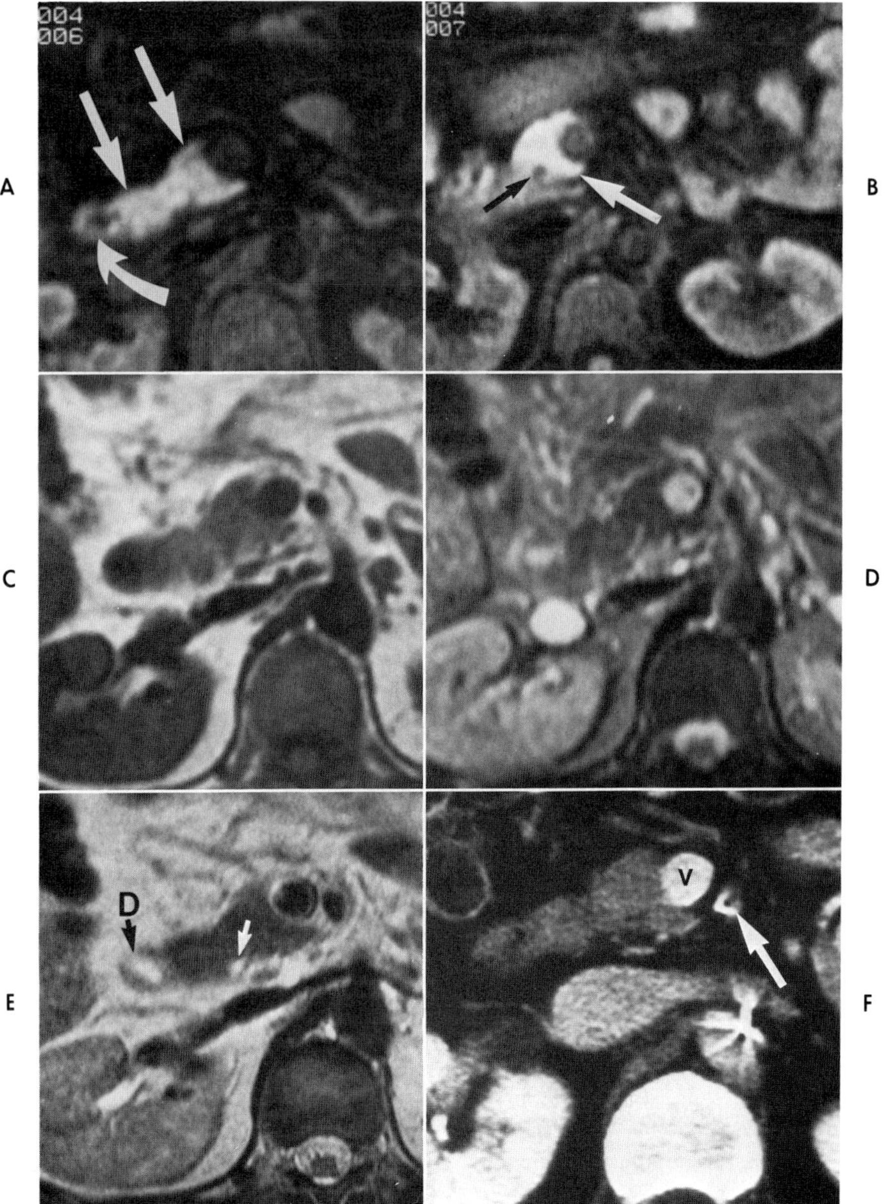

Fig. 21-1 Irregular shape of pancreatic head at 1.5 T: a normal variant. **A** and **B,** Fat suppressed SE 450/13 (combination of saturation and opposed-phase techniques) demonstrates irregular shape of the pancreatic head *(large arrows).* The signal intensity is well within normal limits, excluding a mass lesion as the cause for irregular shape. *Curved arrows =* duodenum, *small black arrow =* common bile duct. **C,** Axial SE 450/11 image without fat suppression, corresponding to **A. D,** Axial SE 2500/100 image. The pancreas is not delineated well. **E,** T2-weighted conjugate (fast) SE image (TR/TE = 6000/102, matrix = 512 × 256, four signals averaged, 19 images obtained in 6:24 [m:s]). Delineation of pancreas is superior to that in **D.** *D =* duodenum, *arrow =* common bile duct. **F,** Images from CT during arterial portography depict inferior contrast between pancreas and duodenum. *Arrow =* catheter in the superior mesenteric artery, *V =* superior mesenteric vein. (From Mitchell, D.G., Shapiro, A., Scharicht, A., et al.: AJR [in press].)

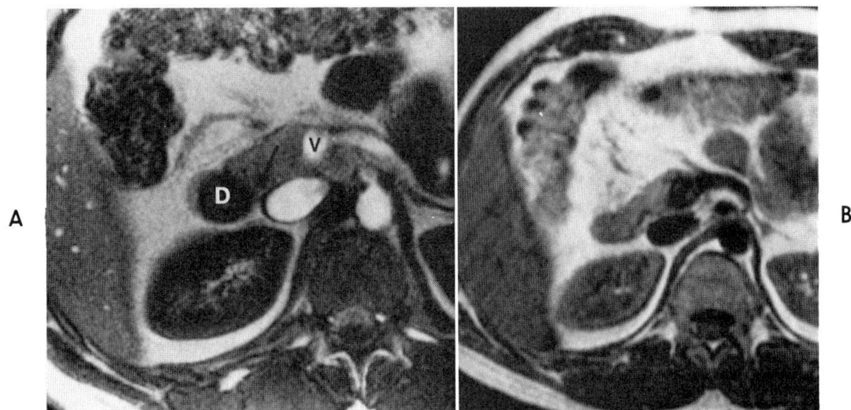

Fig. 21-2   Images in a normal volunteer demonstrate potential of surface coil techniques for imaging the pancreas. **A,** Snapshot inversion recovery image of a normal volunteer using flexible phased-array body coil (TR/TE/TI = 14.5/3.5/550 with centric phase order; matrix = 256 × 256, field of view = 24 cm^2, two signals averaged, acquisition time for six images = 48 sec). D = duodenum, *arrow* = common bile duct, V = confluence of splenic and superior mesenteric veins. **B,** SE 400/11 image using standard body coil (matrix = 256 × 192, 36-cm^2 field of view, two signals averaged, acquisition time for nine images = 2:43). (Acquired as a cooperative venture by investigators from the Hospital of the University of Pennsylvania, Thomas Jefferson University Hospital, and General Electric Medical Systems. From Mitchell, D.G., Shapiro, A., Scharicht, A., et al.: AJR [in press].)

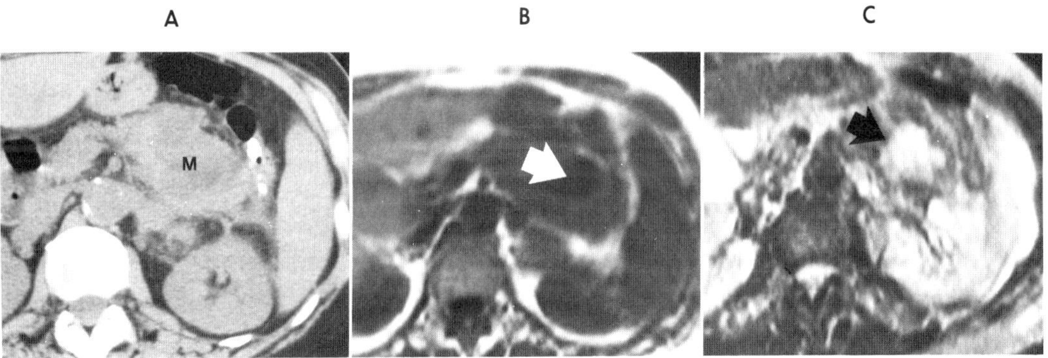

Fig. 21-3   Adenocarcinoma involving the tail of the pancreas. **A,** Unenhanced CT scan shows large mass *(M)* with low attenuation center obliterating the tail of the pancreas. **B** and **C,** Axial T1-weighted (SE 275/14) and T2-weighted (SE 2350/120) axial MR images demonstrate a mass with a necrotic center *(arrow).* The pancreatic head is small and has higher signal intensity on both MR images.

can be seen as a low signal defect within the pancreas (Figs. 21-4 to 21-6). Many tumors, however, are located in the pancreatic head and have caused glandular atrophy before presentation. In these patients the signal intensity of the remainder of the pancreas is abnormally low on T1-weighted images (Figs. 21-7 to 21-9). In some cases a small amount of residual pancreatic tissue with normal signal may be noted at the posterior aspect of the uncinate process (Figs. 21-5, 21-10).

The pancreas should not be considered normal on high field fat suppressed T1-weighted images unless it has signal intensity equal to or greater than that of normal liver. The liver rarely, if ever, has pathologically increased signal on fat-suppressed T1-weighted images, so it serves as a good standard compared with which the pancreas should have increased signal. If the liver has abnormally decreased intensity, such as in patients with iron overload or severe edema, an abnormal pancreas might appear falsely normal. In patients with low-signal livers, the renal cortex is another internal standard that may be used.

Although pancreatic tumors may be depicted as high-signal masses on T2-weighted images (see Fig. 21-6), contrast between pancreatic parenchyma and tumor is usually limited on T2-weighted images, even with fat

Text continues on page 236.

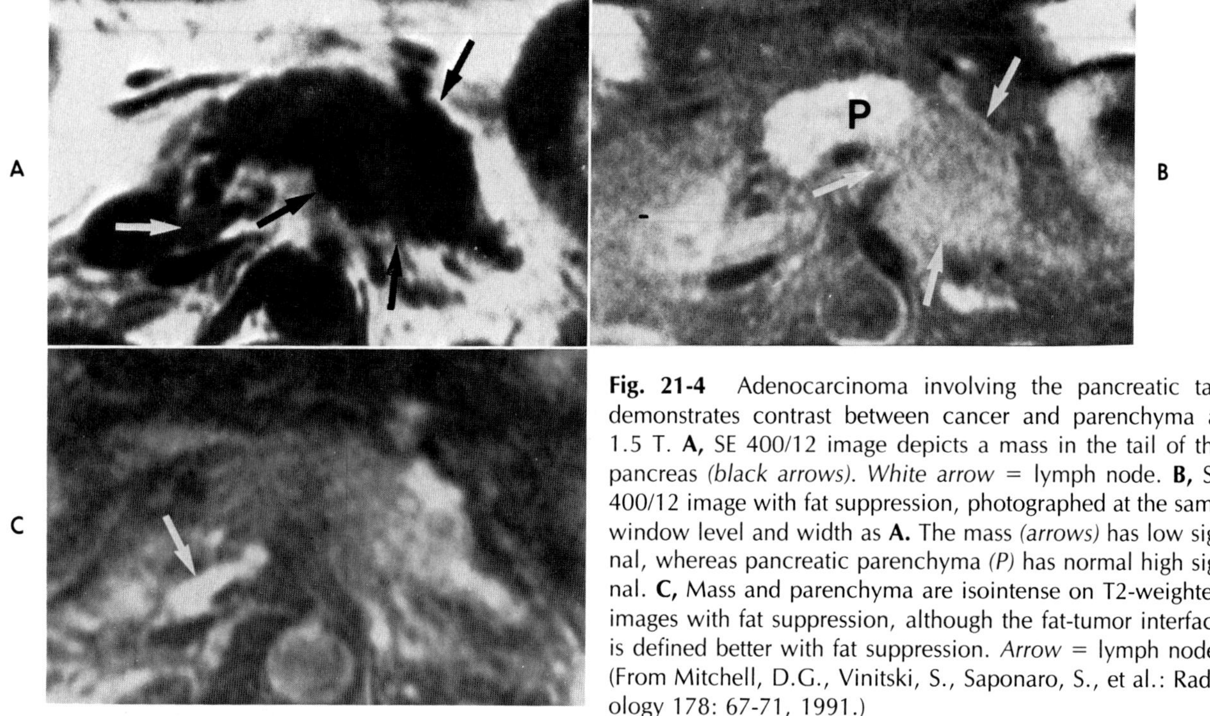

Fig. 21-4 Adenocarcinoma involving the pancreatic tail demonstrates contrast between cancer and parenchyma at 1.5 T. **A,** SE 400/12 image depicts a mass in the tail of the pancreas *(black arrows). White arrow* = lymph node. **B,** SE 400/12 image with fat suppression, photographed at the same window level and width as **A.** The mass *(arrows)* has low signal, whereas pancreatic parenchyma *(P)* has normal high signal. **C,** Mass and parenchyma are isointense on T2-weighted images with fat suppression, although the fat-tumor interface is defined better with fat suppression. *Arrow* = lymph node. (From Mitchell, D.G., Vinitski, S., Saponaro, S., et al.: Radiology 178: 67-71, 1991.)

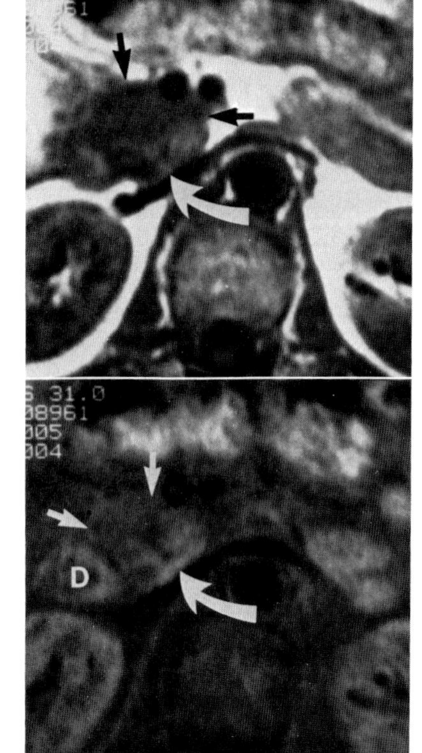

Fig. 21-5 Adenocarcinoma of the pancreatic head with normal signal of the posterior portion of the uncinate process. **A,** SE 400/12 image at 1.5 T reveals a mass in the pancreatic head *(straight arrows)* with apparent sparing of the posterior uncinate process *(curved arrows).* **B,** SE 400/12 image with fat suppression accentuates the contrast between tumor and parenchyma. The separation of duodenum *(D)* from pancreas is more apparent with fat suppression.

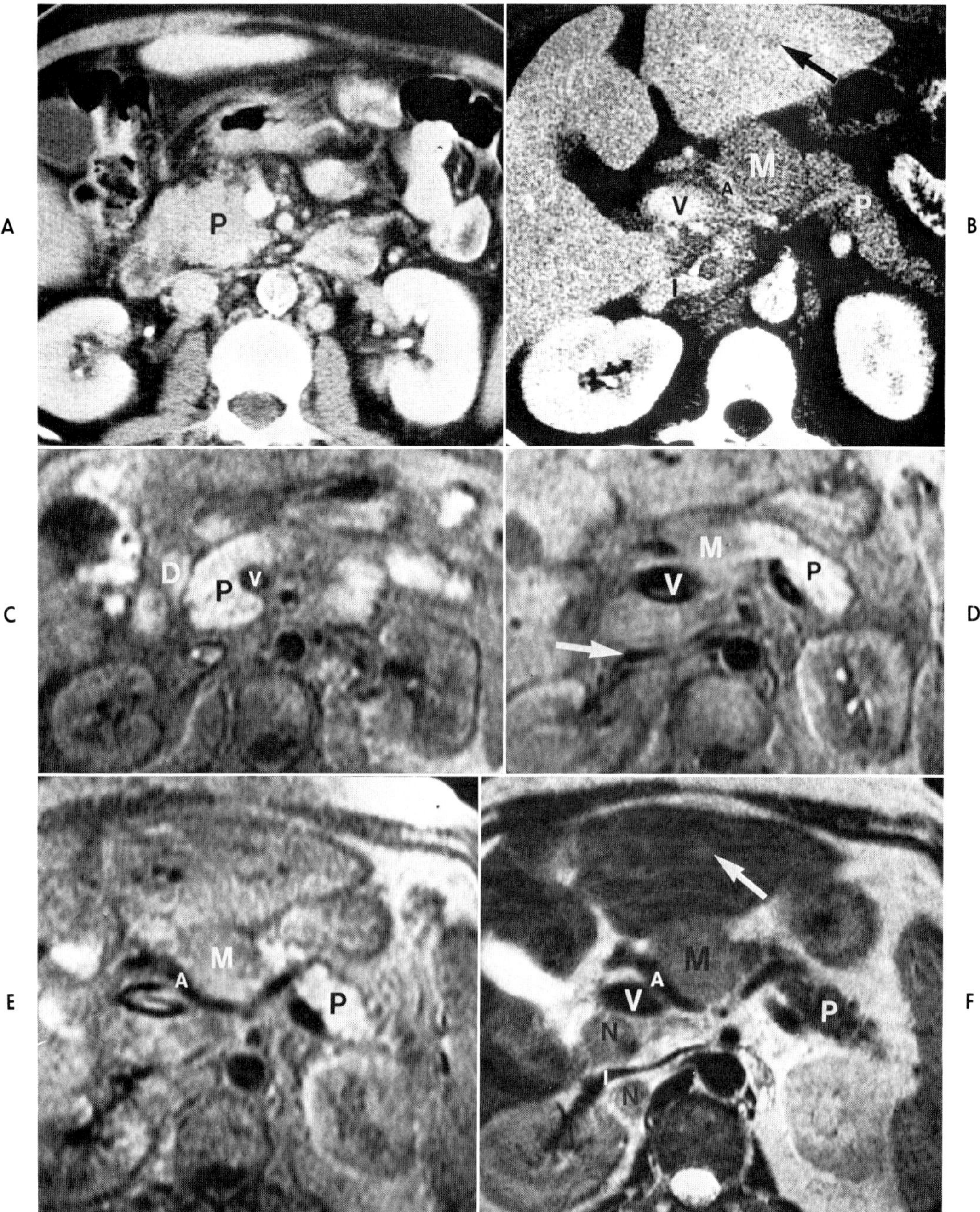

Fig. 21-6 Carcinoma arising from the superior surface of the pancreas. **A,** Image from CT with arterial portography reveals a prominent pancreatic head *(P)* that is not clearly separated from the duodenum. **B,** At a higher level, a large mass *(M)* displaces the hepatic artery *(A)* posteriorly. Additional masses are contiguous with the inferior vena cava *(I)* and portal vein *(V)*. The masses have the same attenuation as the pancreatic tail *(P)*. *Straight arrow =* hepatic metastasis. **C,** Fat suppressed SE 500/11 image slightly above **A** reveals normal signal of the pancreatic head *(P)*. The duodenum *(D)*, isointense with suppressed lipid signal in this image, probably contributed to the impression of enlarged pancreatic head in **A.** *V =* superior mesenteric vein. **D,** At a higher level, the low-signal mass *(M)* is seen adjacent to the pancreatic body and tail *(P)*, which has normal signal intensity. *V =* portal vein. *Arrow* indicates inferior vena cava. **E,** At a higher level, the mass (M) displaces the hepatic artery *(A)* posteriorly. **F,** T2-weighted conjugate (fast) SE image (TR/TE = 7000/102, matrix = 512 × 256, four signals averaged, 21 images obtained in 7:28 (m:s)). *Arrow =* hepatic metastasis. *A =* hepatic artery, *I =* inferior vena cava, *M =* mass, *N =* nodes, *V =* portal vein. At surgery, extensive tumor was noted superior to the pancreas, with a relatively normal gland inferiorly. (From Mitchell, D.G., Shapiro, A., Scharicht, A., et al.: AJR [in press].)

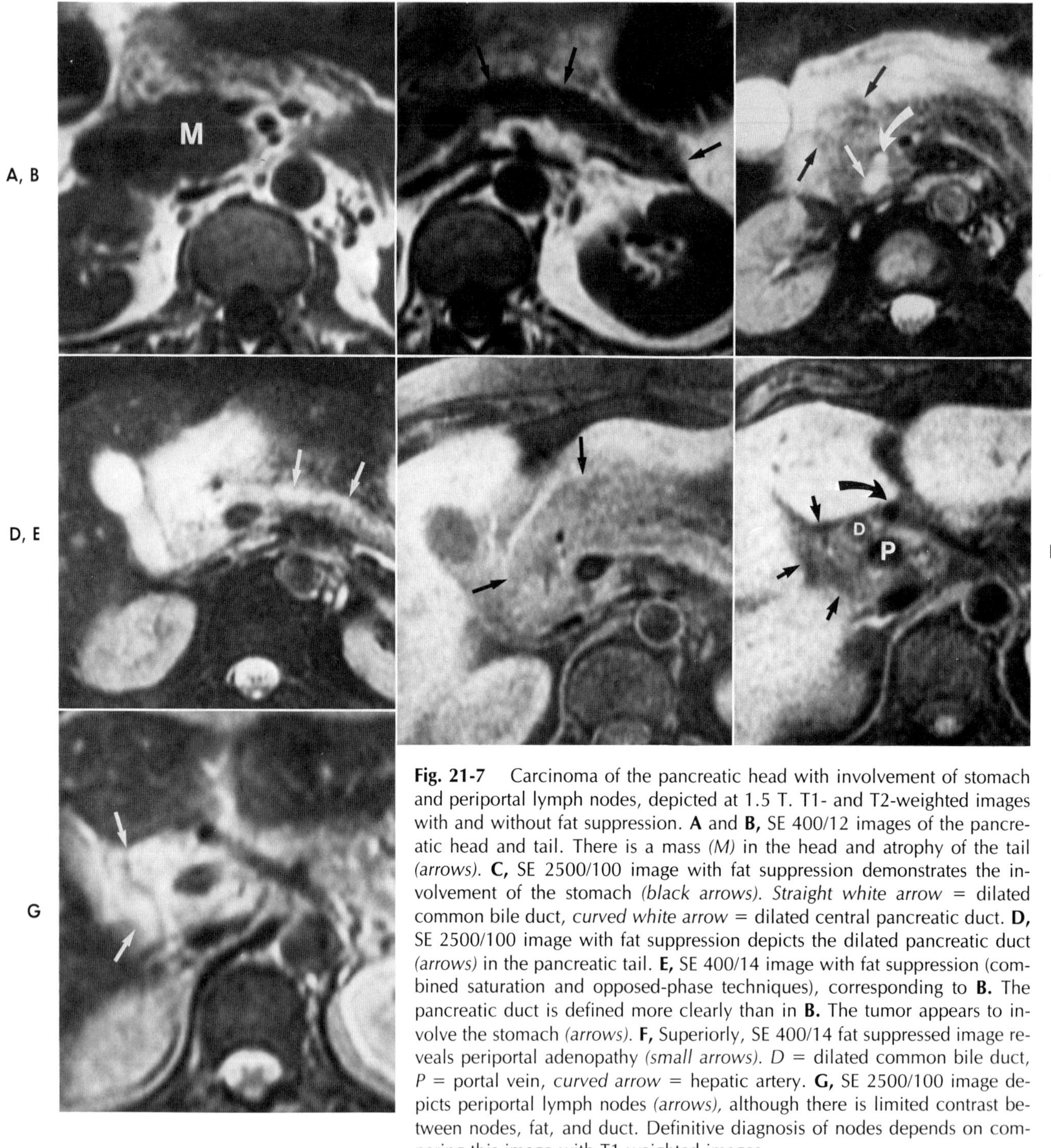

Fig. 21-7 Carcinoma of the pancreatic head with involvement of stomach and periportal lymph nodes, depicted at 1.5 T. T1- and T2-weighted images with and without fat suppression. **A** and **B,** SE 400/12 images of the pancreatic head and tail. There is a mass *(M)* in the head and atrophy of the tail *(arrows).* **C,** SE 2500/100 image with fat suppression demonstrates the involvement of the stomach *(black arrows). Straight white arrow* = dilated common bile duct, *curved white arrow* = dilated central pancreatic duct. **D,** SE 2500/100 image with fat suppression depicts the dilated pancreatic duct *(arrows)* in the pancreatic tail. **E,** SE 400/14 image with fat suppression (combined saturation and opposed-phase techniques), corresponding to **B.** The pancreatic duct is defined more clearly than in **B.** The tumor appears to involve the stomach *(arrows).* **F,** Superiorly, SE 400/14 fat suppressed image reveals periportal adenopathy *(small arrows). D* = dilated common bile duct, *P* = portal vein, *curved arrow* = hepatic artery. **G,** SE 2500/100 image depicts periportal lymph nodes *(arrows),* although there is limited contrast between nodes, fat, and duct. Definitive diagnosis of nodes depends on comparing this image with T1-weighted images.

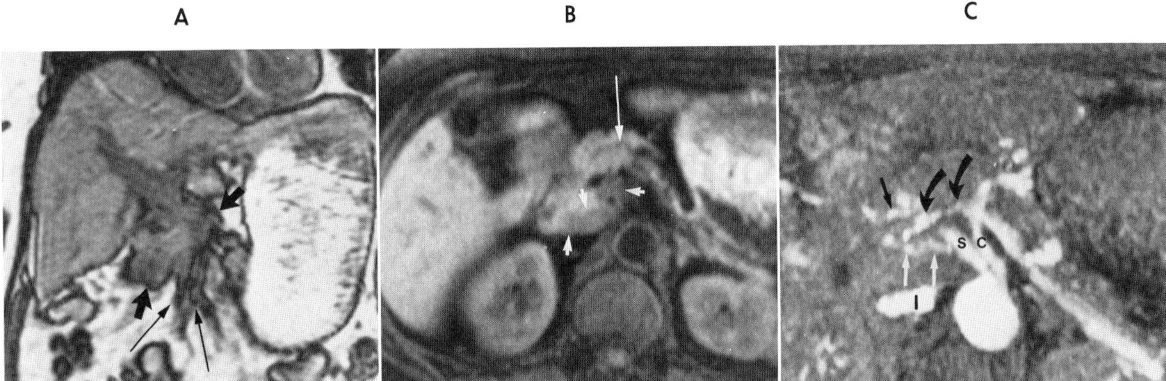

Fig. 21-8 Carcinoma involving the pancreatic head with encasement of the portal vein and hepatic arteries. **A,** Coronal T1-weighted gradient echo image at 1.5 T (TR/TE/flip angle = 101/2.5/90 degrees) reveals a mass at the superior portion of the pancreatic head *(short arrows)*. *Long arrows* = superior mesenteric artery and vein. **B,** SE 500/14 image with fat suppression (combined saturation and opposed-phase techniques) reveals a low-signal mass posteriorly *(short arrows)*. The body of the pancreas has slightly decreased signal intensity, isointense to liver, but otherwise appears within normal limits. *Long arrow* = normal pancreatic duct. **C,** Corresponding MR angiographic slab (TR/TE/flip angle = 27/7.4/20 degrees) reveals encasement of the central splenic and proximal portal veins *(curved arrows)*, hepatic artery *(straight black arrow)*, and replaced right hepatic artery *(white arrows)*. C = celiac trunk, *I* = inferior vena cava, *S* = superior mesenteric artery.

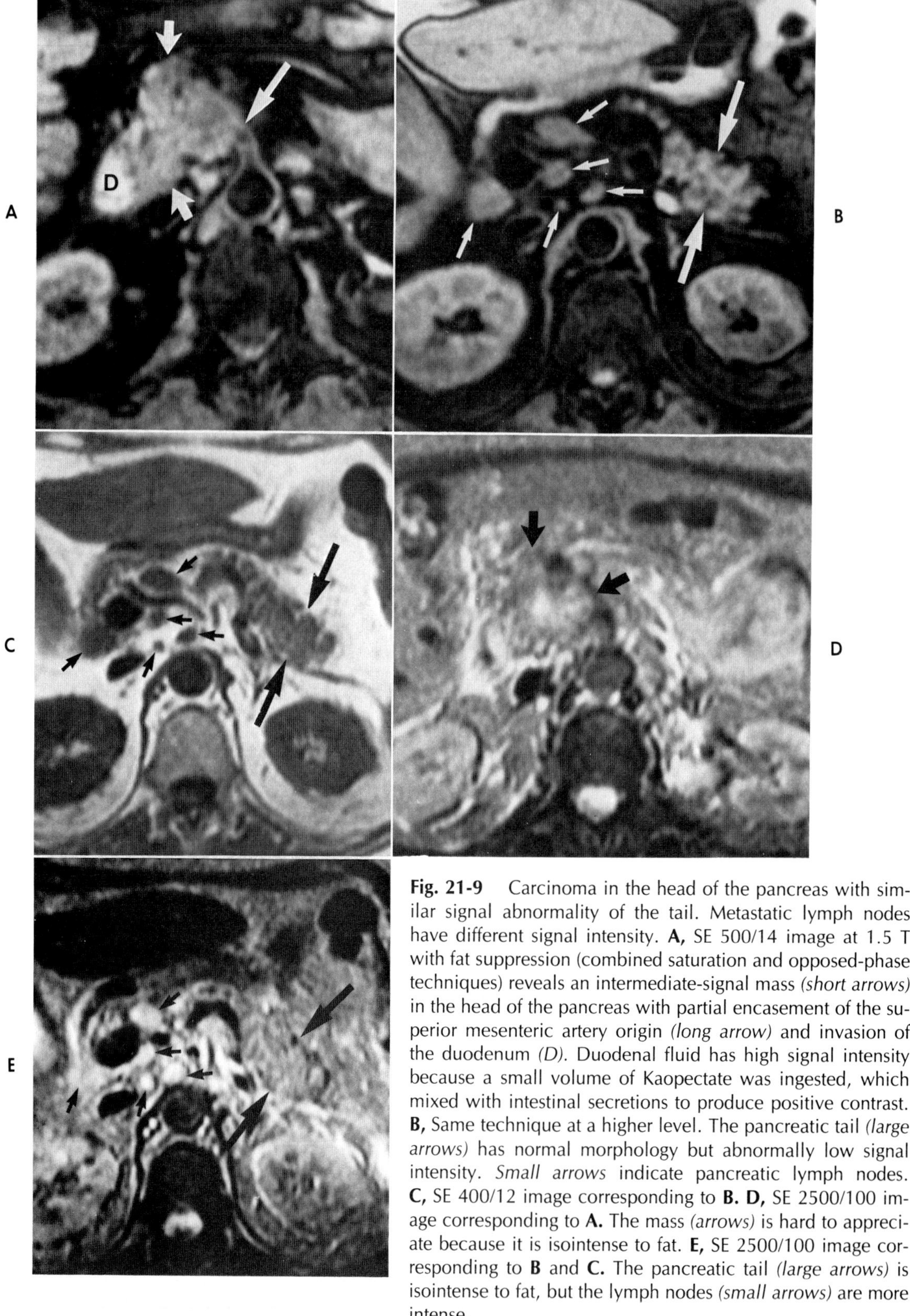

Fig. 21-9 Carcinoma in the head of the pancreas with similar signal abnormality of the tail. Metastatic lymph nodes have different signal intensity. **A,** SE 500/14 image at 1.5 T with fat suppression (combined saturation and opposed-phase techniques) reveals an intermediate-signal mass *(short arrows)* in the head of the pancreas with partial encasement of the superior mesenteric artery origin *(long arrow)* and invasion of the duodenum *(D)*. Duodenal fluid has high signal intensity because a small volume of Kaopectate was ingested, which mixed with intestinal secretions to produce positive contrast. **B,** Same technique at a higher level. The pancreatic tail *(large arrows)* has normal morphology but abnormally low signal intensity. *Small arrows* indicate pancreatic lymph nodes. **C,** SE 400/12 image corresponding to **B. D,** SE 2500/100 image corresponding to **A.** The mass *(arrows)* is hard to appreciate because it is isointense to fat. **E,** SE 2500/100 image corresponding to **B** and **C.** The pancreatic tail *(large arrows)* is isointense to fat, but the lymph nodes *(small arrows)* are more intense.

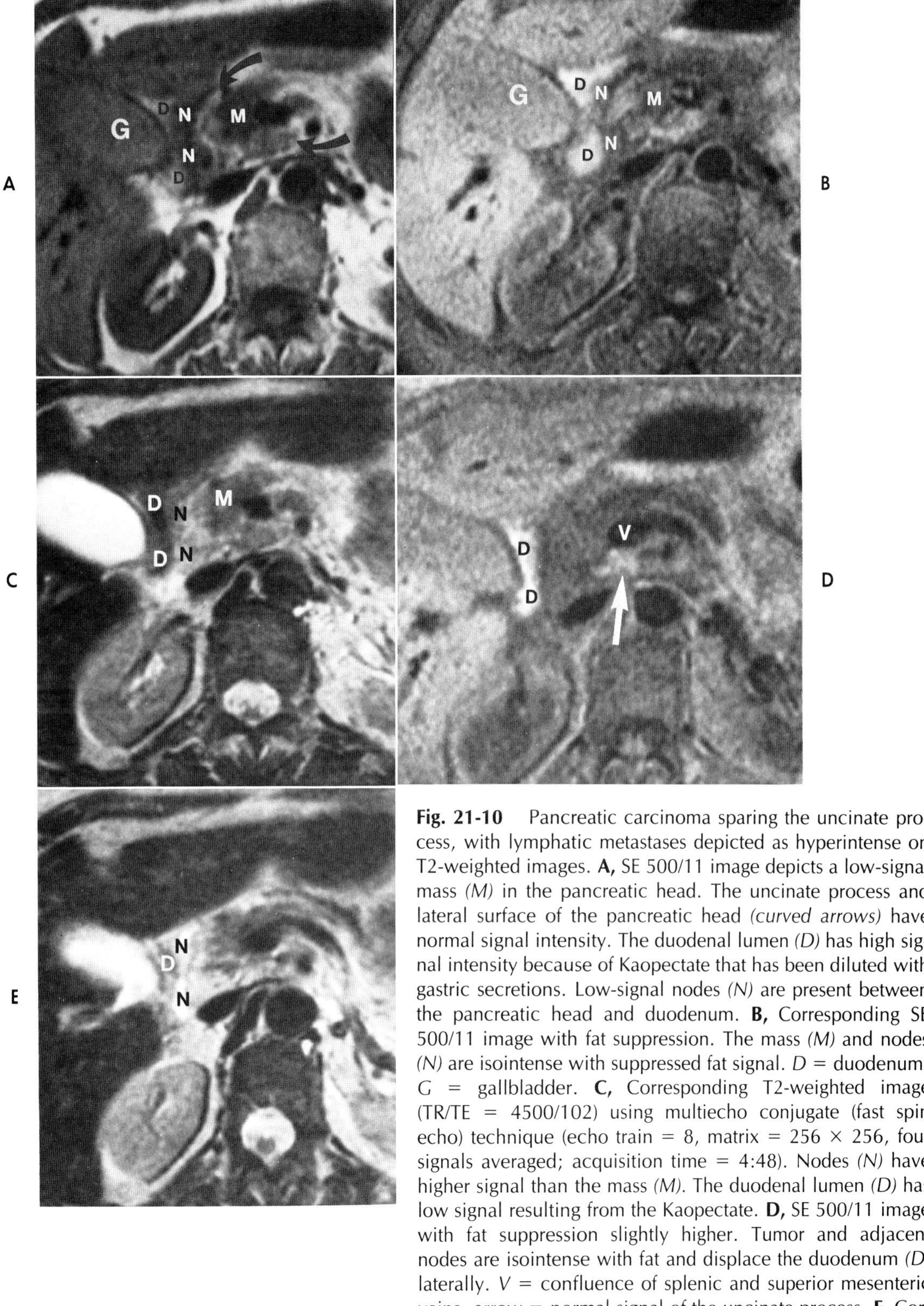

Fig. 21-10   Pancreatic carcinoma sparing the uncinate process, with lymphatic metastases depicted as hyperintense on T2-weighted images. **A,** SE 500/11 image depicts a low-signal mass *(M)* in the pancreatic head. The uncinate process and lateral surface of the pancreatic head *(curved arrows)* have normal signal intensity. The duodenal lumen *(D)* has high signal intensity because of Kaopectate that has been diluted with gastric secretions. Low-signal nodes *(N)* are present between the pancreatic head and duodenum. **B,** Corresponding SE 500/11 image with fat suppression. The mass *(M)* and nodes *(N)* are isointense with suppressed fat signal. D = duodenum, G = gallbladder. **C,** Corresponding T2-weighted image (TR/TE = 4500/102) using multiecho conjugate (fast spin echo) technique (echo train = 8, matrix = 256 × 256, four signals averaged; acquisition time = 4:48). Nodes *(N)* have higher signal than the mass *(M)*. The duodenal lumen *(D)* has low signal resulting from the Kaopectate. **D,** SE 500/11 image with fat suppression slightly higher. Tumor and adjacent nodes are isointense with fat and displace the duodenum *(D)* laterally. V = confluence of splenic and superior mesenteric veins, *arrow* = normal signal of the uncinate process. **E,** Corresponding T2-weighted image (as in **C**). N = nodes.

suppression (Figs. 21-4, 21-7, 21-9, and 21-11). Fat suppression may improve T2-weighted images, however, by improving contrast between tumor and surrounding fat. On multiecho conjugate (fast) SE images, the high signal of fat usually produces clear fat planes in the absence of fat suppression (see Fig. 21-6).

Detection of small pancreatic carcinomas by CT is facilitated by rapid scanning after intravenous bolus injection of iodinated contrast material.[217] Similarly, scanning during the arterial phase after injection of gadopentatate dimeglumine sometimes improves contrast between pancreas and tumor on T1-weighted images, since the cancers are usually less vascular than the pancreas (Fig. 21-12).[73] In some cases, however, pancreatic carcinoma enhances markedly (Fig. 21-13).

Necrosis within tumors of the pancreas has T1 and T2 relaxation times longer than solid tissue and can be readily distinguished from solid pancreatic masses or normal pancreatic tissue (Fig. 21-14). Unfortunately, it is not possible to distinguish fluid within a necrotic tumor from fluid within an inflammatory pseudocyst.

STAGING

MRI has a potential role in staging local spread of pancreatic carcinoma. Because the pancreatic borders are surrounded by retroperitoneal fat, T1-weighted images without fat suppression are best for showing tumor extending beyond the pancreas. This is depicted as foci or strands of intermediate signal intensity extending into the fat (Figs. 21-13, 21-15, and 21-16). In one study, MRI was equal to CT for detecting fat invasion by pancreatic carcinoma.

Vascular patency or occlusion are well demonstrated by MRI (Figs. 21-8, 21-11, 21-14, and 21-17 to 21-22),[125,507,550] but microscopic invasion of the vascular serosa cannot be identified by any imaging technique.

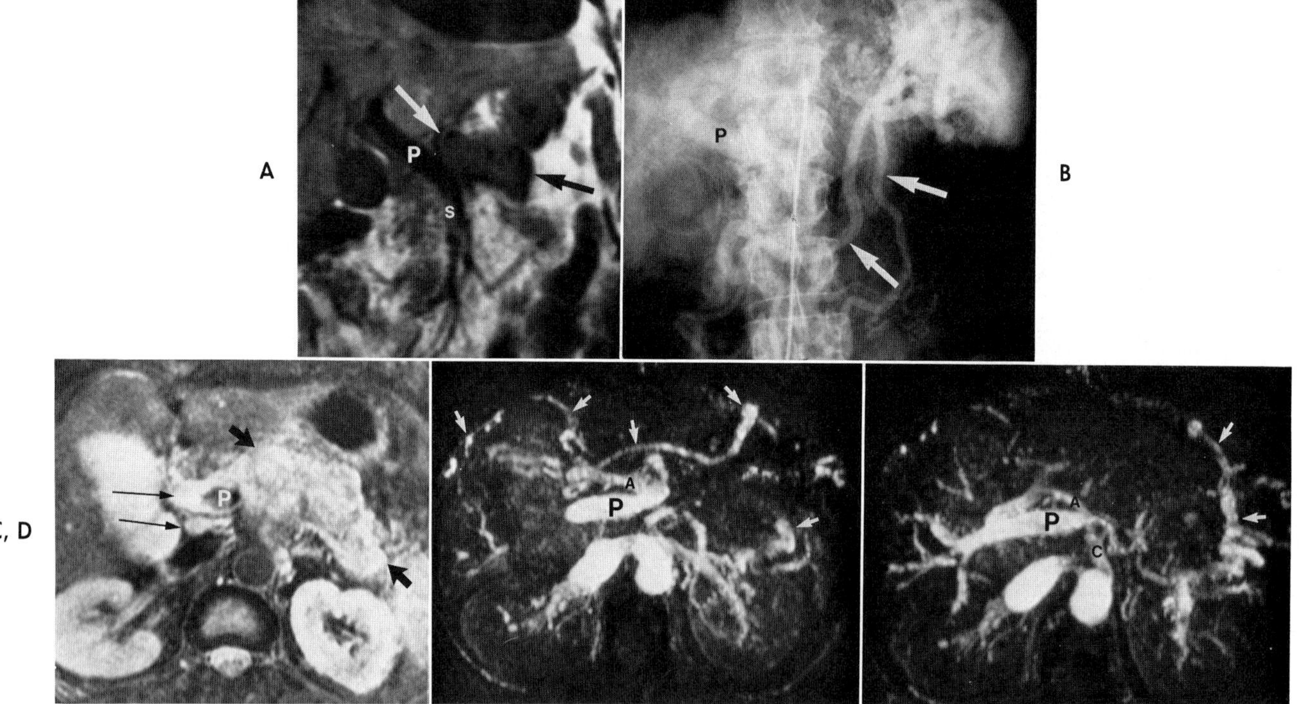

Fig. 21-11   Carcinoma in the body of the pancreas obstructing the splenic vein, depicted at 1.5 T. **A,** Coronal SE 500/20 image reveals a mass *(arrows)* near the origin of the portal *(P)* vein. *S* = superior mesenteric vein. The splenic vein is not visualized. **B,** Venous phase from splenic artery injection. Blood from the spleen drains towards the portal vein *(P)* via dilated gastroepiploic veins *(arrows)*. **C,** Corresponding 2500/100 image with fat suppression. The mass *(short arrows)* is delineated. *Long arrows* = lymph nodes, *P* = portal vein. **D and E,** Axial MR composite MR angiograms inferior to **(D)** and at **(E)** the level of the portal bifurcation, from contiguous 7-mm thick gradient-echo images (TR/TE/flip angle = 27/7.4/20 degrees). The mass is not delineated well, but obstruction of the splenic vein can be seen. *Small arrows* = collateral veins, *A* = hepatic artery, *C* = celiac trunk, *P* = main portal vein.

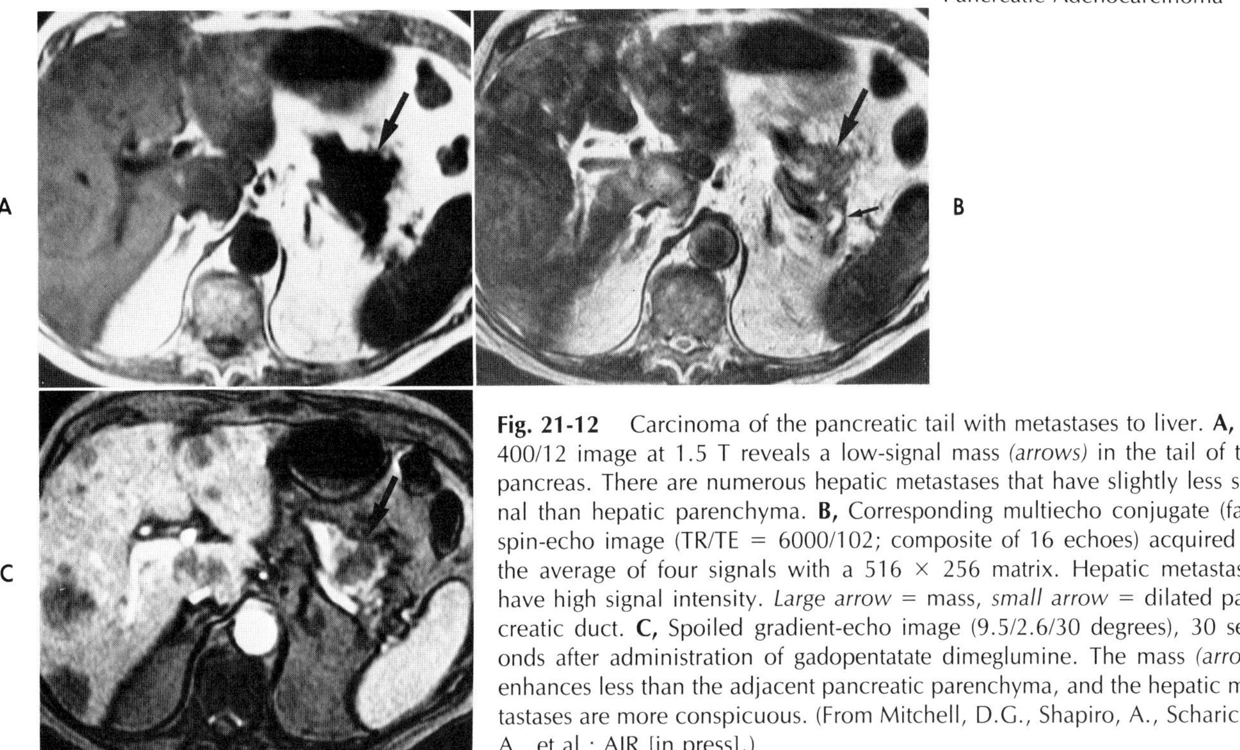

Fig. 21-12 Carcinoma of the pancreatic tail with metastases to liver. **A,** SE 400/12 image at 1.5 T reveals a low-signal mass *(arrows)* in the tail of the pancreas. There are numerous hepatic metastases that have slightly less signal than hepatic parenchyma. **B,** Corresponding multiecho conjugate (fast) spin-echo image (TR/TE = 6000/102; composite of 16 echoes) acquired as the average of four signals with a 516 × 256 matrix. Hepatic metastases have high signal intensity. *Large arrow* = mass, *small arrow* = dilated pancreatic duct. **C,** Spoiled gradient-echo image (9.5/2.6/30 degrees), 30 seconds after administration of gadopentatate dimeglumine. The mass *(arrow)* enhances less than the adjacent pancreatic parenchyma, and the hepatic metastases are more conspicuous. (From Mitchell, D.G., Shapiro, A., Scharicht, A., et al.: AJR [in press].)

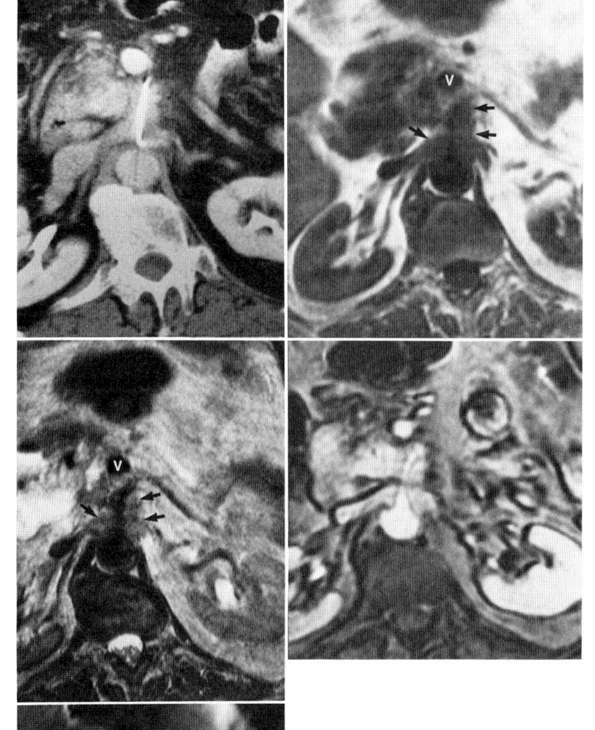

Fig. 21-13 Carcinoma of the pancreatic head and vascular encasement at 1.5 T with marked enhancement. **A,** Image from CT with arterial portography reveals encasement of the superior mesenteric artery (SMA), which is identified by the catheter. **B,** SE 500/11 images demonstrate abnormal low intensity tissue encasing the SMA origin *(arrows)*. V = superior mesenteric vein. **C,** T2-weighted conjugate (fast) SE image (TR/TE = 7000/102, matrix = 512 × 256, four signals averaged, 21 images obtained in 7:28 [m:s]). *Arrows* = high-signal tumor encasing SMA, V = superior mesenteric vein. **D,** T1-weighted gradient-echo images (TR/TE/flip angle = 102/2.3/90 degrees less than 1 minute after administration of gadopentatate dimeglumine demonstrates enhancement of tumor and delineation of vessels. **E,** SE 500/11 images with fat suppression obtained 5 minutes after contrast administration depicts persistent hyperintensity of tumor. (From Mitchell, D.G., Shapiro, A., Scharicht. A., et al.: AJR [in press].)

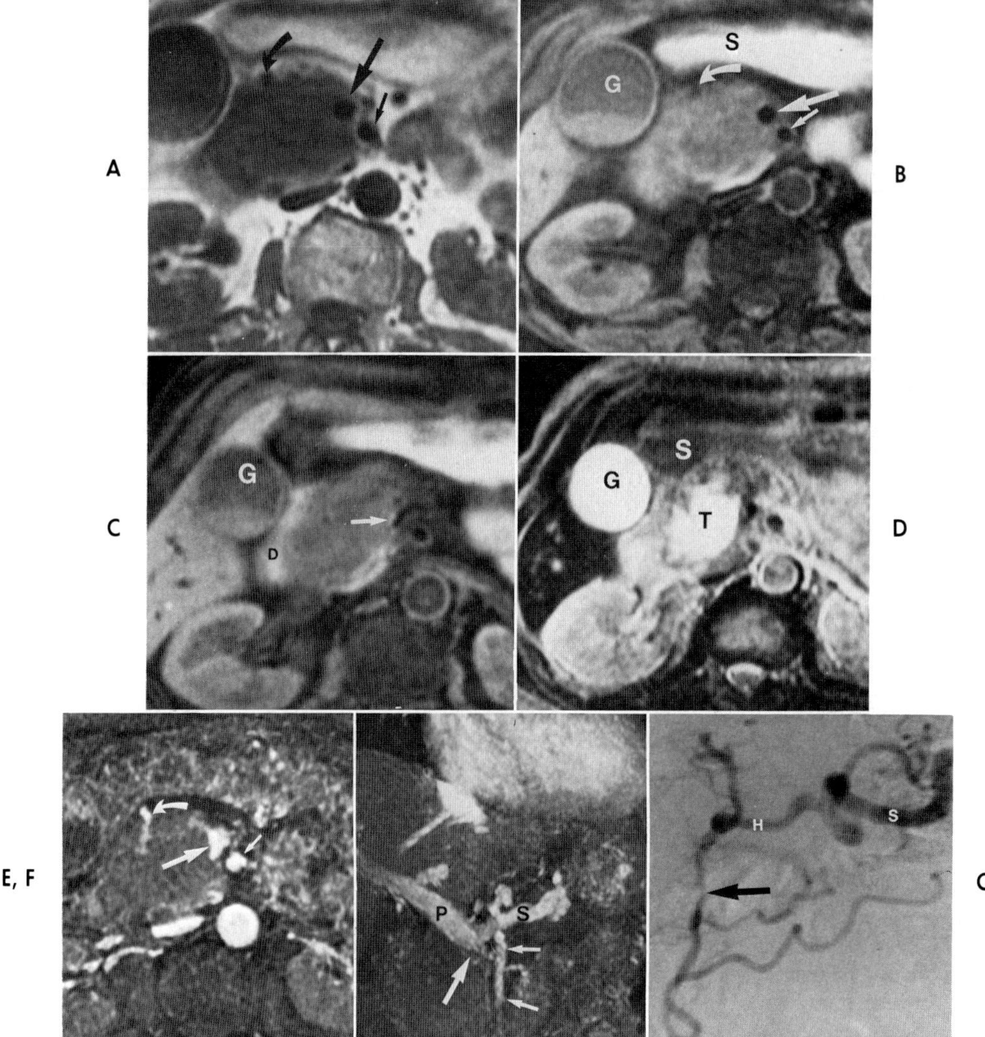

Fig. 21-14 Necrotic pancreatic carcinoma with encasement of the superior mesenteric vein *(large arrow)* and partial encasement of the superior mesenteric *(small arrow)* and gastroduodenal *(curved arrow)* arteries. Kaopectate, diluted with gastric secretions, has produced "positive" contrast on T1-weighted images and "negative" contrast on T2-weighted and gradient-echo images. **A,** SE 400/12 image at 1.5 T. **B,** SE 500/14 image with fat suppression (combined saturation and opposed-phase techniques) depicts the tumor as much less intense than liver. *G* = gallbladder, *S* = stomach. **C,** As in **B,** one section higher. The cephalad portion of the superior mesenteric vein is narrowed *(arrow)*. *D* = duodenum. **D,** SE 2500/100 image corresponding to **C.** Much of the tumor *(T)* appears necrotic. *G* = gallbladder, *S* = stomach. **E,** Axial composite MR angiogram and **F,** Coronal composite MR angiogram show encasement of the superior mesenteric vein *(large arrow)* and gastroduodenal artery *(curved arrow)*. *Small arrows* = superior mesenteric artery. *P* = portal vein, *S* = splenic vein. **G,** Digital subtraction arteriogram confirming encasement of the gastroduodenal artery *(arrow)*. *H* = common hepatic artery, *S* = splenic artery. The venous phase was not technically adequate. (From Mitchell, D.G., Shapiro, A., Scharicht, A., et al.: AJR [in press].)

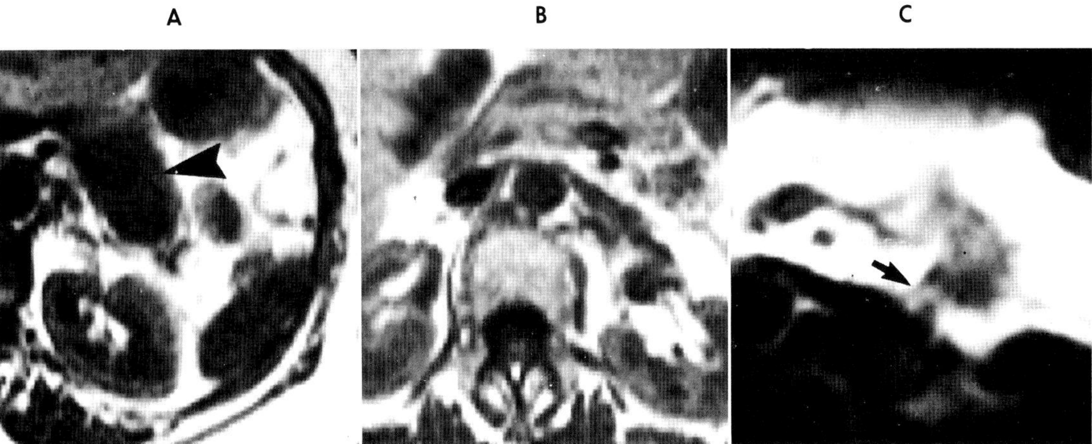

Fig. 21-15   Carcinoma of the pancreatic tail. **A,** Tumor is seen as a focal enlargement *(arrowhead)* with low signal intensity relative to the liver. **B,** Body coil image 1 cm caudal to **A.** Retroperitoneal tissue planes appear intact. **C,** Surface coil at same level as **B** shows retroperitoneal extension of tumor *(arrows)* involving the left renal vein. This finding was confirmed at surgery.

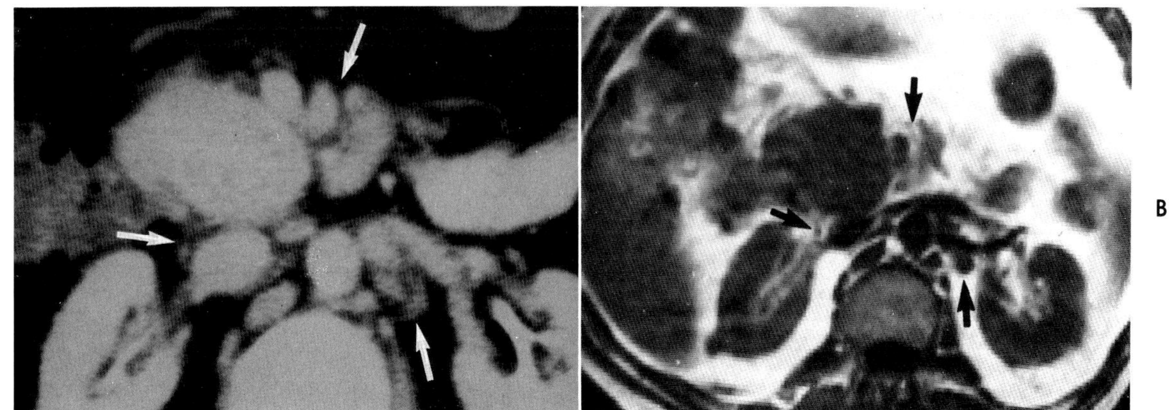

Fig. 21-16   Pancreatic adenocarcinoma. **A,** CT scan shows a 4-cm pancreatic head mass. Lymphadenopathy and infiltration of retroperitoneal fat *(arrows)* indicate nonresectability. **B,** SE 3400/14 image shows the pancreatic head cancer and retroperitoneal infiltration.

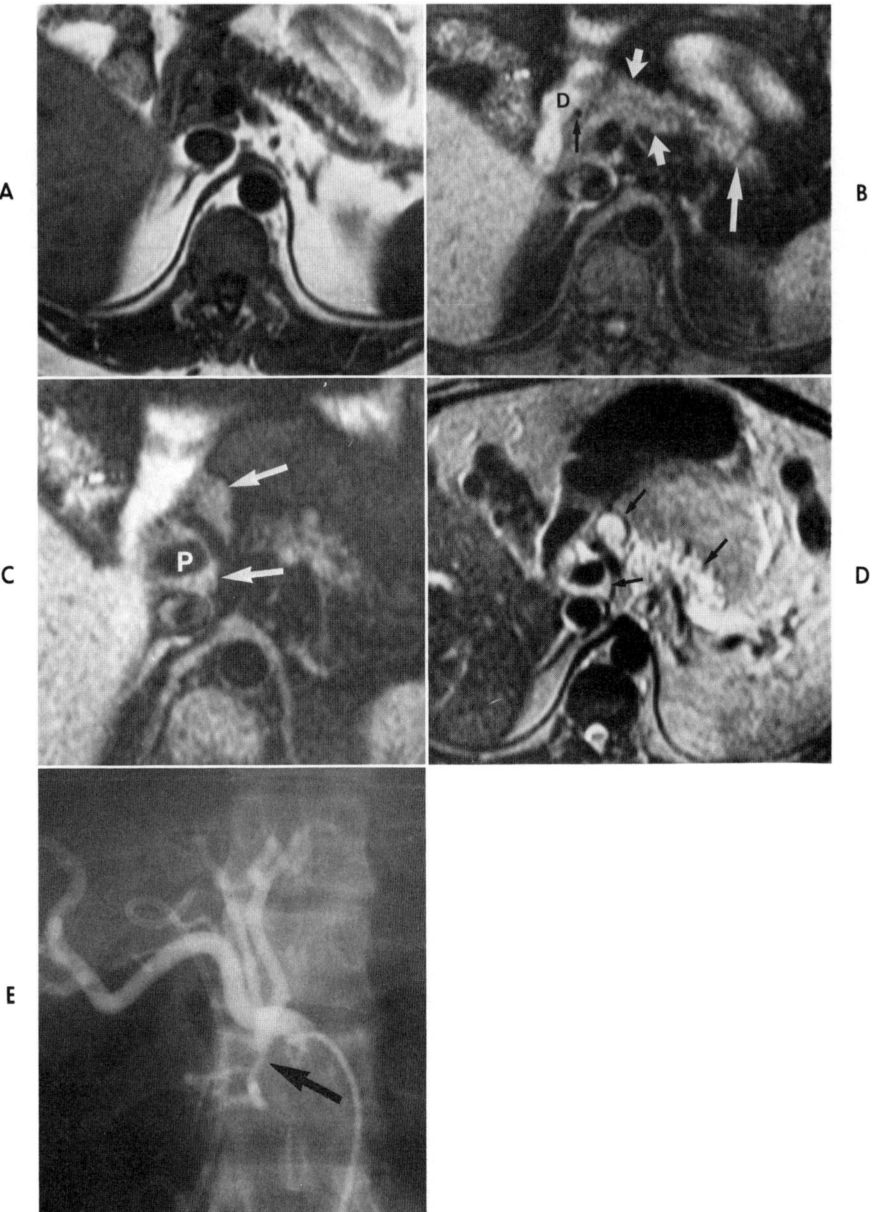

Fig. 21-17 Pancreatic carcinoma with peripancreatic lymph nodes and gastroduodenal artery encasement. **A,** SE 400/12 image at 1.5 T. The pancreas appears grossly normal. **B,** Corresponding SE 500/14 image with fat suppression (combined saturation and opposed-phase techniques) shows that the pancreatic head and body *(short arrows)* are less intense than the liver. Signal intensity of the pancreatic tail *(large arrow)* may be normal. Additionally, the pancreatic tail has a normal marbled texture, different from the homogeneous texture of the remainder of the gland. Improved dynamic range allows clear depiction of the gastroduodenal artery *(black arrow),* which is encased by tumor. The duodenum *(D)* appears invaded. **C,** Fat-suppressed SE 500/14 image one section higher reveals suprapancreatic lymph nodes *(arrows)* that are less intense than liver. *P* = portal vein. **D,** SE 2500/100 image at a level between that of **B** and **C.** The pancreas and lymph nodes *(arrows)* are hyperintense. **E,** Hepatic arteriogram demonstrates encasement of the gastroduodenal artery *(arrow).*

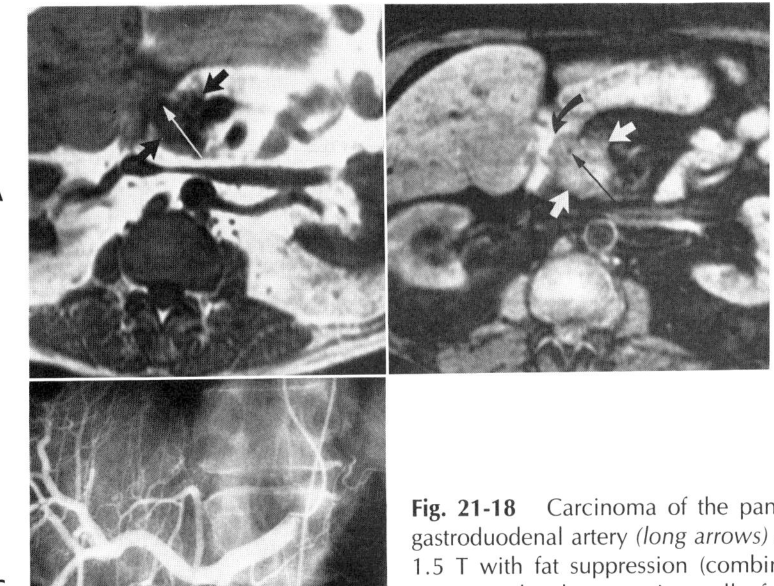

Fig. 21-18   Carcinoma of the pancreatic head *(short arrows)* with encasement of the gastroduodenal artery *(long arrows)* at 1.5 T. **A,** SE 400/12 image. **B,** SE 500/14 image at 1.5 T with fat suppression (combined saturation and opposed-phase techniques). The mass invades the posterior wall of the gastric antrum *(curved arrow).* **C,** Arterial phase radiographic angiogram from selective hepatic artery injection confirms the encasement *(arrow)* of the gastroduodenal artery.

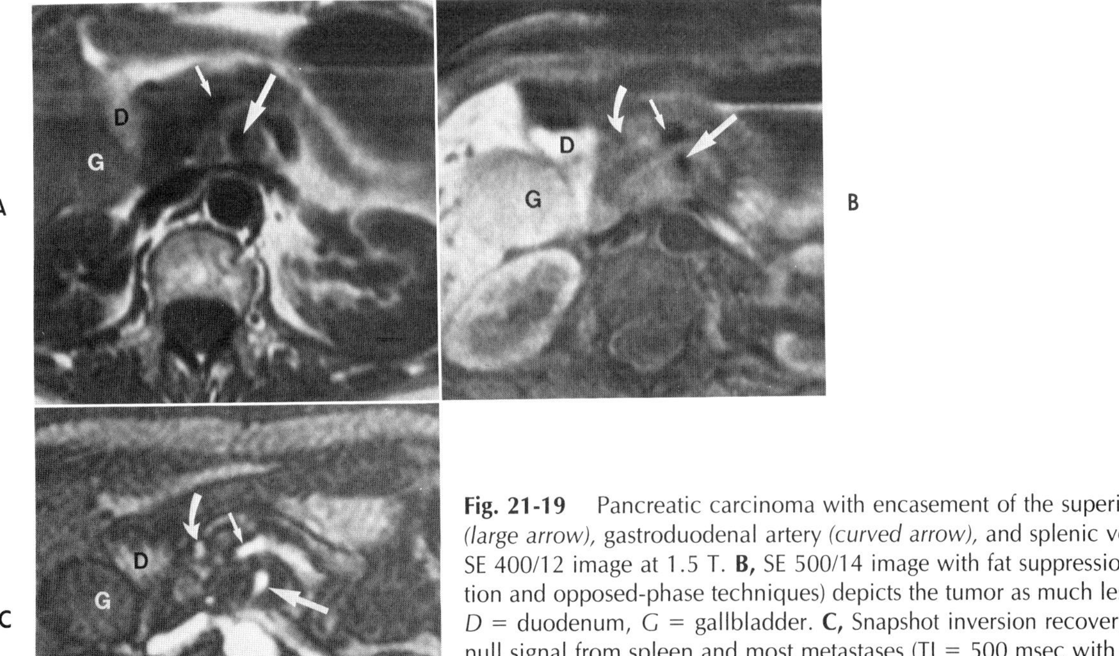

Fig. 21-19   Pancreatic carcinoma with encasement of the superior mesenteric artery *(large arrow),* gastroduodenal artery *(curved arrow),* and splenic vein *(small arrow).* **A,** SE 400/12 image at 1.5 T. **B,** SE 500/14 image with fat suppression (combined saturation and opposed-phase techniques) depicts the tumor as much less intense than liver. *D* = duodenum, *G* = gallbladder. **C,** Snapshot inversion recovery image designed to null signal from spleen and most metastases (TI = 500 msec with centric phase order) depicts the tumor as a virtual signal void. Blood vessels have high signal intensity because of the wash-in effect on this single-slice acquisition.

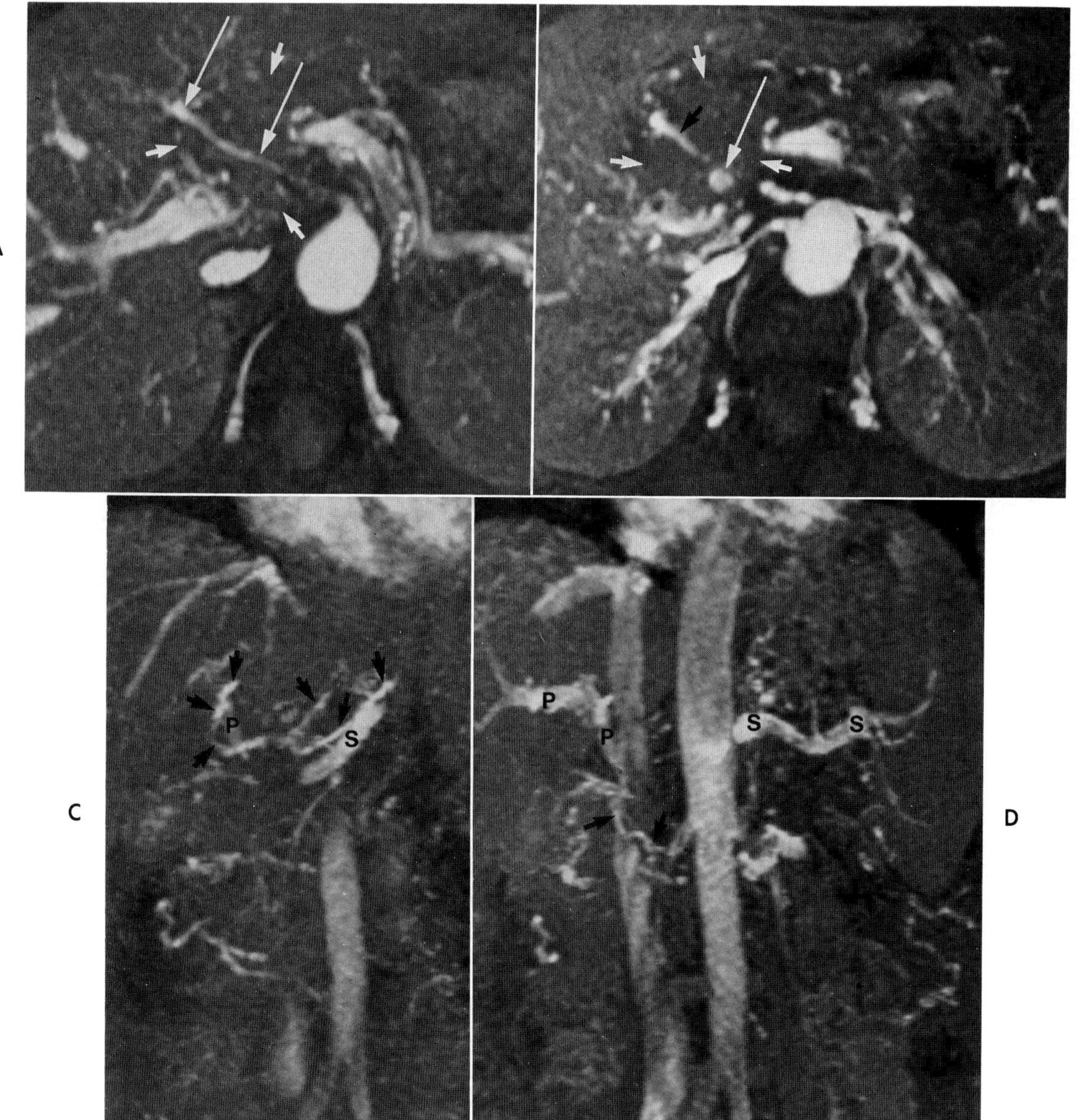

Fig. 21-20   MR angiographic depiction at 1.5 T of portal vein encasement by pancreatic carcinoma. **A,** Axial MR angiographic slab depicts a mass *(short arrows)* that splays the hepatic artery *(long arrows).* **B,** At a lower level, the mass *(short white arrows)* encases the main portal vein *(long arrow). Black arrow* = hepatic artery **C,** Coronal MR angiographic slab depicts the mass interrupting the portal *(P)* and splenic *(S)* veins. *Arrows* = celiac axis. **D,** Coronal MR image posterior to **C** depicts a pancreatoduodenal collateral vein *(arrows)* reconstituting the portal vein *(P). S* = splenic vein.

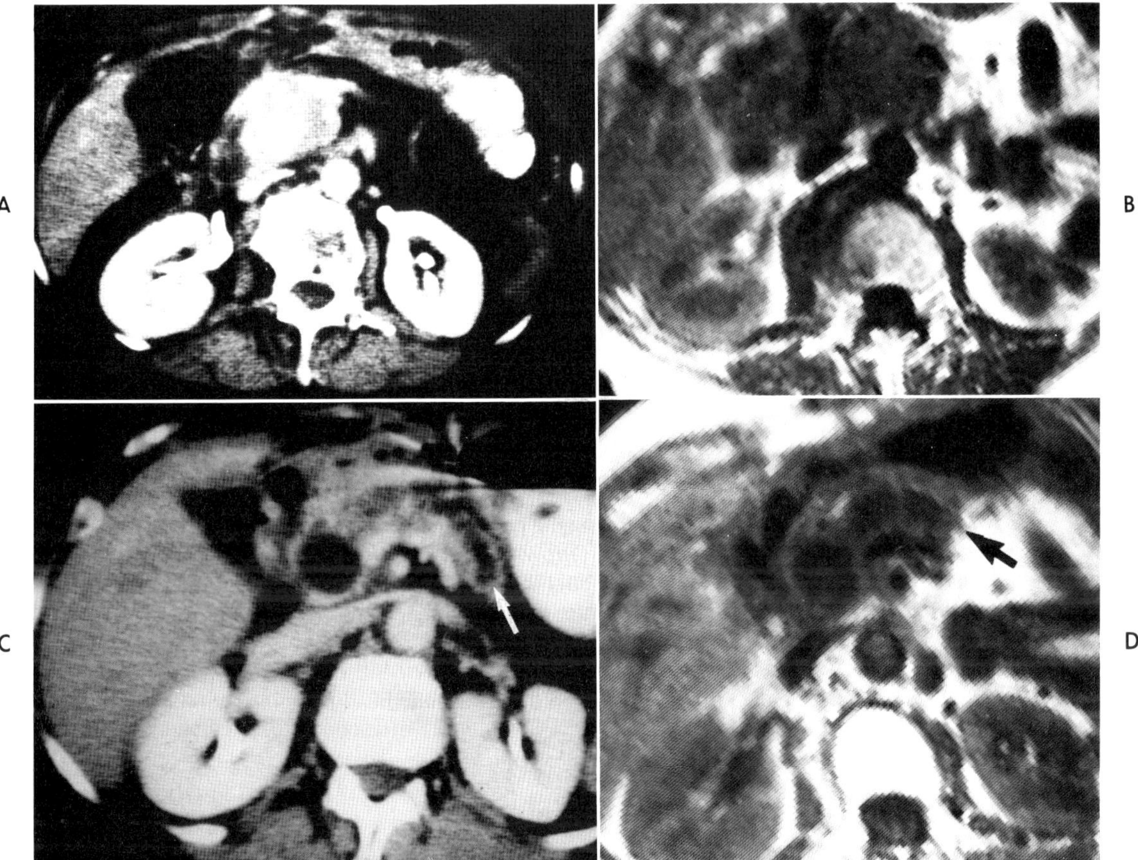

Fig. 21-21   Carcinoma of the pancreatic head and dilated pancreatic duct. **A,** CT scan shows a pancreatic head mass encasing the superior mesenteric artery and vein. **B,** SE 500/20 high-resolution image acquired with a 7-mm thick slice and 192 phase-encoding steps (1.8 × 2.7 × 7.0 mm voxel size). Pancreatic tumor encases the superior mesenteric artery and vein. **C,** CT scan 1.5 cm cephalad to **A** shows dilated common bile duct and dilated pancreatic duct *(arrow)*. **D,** SE 500/20 high-resolution image shows the double-duct sign of pancreatic cancer.

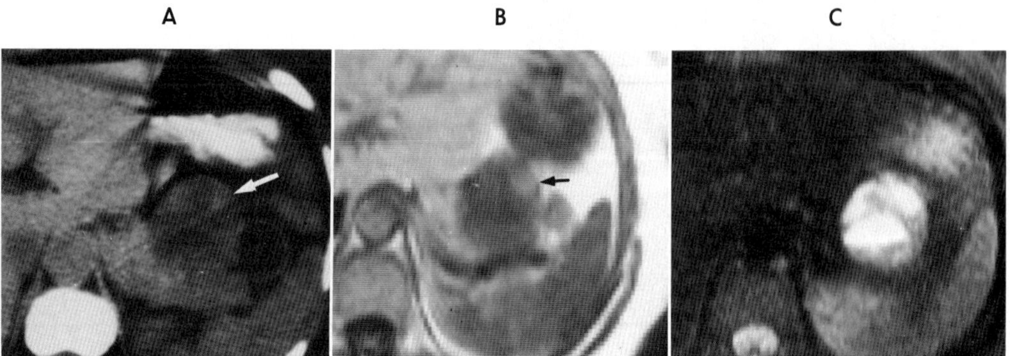

Fig. 22-7 Pancreatic gastrinoma. **A,** CT scan shows hypodense mass anterior to pancreatic tail. Heterogeneous density is seen within mass *(arrow).* **B,** SE 260/15 image shows the x-ray dense portion of mass to have high signal intensity or short T1. **C,** SE 2000/180. Portions of the mass have extremely high signal intensity.

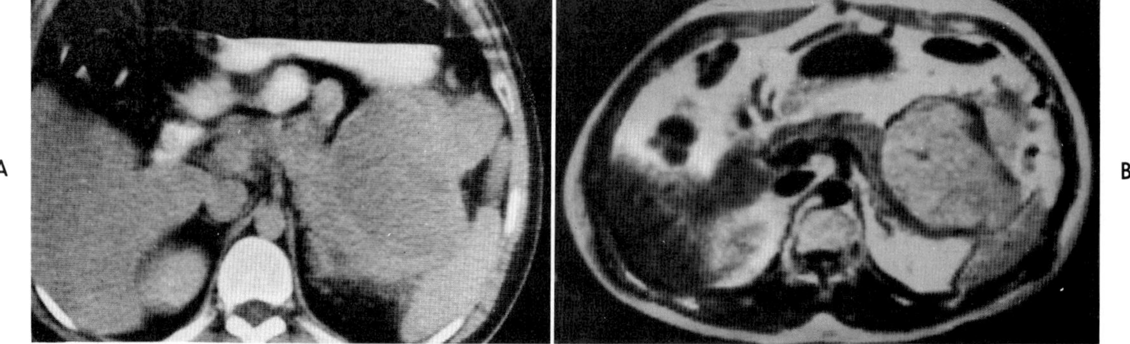

Fig. 22-8 Nonfunctioning islet cell tumor of the pancreatic tail. **A,** CT scan shows a large mass, slightly hypodense relative to the pancreas. **B,** SE 1500/28 image shows a sharply circumscribed mass in the pancreatic tail.

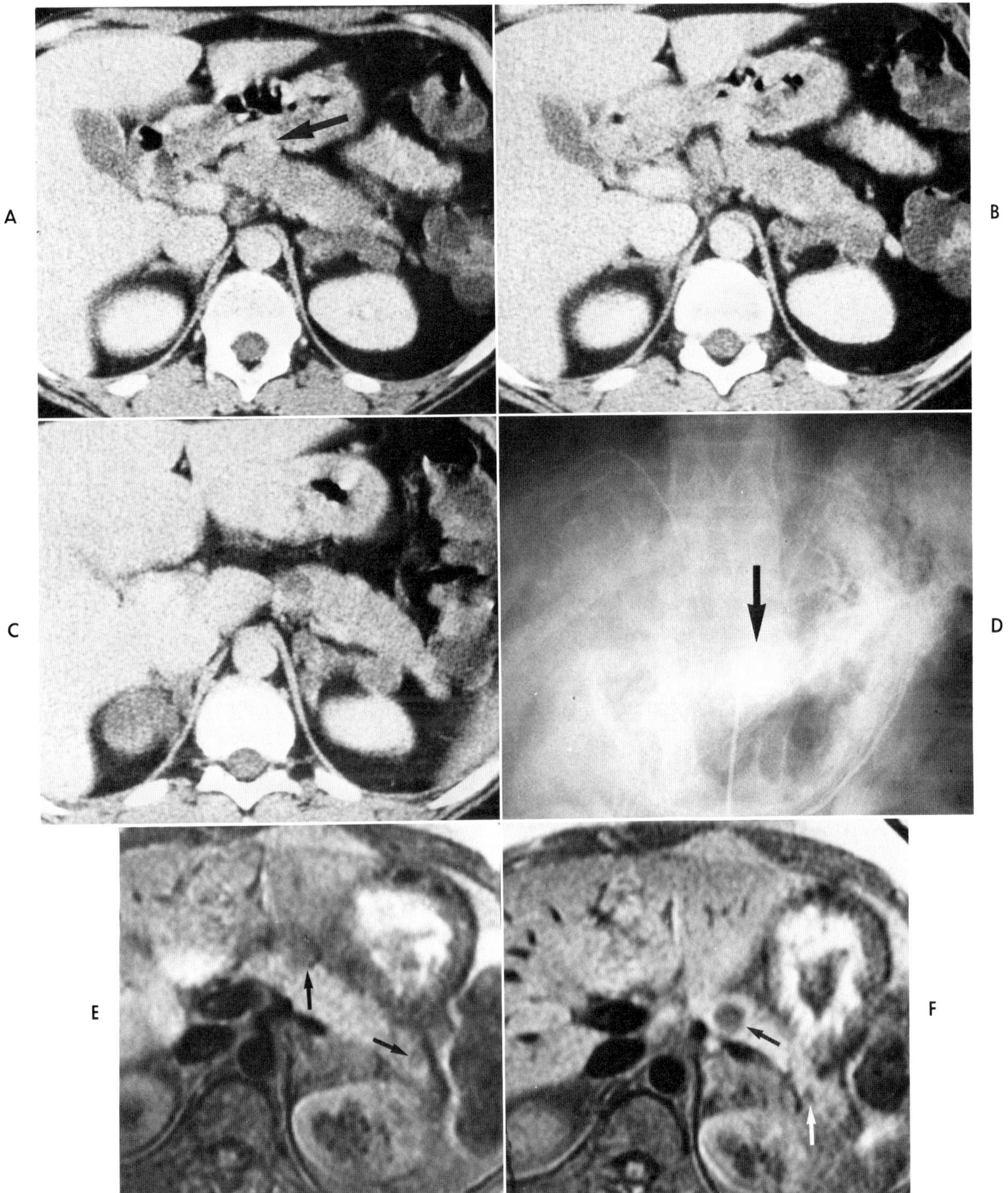

Fig. 22-9   Multiple gastrinomas in a patient with Multiple Endocrine Neoplasia, Type I. **A** to **C,** Contrast-enhanced CT images depict a solitary 2-cm enhancing lesion in the neck of the pancreas. **D,** Delayed arteriographic image after celiac injection reveals a 2-cm hypervascular mass in the pancreatic neck *(arrow)*. Contrast enhancement of the gastric mucosa obscures visualization of the pancreatic tail. **E** and **F,** Fat suppressed SE 500/11 images depict four low signal lesions *(arrows)*. *Figure continues.*

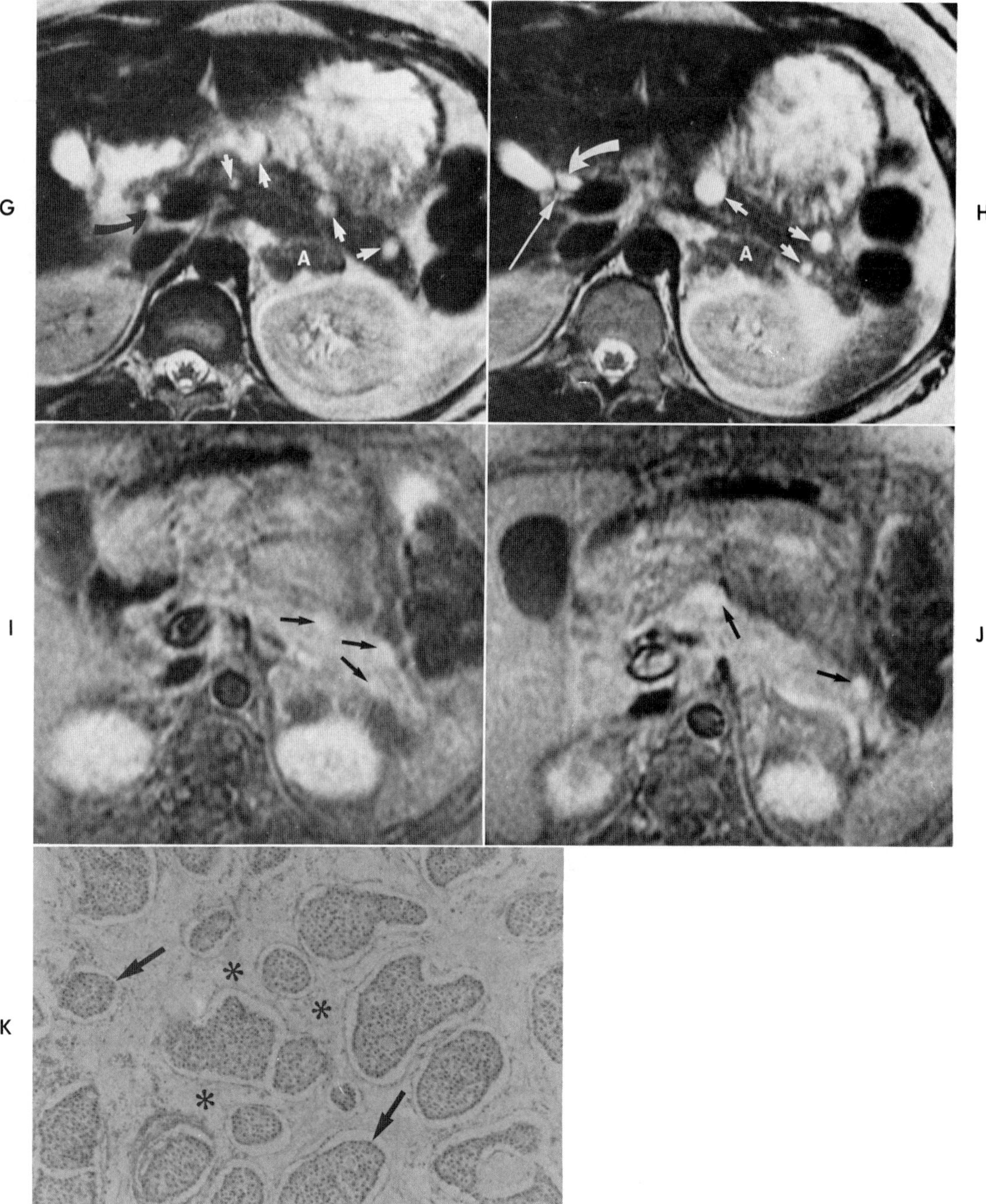

Fig. 22-9, cont'd   **G** and **H,** T2-weighted images using multiecho conjugate ("fast spin echo") technique (TR/TE = 5000/102, echo train = 16, matrix = 512 × 256, four signals averaged) shows the lesions to have extremely high signal intensity, similar to that of cysts. Seven lesions *(straight arrows)* are visible. *Curved arrow* = common bile (or common hepatic) duct, *thin arrow* = cystic duct. *A* = nodular hypertrophy of left adrenal gland. **I** and **J,** Fat suppressed SE 500/11 images approximately 20 minutes after administration of gadopentetate dimeglumine demonstrate enhancement of the lesions *(arrows),* proving that they are not cysts. MRI was used to guide resection of the pancreatic body and tail. No lesions were seen in the head by MRI or surgical inspection. **K,** Histologic specimen (H & E × 200) reveals broad bands of edematous stroma *(asterisks)* separating clumps of pancreatic islet cells *(arrows).* (**A, E, G,** and **J** from Mitchell, D.G., Cravella, M., Eschelman, D.J., et al.: J Comput Assist Tomogr [in press]. **F, H,** and **I** from Mitchell, D.G., Shapiro, M., Schuricht, A., et al.: AJR [in press].)

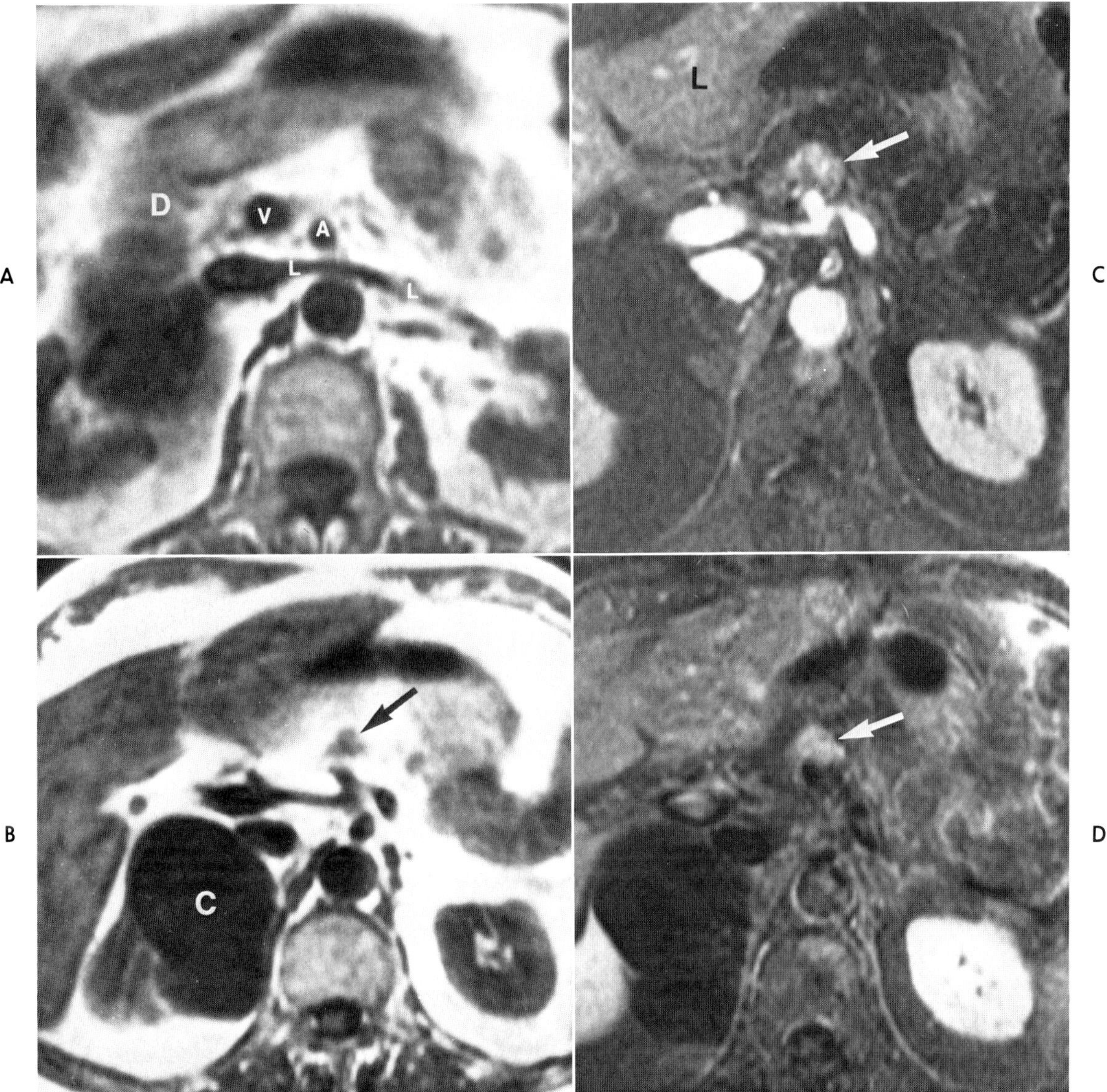

Fig. 22-10   Insulinoma in an elderly man with fatty replacement of the pancreas. **A,** SE 500/11 image at the level of the pancreas. There is near total replacement by fat of the pancreas. Anatomic landmarks include the first part of the duodenum (*D*), the superior mesenteric artery *(A)* and vein *(V)* and the left renal vein *(L)*. **B,** SE 500/11 image at the level of the pancreatic body depicts a homogeneous mass *(arrow)*. C = renal cyst. **C,** Fat suppressed T1-weighted spoiled gradient-echo image (TR/TE/flip angle = 50/5/60 degress) obtained approximately 45 seconds after administration of gadopentatate dimeglumine reveals enhancement of the mass *(arrow)* greater than that of the liver *(L)*. The high signal of vessels allows differentiation of the mass from branches of the celiac axis which are located posteriorly. **D,** Corresponding fat suppressed SE 500/11 image approximately 5 minutes after contrast administration depicts persistent hyperintensity of the mass *(arrow)*.

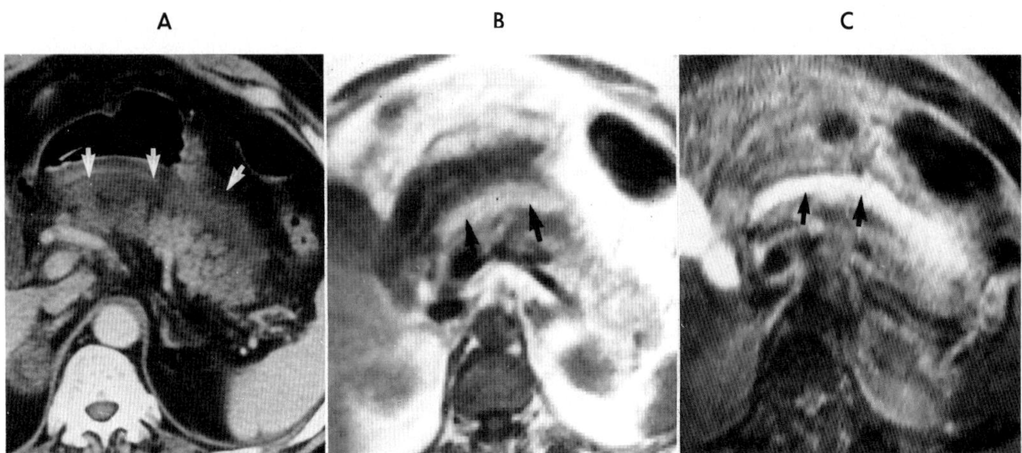

Fig. 22-11 Hemorrhagic pancreatitis. **A,** CT scan shows inflammation of peripancreatic fatty tissues, duodenal wall thickening, fluid in the anterior pararenal space, and a fluid collection in the lesser sac *(arrows)*. A low-density right adrenal mass is incidentally noted. **B,** SE 300/14 image shows duodenal wall thickening and infiltration of the peripancreatic tissues. The lesser sac fluid collection *(arrows)* has a relatively high signal intensity. **C,** SE 2350/120 image shows relatively poor contrast between pancreatic tissue (P) and retroperitoneal fat. The lesser sac collection shows a high signal intensity *(arrows)* consistent with a long T2 relaxation time. Correlated with the high signal intensity on the T1-weighted image, this finding is diagnostic of hemorrhage. Paramagnetic hemoglobin degradation products shorted T1-relaxation sufficiently to produce a high signal intensity on T1-weighted images.

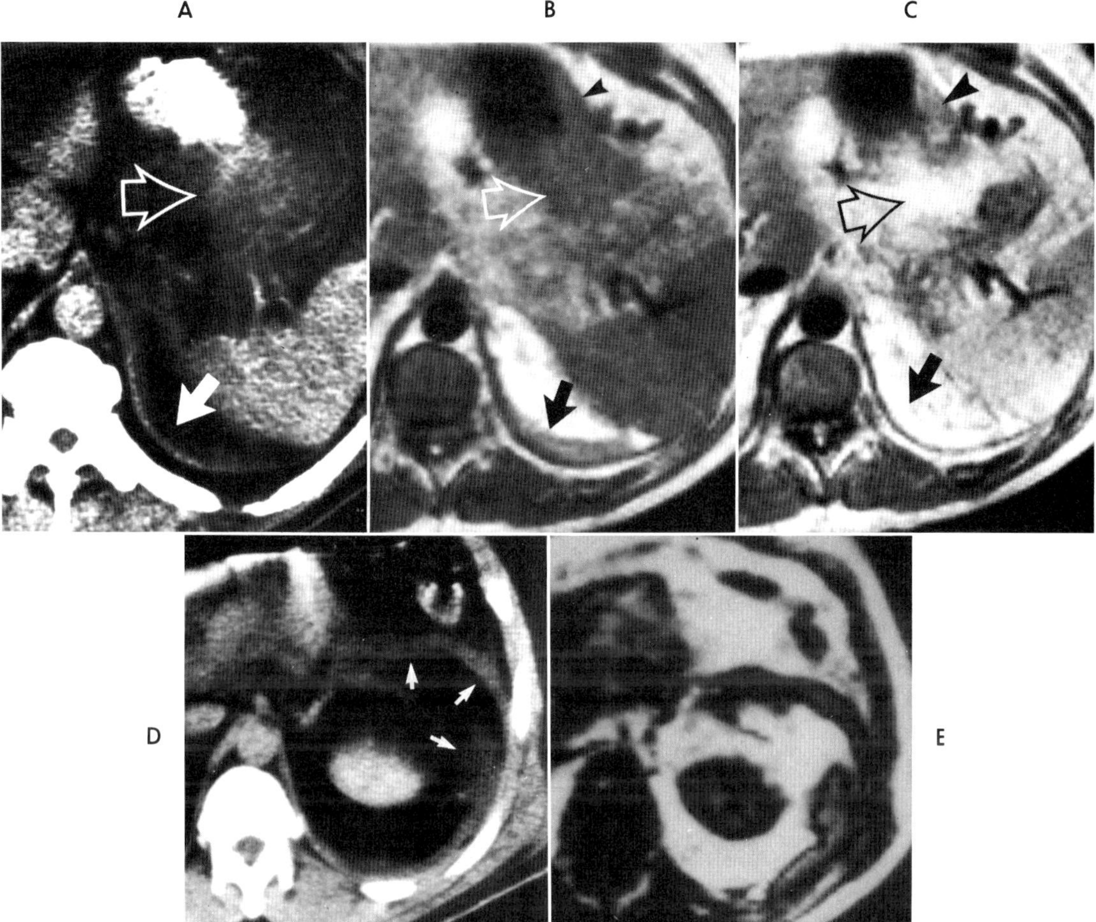

Fig. 22-12   Acute pancreatitis extending into the lesser peritoneal sac and pararenal and perinephric spaces. **A,** CT scan shows increased soft tissue density in the region of the lesser sac *(open arrow)*. Posteriorly, fluid is seen in the left subphrenic space *(solid arrow)*. **B,** SE 500/28 image shows findings similar to CT. The fatty gastrolienal ligament is effaced by edema. Thickening of the gastric wall is present *(arrowhead)*. **C,** SE 2000/28 shows the lesser sac collection to increase in intensity relative to fat, indicating a long T2, consistent with fluid. **D,** CT scan caudal to **A.** Thickening of Gerota's fascia and infiltration of the perinephric space are seen *(arrows)*. **E,** IR 1500/280/28. Note bounce-point artifact at border between fluid (below null point) and fat (above null point).

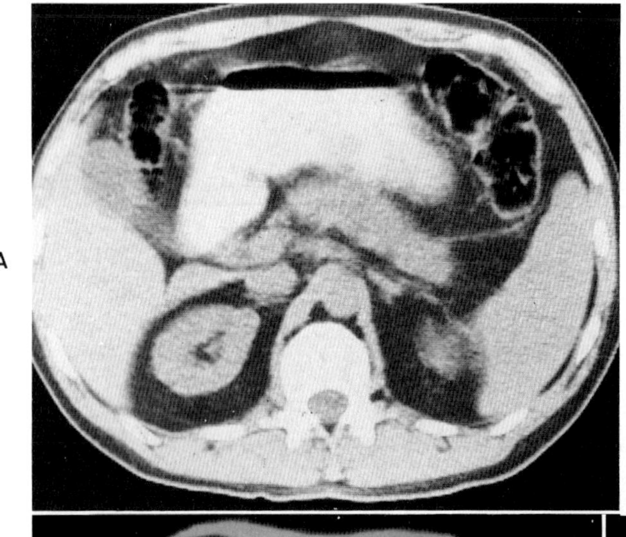

Fig. 22-13 Mild pancreatitis based on clinical and serologic criteria. **A,** CT scan shows normal findings. **B,** IR 1800/280/28 image shows the pancreas to produce a lower signal intensity than the liver and a signal intensity similar to that for the spleen. The normal pancreas would show a signal intensity similar to that of the liver on all pulse sequences, reflecting similar T1 and T2 relaxation times. In the present case, prolongation of T1 into the range of splenic tissue suggests a diffuse pancreatic abnormality with increased T1. **C,** SE 2000/28 image also shows the pancreas to produce greater signal intensity than liver and that the pancreas resembles splenic tissue, an abnormality consistent with prolonged T2.

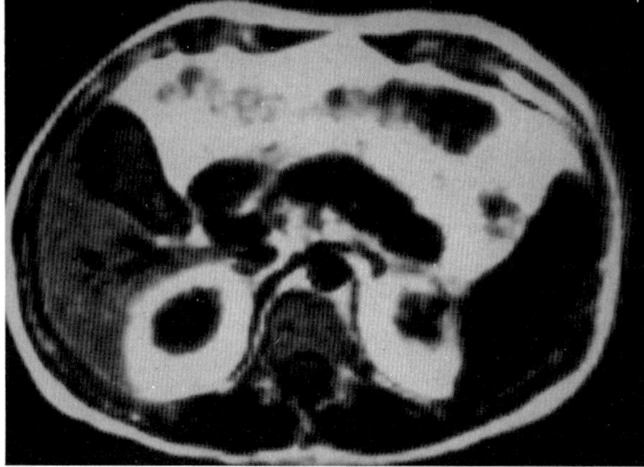

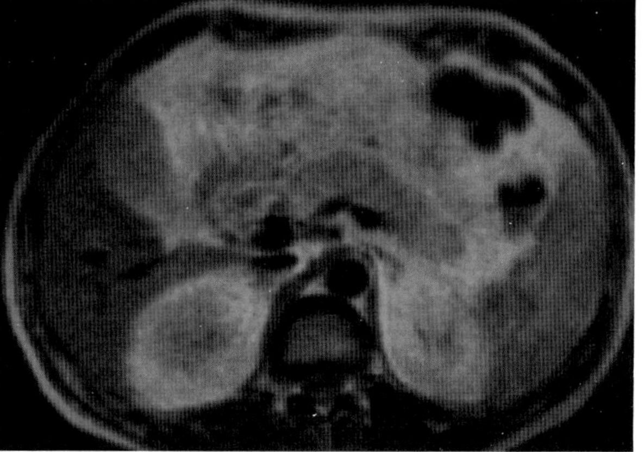

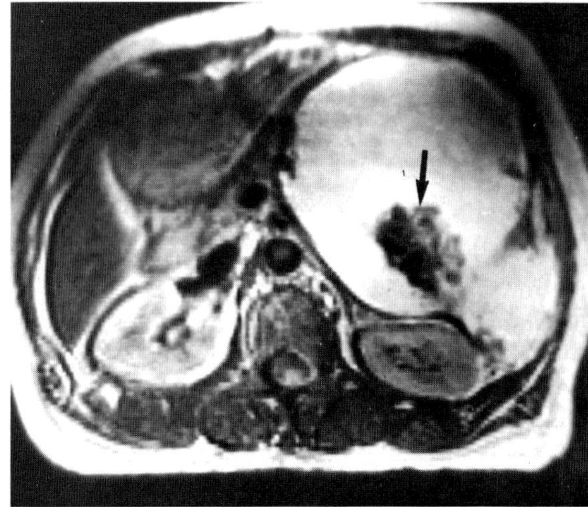

Fig. 22-14 Pancreatic pseudocyst. SE 1600/70 image at 1.5 T shows a large, high signal intensity lesion with thin wall. Low signal intensity material *(arrow)* projecting posteriorly into the main cystic component was found at surgery to be necrotic debris. (Courtesy Y. Itai.)

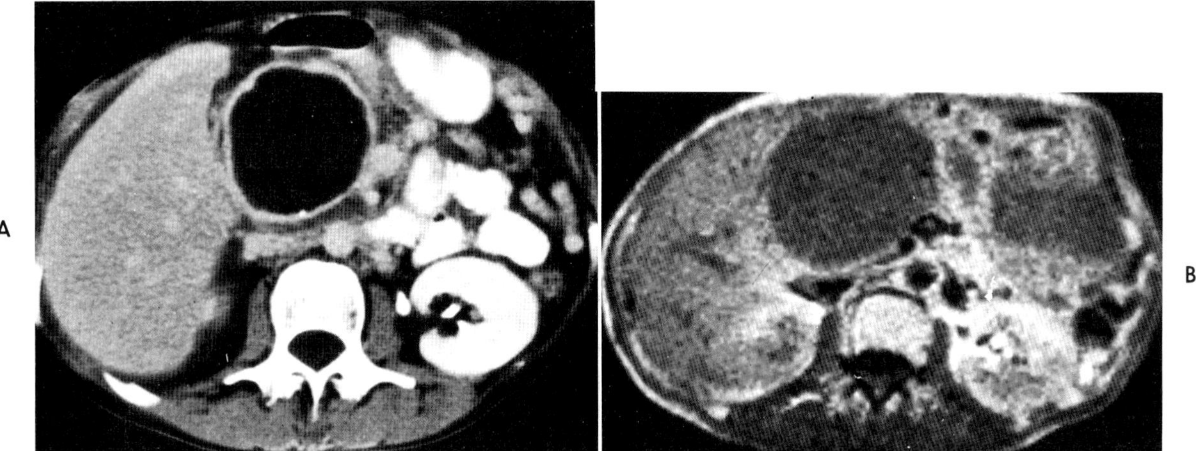

Fig. 22-15   Pancreatic pseudocyst. **A,** A mature cyst with a sharply defined wall is demonstrated by CT. **B,** SE 1000/28 MR shows the cyst fluid as having a relatively low signal intensity, reflecting its long T1, relatively pure water content, and lack of inflammatory debris.

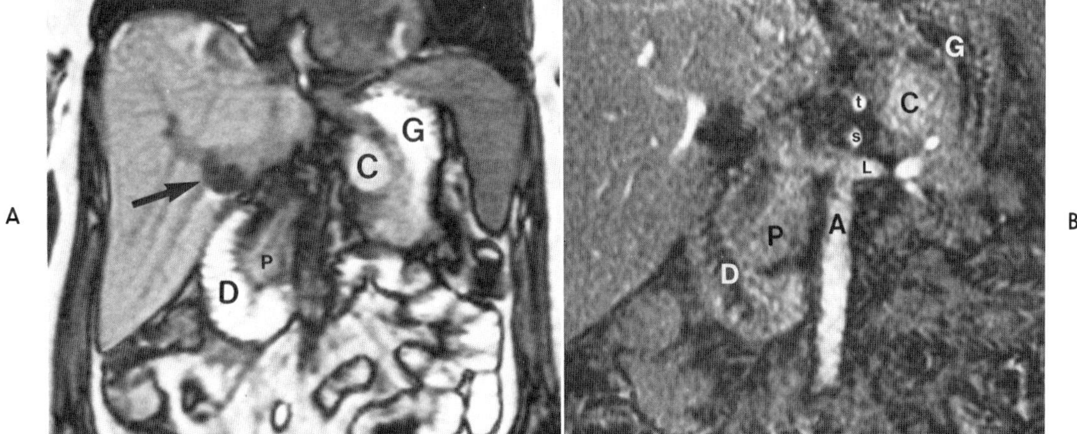

Fig. 22-16   Images obtained at 1.5 T in a patient with pancreatic pseudocysts after acute pancreatitis. Kaopectate has been administered as oral contrast. **A,** Coronal T1-weighted gradient-echo image (TR/TE/flip angle = 101/ 2.3/90 degrees). Kaopectate within the gastric *(G)* and duodenal *(D)* lumens has high signal, allowing clear depiction of the mural folds of both structures. A high-signal pseudocyst *(C)* is adjacent to but separate from the lesser curvature of the stomach. The pancreatic head *(P)* is prominent. *Black arrow* indicates susceptibility artifact from metallic clips in the gallbladder fossa. **B,** Coronal gradient-echo image (TR/TR/flip angle = 27/7.4/20 degrees) corresponding to **A.** Kaopectate within the gastric *(G)* and duodenal *(D)* lumens has low signal. C = pseudocyst, P = large pancreatic head. The aorta *(A)*, celiac trunk *(t)*, superior mesenteric artery *(s)*, left renal vein *(L)*, and other vessels are depicted as high intensity.   *Figure continues.*

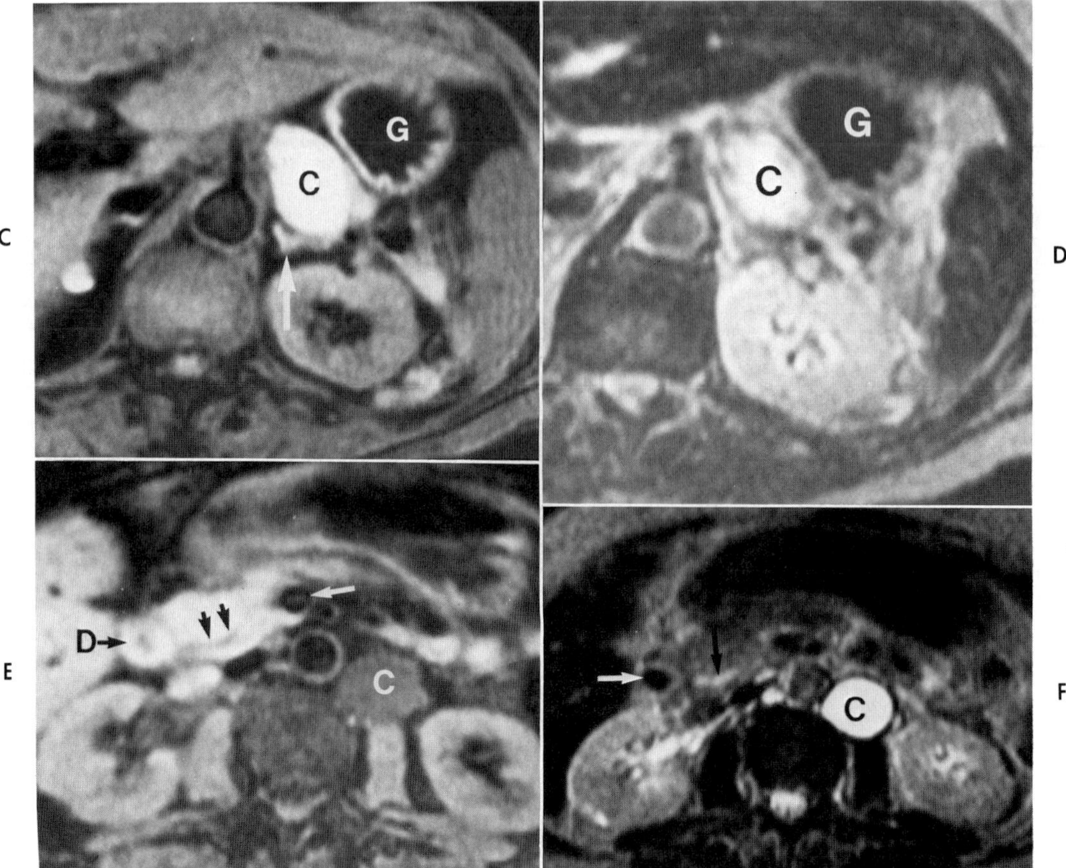

Fig. 22-16, cont'd **C,** Axial fat suppressed SE 400/14 image (combined saturation and opposed-phase techniques). Kaopectate within the gastric lumen *(G)* has low signal, allowing clear depiction of the gastric wall by "double contrast" relative to lumen and fat. The high signal pseudocyst *(C)* can be clearly separated from the stomach and the left adrenal gland *(arrow)*. **D,** Axial SE 2500/100 image corresponding to **D** reveals a signal void within the gastric lumen *(G)*. The pseudocyst *(C)* has high signal that is heterogeneous peripherally. **E,** Axial fat-suppressed image at a lower level reveals a low-signal pseudocyst *(C)* anterior to the left psoas muscle. *D* = duodenum. The superior mesenteric vein *(white arrow)* and duodenum *(D)* mark the lateral borders of the enlarged pancreatic head between them. *Black arrows* indicate the pancreatic duct within the pancreatic head. **F,** Axial SE 2500/100 image corresponding to **E** reveals a signal void within the duodenum *(white arrow)* and stomach. *Black arrow* indicates the pancreatic duct. The pseudocyst *(C)* has high signal. (From Mitchell, D.G., Vinitski, S., Haidet, K., et al.: Radiology 181:475-480, 1991.)

identified morphologcially or by alterations in MR tissue characteristics. As with pseudocyst fluid, these extrapancreatic collections have markedly prolonged T1 and T2 relaxation times and can be readily differentiated from bowel or fat. In cases of pancreatic hemorrhage or hemorrhagic pancreatitis, fluid collections can show T1 shortening because of paramagnetic effects of hemoglobin degradation products (Figs. 22-11, 22-17 and 22-18). In at least some occasions, the signal of blood mixed with pancreatic enzymes and necrotic cellular debris may differ from that of simple hematoma (Fig. 22-19).

During an episode of severe acute pancreatitis, retroperitoneal fat may develop T1 and T2 relaxation times similar to pancreatic tissue, obscuring the margins between pancreas and inflamed retroperitoneal tissue. When this happens, neither MRI nor plain CT depicts the pancreatic margins or discriminates viable from necrotic pancreatic tissue. This distinction can probably be made with CT or MRI after a rapid intravenous bolus of contrast material.[20] Limited experience with both modalities indicates that CT remains superior in this seriously ill group of patients because of shorter examination times, less motion artifact and finer resolution.

Carcinoma of the pancreas can coexist with pancreatitis (Fig. 22-20), either causing secondary inflammation

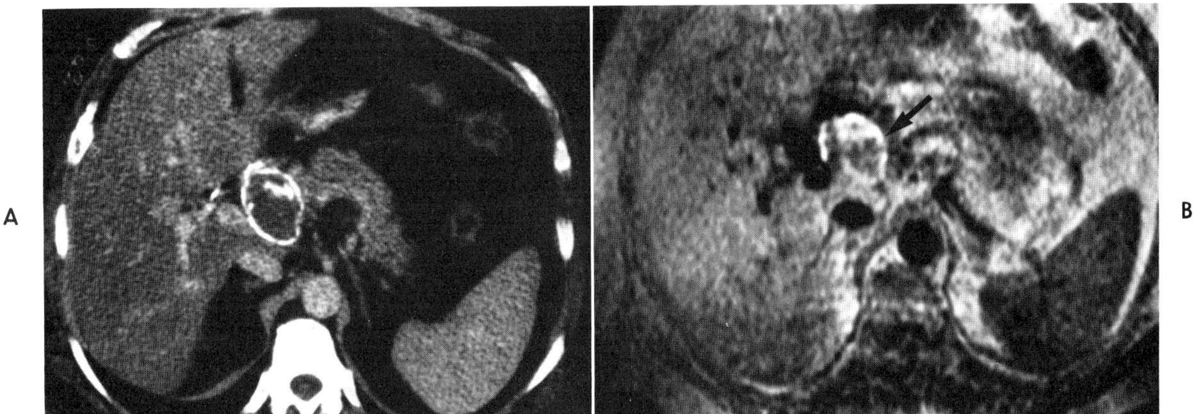

Fig. 22-17   Posttraumatic rim calcified hematoma of the neck of the pancreas. **A,** CT scan demonstrating a rim calcified mass just anterior to the portocaval space. **B,** T1-weighted axial image at 1.5 through the same level as **A,** demonstrating a ring *(arrow)* of increased signal attributed to methemoglobin within the hematoma. Persistence of the short T1 methemoglobin is variable and has been reported as late as 11 months after intraabdominal hemorrhage.

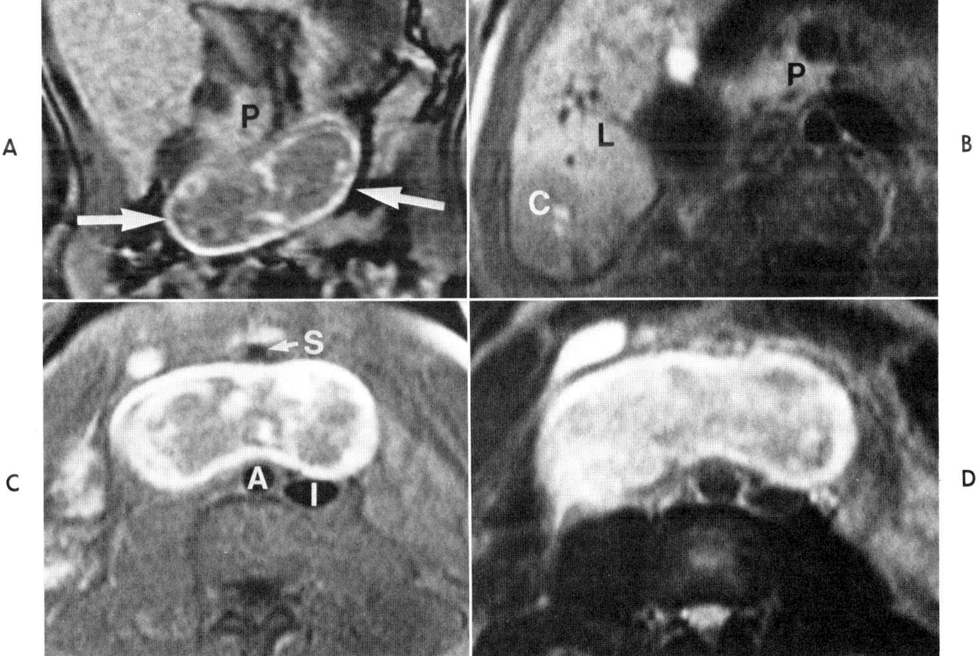

Fig. 22-18   Chronic pancreatitis with surgically proven hemorrhagic collection inferior to the pancreas. **A,** Coronal T1-weighted spoiled gradient-echo image (TR/TE/flip angle = 57/2.4/90 degrees) reveals a large oblong collection with a high-signal peripheral rim *(arrows)* inferior to the pancreatic head *(P)*. **B,** Axial fat-suppressed T1-weighted image (SE 500/11) reveals mildly decreased signal of the pancreatic head *(P)*, which is isointense to the liver *(L)*. There is hepatic cirrhosis and an hepatocellular carcinoma *(C)* posteriorly. **C,** Inferiorly, as in **B,** the hemorrhagic collection is seen between the aorta *(A)* and the superior mesenteric artery *(S)*. *I* = anomalous left-sided inferior vena cava. **D,** SE 2500/100 image.

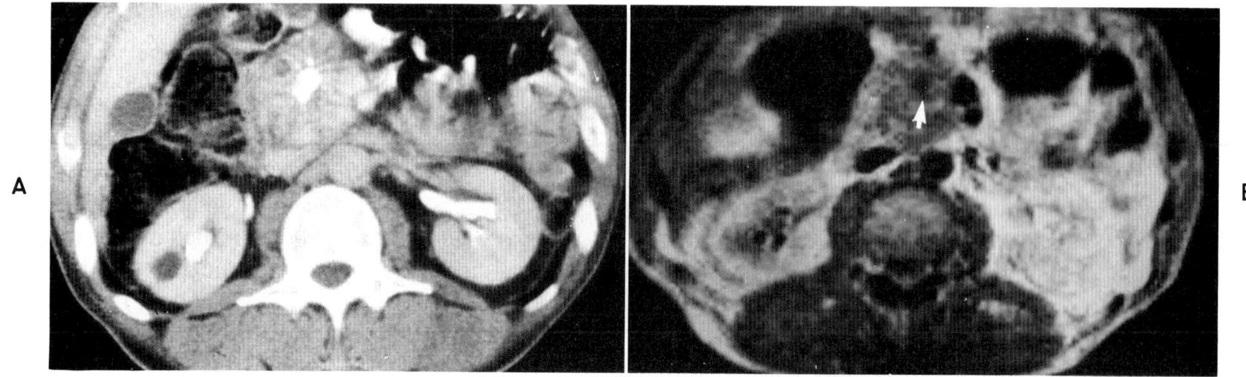

Fig. 22-22 Chronic pancreatitis. **A,** CT shows an inflammatory mass involving the pancreatic head with a large central calcification and small peripheral pseudocysts. **B,** MRI faintly shows the calcification as a low signal intensity zone *(arrow)*. Patency of the superior mesenteric vein and artery is more easily determined by MRI.

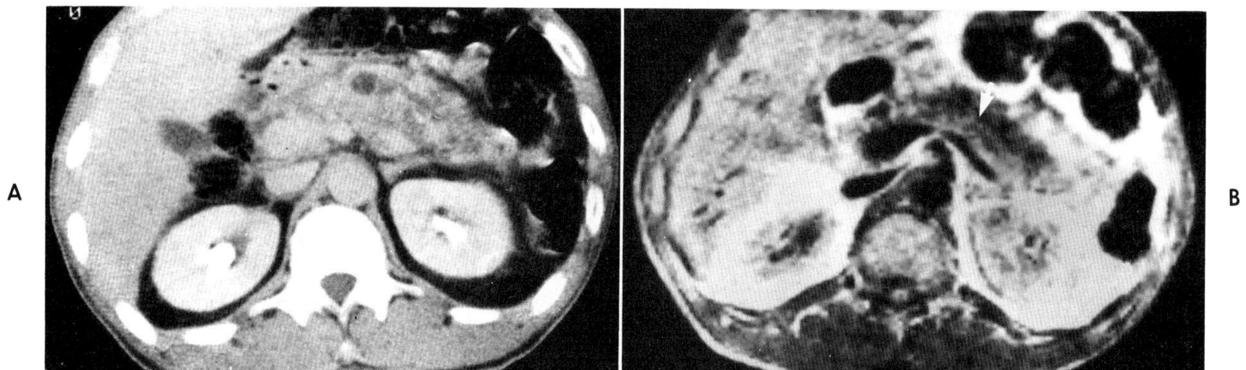

Fig. 22-23 Pancreatic duct dilatation in a patient with acute and chronic pancreatitis. **A,** CT scan shows diffuse enlargement of the pancreatic body. Low-attenuation fluid is seen within the dilated duct. **B,** SE 1000/28 MRI also demonstrates the dilated duct; however, anatomic resolution is reduced, in part because of blurring from respiratory motion.

lated ducts often contain viscous fluid and debris, which reduce the T1 and T2 relaxation times of associated fluid, rendering it isointense relative to inflamed pancreatic tissue.

Vascular complications of pancreatitis include venous thrombosis and arterial pseudoaneurysm formation. Pseudoaneurysms complicate up to 10% of severe cases of pancreatitis, usually involving the splenic artery (Fig. 22-24). (See also Color Plate XV) Differentiation of pseudoaneurysms from pseudocysts may be difficult by using SE images,[345] but flow-sensitive techniques may be helpful. Unfortunately, it is difficult to distinguish pseudoaneurysms from incidental atherosclerotic aneurysms. This differentiation is important clinically because pseudoaneurysm rupture is associated with a high mortality, whereas atherosclerotic aneurysms rarely hemorrhage.

Pancreatic disease is the most common cause of splenic vein thrombosis. Splenic vein thrombosis has been demonstrated by splenoportography in 45% of cases of chronic alcoholic pancreatitis.[168] Although isolated splenic vein thrombosis is often silent clinically, hemorrhage can result from gastric varices. Hemorrhagic thrombus in the splenic vein can produce T1 shortening and signal visible within the vein, but MR diagnosis relies on flow techniques that show an absence of flow in the splenic vein, coupled with a demonstration of collaterals. Although left gastric and esophageal varices are nonspecific, the pattern of other collateral varices tends to be different from that seen with portal hypertension. Large gastroepiploic veins are commonly associated with splenic vein occlusion, whereas a patent paraumbilical vein indicates portal hypertension.[313]

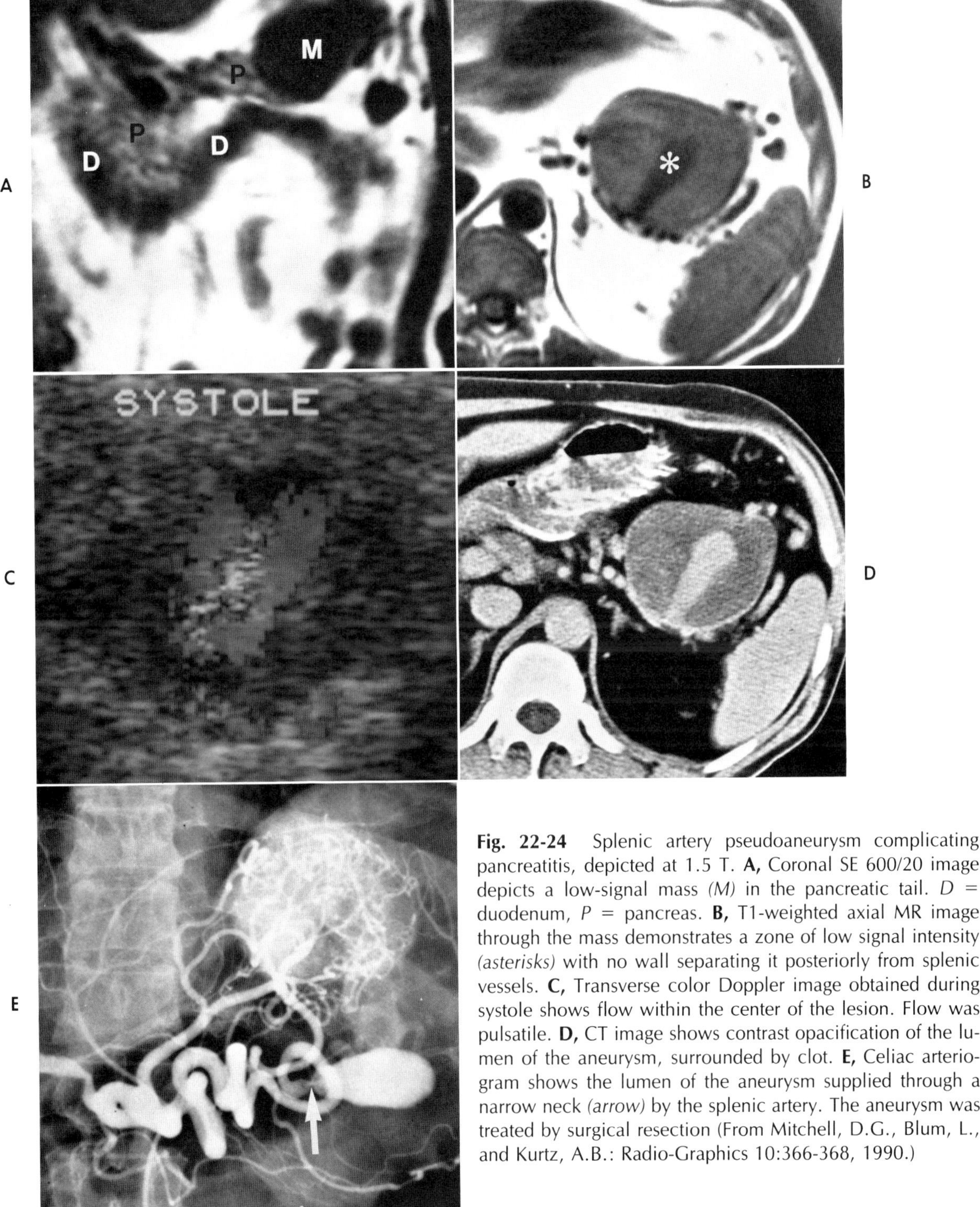

Fig. 22-24 Splenic artery pseudoaneurysm complicating pancreatitis, depicted at 1.5 T. **A,** Coronal SE 600/20 image depicts a low-signal mass *(M)* in the pancreatic tail. *D =* duodenum, *P =* pancreas. **B,** T1-weighted axial MR image through the mass demonstrates a zone of low signal intensity *(asterisks)* with no wall separating it posteriorly from splenic vessels. **C,** Transverse color Doppler image obtained during systole shows flow within the center of the lesion. Flow was pulsatile. **D,** CT image shows contrast opacification of the lumen of the aneurysm, surrounded by clot. **E,** Celiac arteriogram shows the lumen of the aneurysm supplied through a narrow neck *(arrow)* by the splenic artery. The aneurysm was treated by surgical resection (From Mitchell, D.G., Blum, L., and Kurtz, A.B.: Radio-Graphics 10:366-368, 1990.)

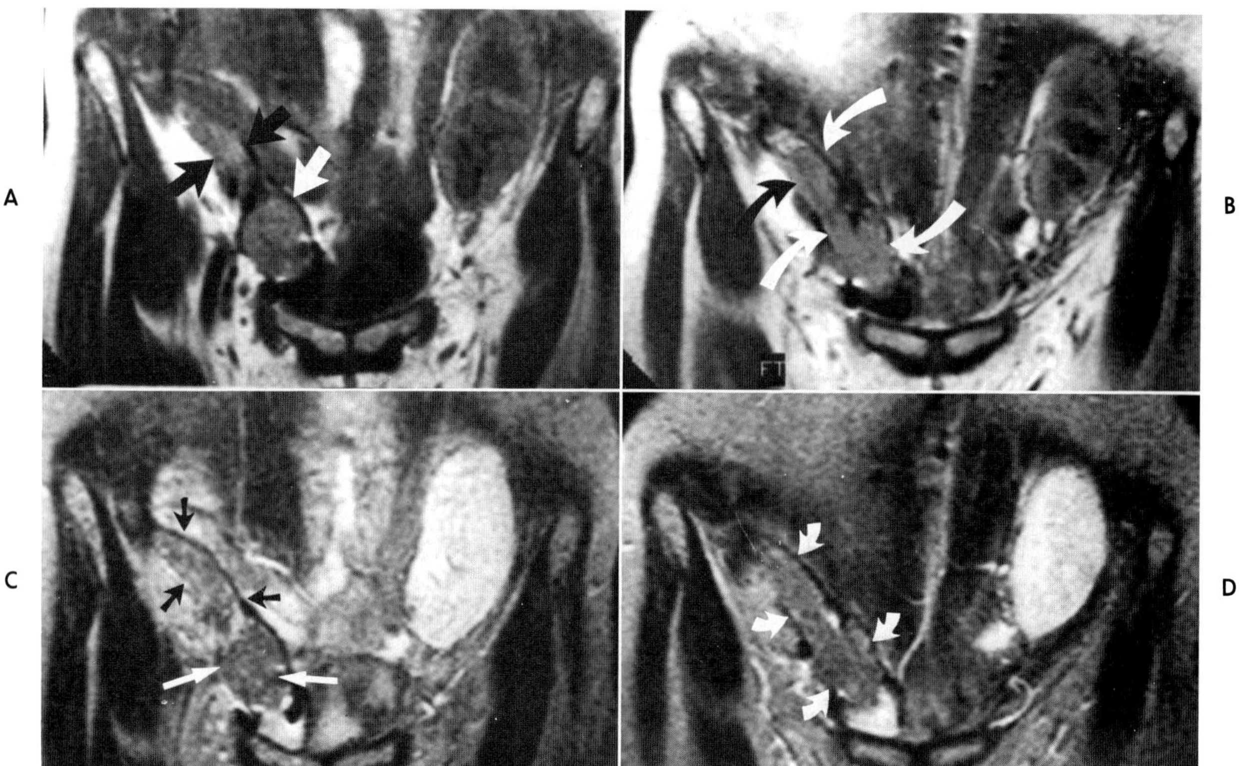

Fig. 22-25 Normal pancreatic allograft, which is 6 months old. **A,** Coronal T1-weighted image (SE 683/20, 0.5 T) shows allograft body *(black arrows)* and head *(white arrow)* in right iliac fossa. **B,** A more anterior image again shows the allograft *(arrows),* hyperintense to muscle and isointense to the cortex of the healthy renal allograft in the contralateral side. **C** and **D,** Corresponding T2-weighted images (SE 2000/100). The pancreas *(arrows)* has signal intensity, similar to that of fat on this pulse sequence but less than urine in the bladder at the inferomedial margin of the pancreas in **D.** (From Yuh, W.T.C., Hunsicker, L.G., Nghiem, D.D., et al.: Radiology 170:171-177, 1989.)

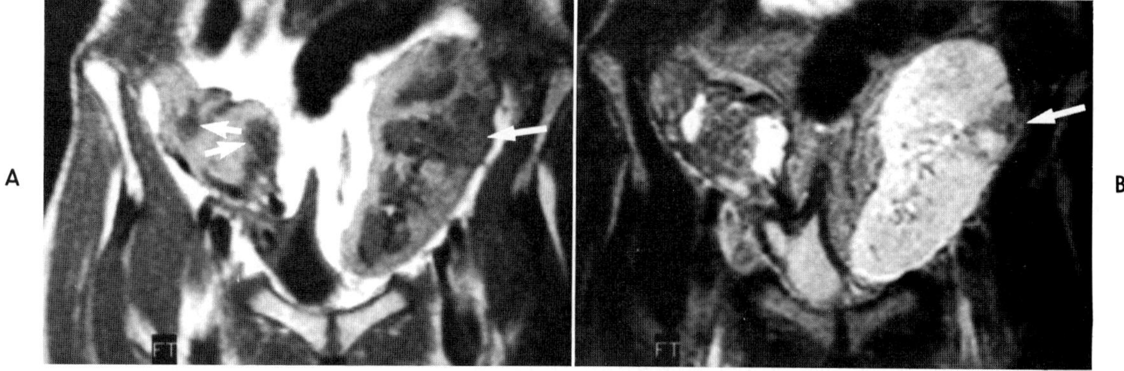

Fig. 22-26 Acute rejection of pancreatic allograft. **A,** Recovery phase image with relative T1 weighting (SE 680/20, 0.5 T) shows well-defined areas *(short arrows)* of prolonged T1, probably indicating pseudocyst formation. **B,** On corresponding T2-weighted image (SE 2000/100), these areas have a high signal intensity, like bladder urine. These zones develop from patchy foci of poorly defined relaxation time prolongation seen earlier in the rejection process. Note renal infarct *(long arrow)* in contralateral renal allograft. (From Yuh, W.T.C., Hunsicker, L.G., Nghiem, D.D., et al.: Radiology 170:171-177, 1989.)

HEMOCHROMATOSIS

In patients with hemochromatosis (see Chapter 17), excessive iron accumulates within pancreatic acinar cells and in islet B cells. For uncertain reasons, other islet cells are usually spared (see Fig. 17-2I), so pancreatic endocrine defects are usually restricted to deficient insulin production, resulting in insulin-dependent diabetes mellitus. Pancreatic exocrine function is usually spared.

MRI shows decreased intensity of iron-overloaded pancreatic tissue that is most marked on gradient-echo and T2-weighted spin-echo sequences, similar to that seen in the liver. Changes in the pancreas may be less marked than changes in the liver and depend on pancreatic iron levels. Therefore MRI may be useful in detecting pancreatic iron and assessing the risk for diabetes in patients with iron overload.[243,483,492,497]

PANCREATIC TRANSPLANTATION

Pancreatic transplantation is performed most often in conjunction with renal transplantation in patients with end-stage diabetic nephropathy.[298] The pancreatic allograft is placed into the contralateral iliac fossa with blood supply furnished by the iliac artery. Exocrine drainage is into the bowel (pancreaticoduodenojejunostomy) or into the bladder (pancreaticoduodenocystostomy). The distinction is important because only in the latter can pancreatic exocrine function be monitored by urinary pH, bicarbonate, and amylase levels. A third technique, duct-occluded partial pancreatic allotransplantation, leaves no outlet for exocrine secretions, and the graft undergoes progressive fibrous atrophy.[470]

Pancreatic transplant rejection is the major cause of graft loss. Clinical manifestations of rejection may be subtle and are not sensitive for rejection or its resolution. Although acute rejection can be treated with immunosuppressive drugs, these increase the risk of infection, nephrotoxicity, and marrow suppression. Pancreatic graft biopsy is associated with greater risk of morbidity (pancreatitis) than renal graft biopsy. Moreover, rejection can be focal, multifocal, or diffuse, so sampling error may occur. Therefore the ability of MRI to provide diagnostic information about pancreatic allografts is of considerable interest.

Locating the allograft may be difficult, requiring historical and imaging information. Both axial and coronal T1-weighted images should be employed to demonstrate the gland. Coronal images are particularly useful because they permit simultaneous visualization of muscle, fat, bladder, and renal graft along with the pancreas. If available, breath-hold techniques should be used for coronal images because of the severe respiratory blurring that occurs in the coronal plane. Coronal T2-weighted images should also be obtained.

If MRI is used to follow pancreatic allografts, baseline images should be obtained. These should be acquired at least 4 weeks after transplantation. Size can be assessed only on sequential images, since the initial size of the donor pancreas is variable. During the first 4 weeks, the pancreas decreases 20% to 40% in size and loses its heterogeneity on T2-weighted images, becoming isointense to renal cortex on T1-weighted images and less intense than urine but similar to fat on T2-weighted images. Fluid collections, including short T1 hemorrhage, should disappear after approximately 4 weeks. Borders of a healthy graft are sharply defined (Fig. 22-25).

Features of acute rejection after 4 weeks usually include increased graft size, diffuse or focal prolongation of T1 and T2, parenchymal hemorrhage (30%) or liquefaction (20%), and recurrence of peripancreatic fluid collections (60%).[559] After the acute phase of rejection, the zones of prolonged T2 either resolve or progress to pseudocyst formation (Fig. 22-26). Intraparenchymal hemorrhage and fluid may resolve or progress to foci of low signal intensity, either from iron deposition or fibrosis.

In initial studies, the sensitivity of MRI approaches 100% for the diagnosis of acute pancreatic allograft rejection.[623] Diagnosis can be based on a combination of signal intensity and morphologic changes. In a study at 0.35 T, calculation from images showed that T2 of healthy grafts averaged 59 ± 6 msec (n = 4), acutely rejecting grafts 86± 15 msec (n = 8); T2 of 70 msec separated the healthy transplants from the rejecting ones.[123]

MRI may actually be overly sensitive, detecting clinically occult focal areas of rejection that may resolve without treatment. On the other hand, MRI can detect other problems, such as vascular occlusions, pseudocysts, hematomas, abscesses, or lymphoceles at the same time that the possibility of rejection is evaluated.[622]

The chronically rejecting graft is small and looks like muscle, with relatively low signal intensity on both T1- and T2-weighted images. Even lower signal intensity may indicate fibrotic replacement. Duct-occluded allotransplants undergo progressive decrease in size for several years after placement. MRI may be complementary to CT in demonstrating and measuring these small structures on the dome of the bladder or fundus of the uterus.

In a more recent study at 1.5 T, T2 was not significantly elevated with rejection unless it was complicated by pancreatic infarction.[131] These investigators also administered gadopentetate dimeglumine, however, and noted that normal grafts enhanced 98% ± 23%, compared with only 42% ± 20% for acute rejection. In four of six cases of rejection, decreased enhancement preceded a drop in urinary amylase, suggesting a role for enhanced MRI in the early diagnosis of pancreatic allograft dysfunction.

Spleen

The spleen is affected by a variety of neoplastic and other diseases, but there is no noninvasive imaging modality that detects disease in the spleen reliably. Moreover, compared with the relatively safe and frequently performed percutaneous liver biopsy, splenic biopsy is uncommon and restricted to the use of fine needles.[516] Our understanding of splenic disease is based on decades-old autopsy series or highly selected series of splenectomies. It is likely that the prevalence and importance of splenic disease has been underestimated. A noninvasive method of detecting splenic disease would make an important contribution to diagnostic imaging. MRI of the spleen promises to furnish new insights into the pathology of this important organ.

MALIGNANT LESIONS

Two thirds of spleens with metastatic disease have grossly visible lesions at autopsy,[317] yet their detection by ultrasound and CT is infrequent and unreliable.[32,488] The spleen is involved by metastases less commonly than the liver. In an old autopsy series of cancer patients, most splenic metastases occurred in patients with widespread metastatic disease.[575] When metastases were present above and below the diaphragm, however, more than half of patients had splenic involvement.[196] It has been argued on this basis that detection of focal splenic disease is of little clinical significance because metastasis to the spleen is a premorbid event. However, these data are more than 50 years old and may not apply to patients undergoing aggressive cancer therapy. More recently, it has been shown that treated cancer patients are more likely to have metastases to the spleen than are untreated patients.[577] This fact suggests that as better treatment methods permit patients to outlive their primary tumor, the spleen may assume greater importance as a site of secondary disease.

Detection of focal splenic lesions is rarely based on distortion of splenic architecture (Fig. 23-1). Splenic contours are highly variable, so that a focal bulge is more likely to be a normal variant than a tumor. Spleen differs from the liver in having no internal structures such as fissures, blood vessels, or bile ducts to be splayed or obliterated by a space-occupying mass. Therefore detection of focal splenic lesions depends on

differences in signal intensity between tumor and normal splenic tissue.

Spectrometer-determined relaxation measurements on animals bearing tumors remote from the spleen suggest slight prolongation of splenic T1 by tumor.[39] There is no clinical evidence, however, that in vivo MR imaging of the spleen can be used to screen patients for malignancy.

The close resemblence of splenic MRI characteristics to those of most tumors (see Table 7-1, p. 56) limits de-

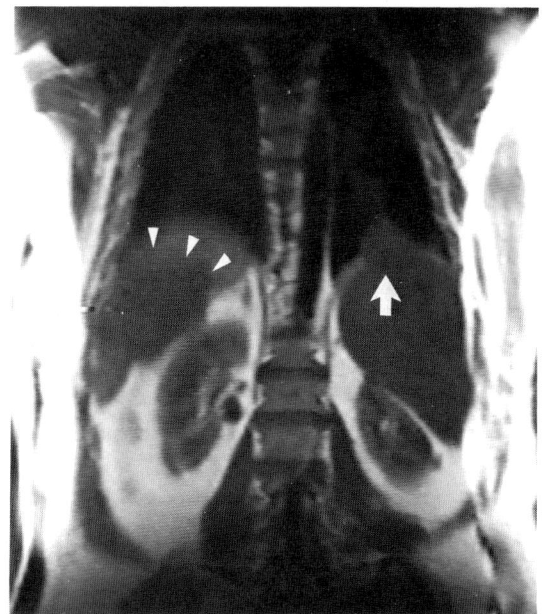

Fig. 23-1 Hepatosplenic lymphoma. Coronal T1-weighted image (SE 310/20, 0.6 T) shows lymphomatous nodule arising from the dome of the spleen (arrow). Although the tumor is isointense to the remainder of the spleen, the lesion is detected because of the resulting deformity of the splenic contour. Normal splenic contour is sufficiently variable so that lesions are rarely detected in the spleen because they deform its contour. Focal hepatic lesion (arrowheads) is readily detected on the basis of lesion signal intensity lower than that of surrounding liver tissue. (From Hahn, P.F., Weissleder, R., Stark, D.D., et al.: AJR 150:823-827, 1988.)

tection of splenic tumors. No pulse sequence reliably distinguishes tumor from spleen because there is no determinant of signal intensity in which spleen and tumor consistently differ. Moreover, when splenic tumors are visible, it is not always possible to predict their appearance or what pulse sequence will best display them.

There are four situations in which focal splenic tumors can be depicted. This can occur when tissue water and relaxation times within the tumor are increased by liquefactive necrosis (Fig. 23-2). This is most common in large masses such as in histocytic lymphomas. Necrotic masses such as these can usually be detected by other imaging modalities (Fig. 23-3). T2-weighted images display best the central necrosis as an area of increased signal intensity. MRI often underestimates the size of lesions detected on the basis of necrosis because only the centrally liquefied zone is readily visible (Fig. 23-4). With improved artifact suppression, however, morphologic differences between tumor and spleen may become evident (Fig. 23-5).

Focal hemorrhage within a tumor can also increase contrast between tumor and spleen. As in hemorrhagic lesions elsewhere, the T1 shortening of hemoglobin degradation products increases signal intensity (Fig. 23-6). Unlike homoeneous space-occupying hematomas in muscle or in potential spaces like the subcapsular zone of spleen, intratumoral splenic hemorrhage usually appears as high-intensity streaks on T1-weighted images within tissue that may be indistinguishable from normal spleen.

In principle, other paramagnetic substances besides hemorrhage could produce T1 shortening within splenic tumors. Melanoma is the most common solid neoplasm found in splenic metastases, and melanotic melanoma is often associated with T1 shortening. However, we have not seen melanoma metastases to the spleen exhibit T1 shortening, even when the same patient's liver metastases had short T1.

Fibrosis can occur in association with splenic Hodgkin's disease.[384] Fibrosis produces zones of reduced proton density and T2 in the spleen, depicted as low signal intensity on motion-compensated T2-weighted images.

Contrast between spleen and tumor can also be increased when there is splenic iron overload, such as in transfusional siderosis (see Chapter 17, Transfusional siderosis). When present, the iron shortens the T2 of the splenic tissue, reducing the signal intensity on T2-weighted images. Splenic neoplasms lack phagocytic capacity and displace splenic tissue capable of phagocytosis, so that excess iron is not present in tumors. Consequently, tumors are displayed as a region of high signal intensity within a low-signal spleen (Fig. 23-7).

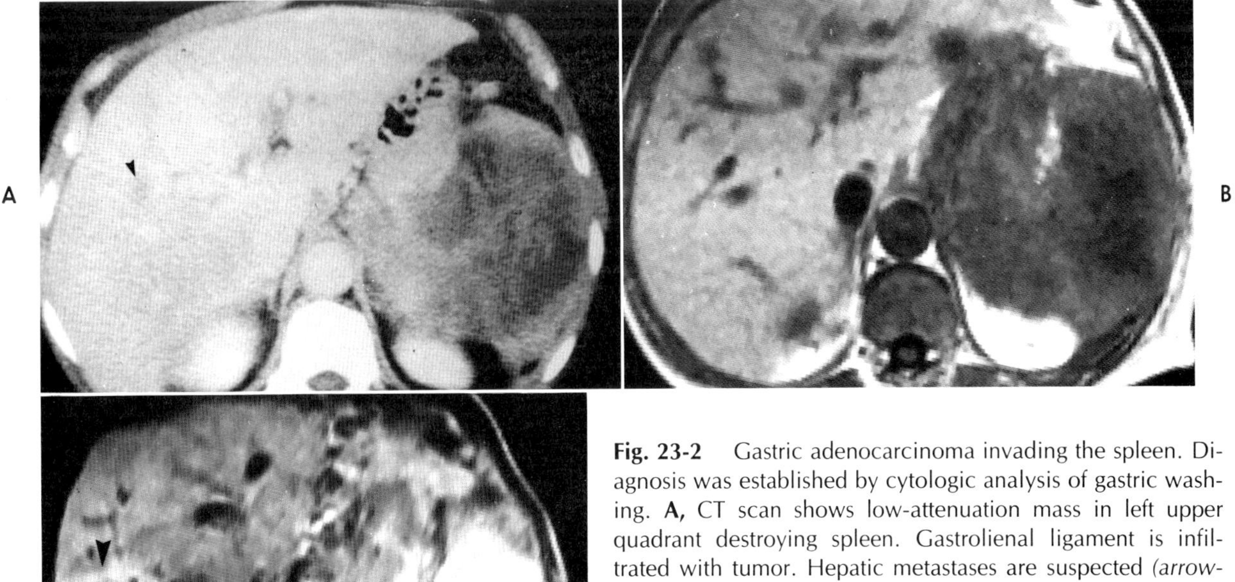

Fig. 23-2   Gastric adenocarcinoma invading the spleen. Diagnosis was established by cytologic analysis of gastric washing. **A,** CT scan shows low-attenuation mass in left upper quadrant destroying spleen. Gastrolienal ligament is infiltrated with tumor. Hepatic metastases are suspected *(arrowhead).* **B,** SE 300/14 images shows confluent mass extending from gastric fundus to spleen. Central spleen has a lower signal intensity than periphery. Multiple hepatic metastases are confirmed. **C,** SE 2400/60 image shows high signal intensity abnormality in spleen. Zones of edema *(arrowheads)* are seen in liver.

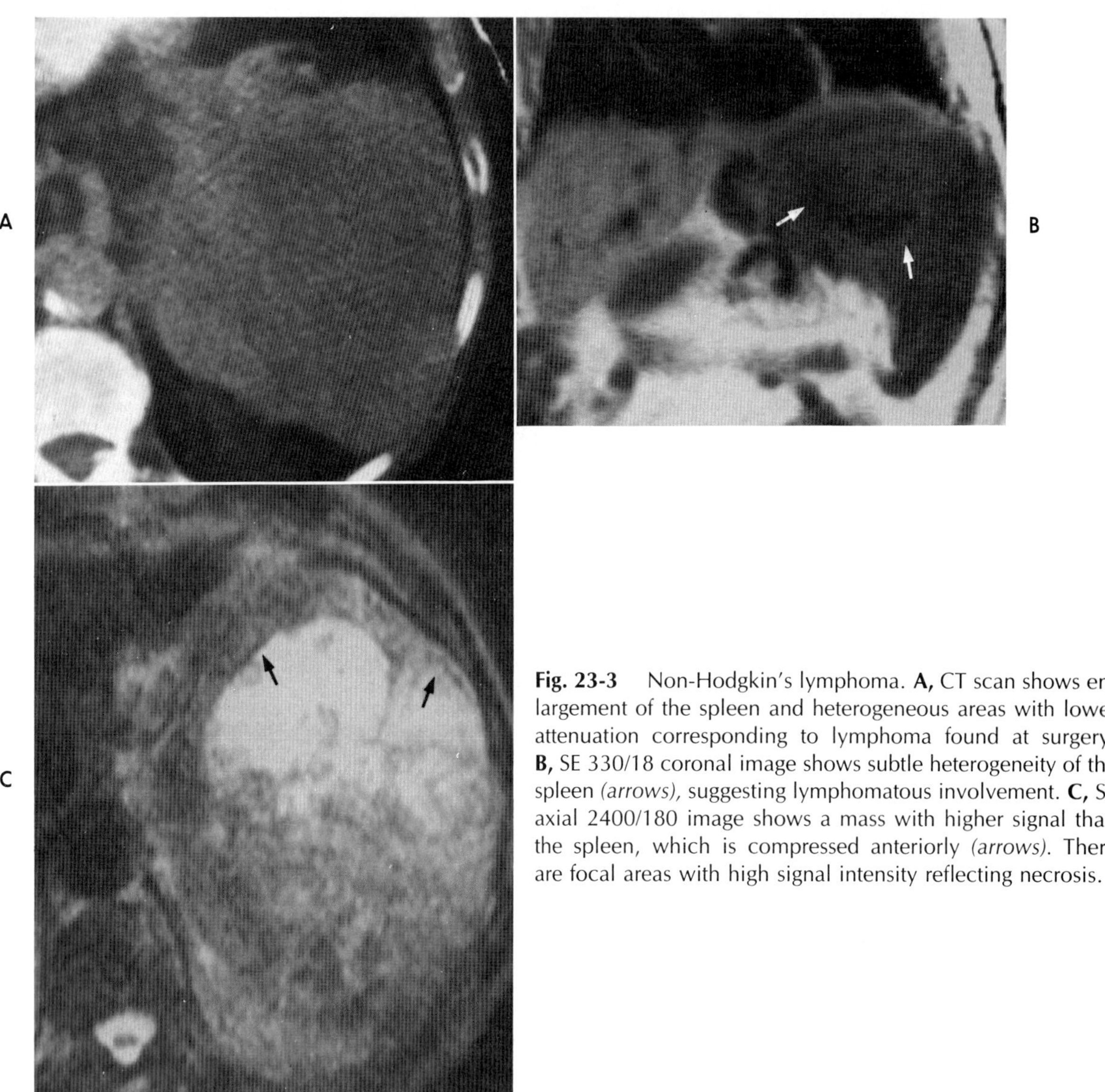

Fig. 23-3   Non-Hodgkin's lymphoma. **A,** CT scan shows enlargement of the spleen and heterogeneous areas with lower attenuation corresponding to lymphoma found at surgery. **B,** SE 330/18 coronal image shows subtle heterogeneity of the spleen *(arrows),* suggesting lymphomatous involvement. **C,** SE axial 2400/180 image shows a mass with higher signal than the spleen, which is compressed anteriorly *(arrows).* There are focal areas with high signal intensity reflecting necrosis.

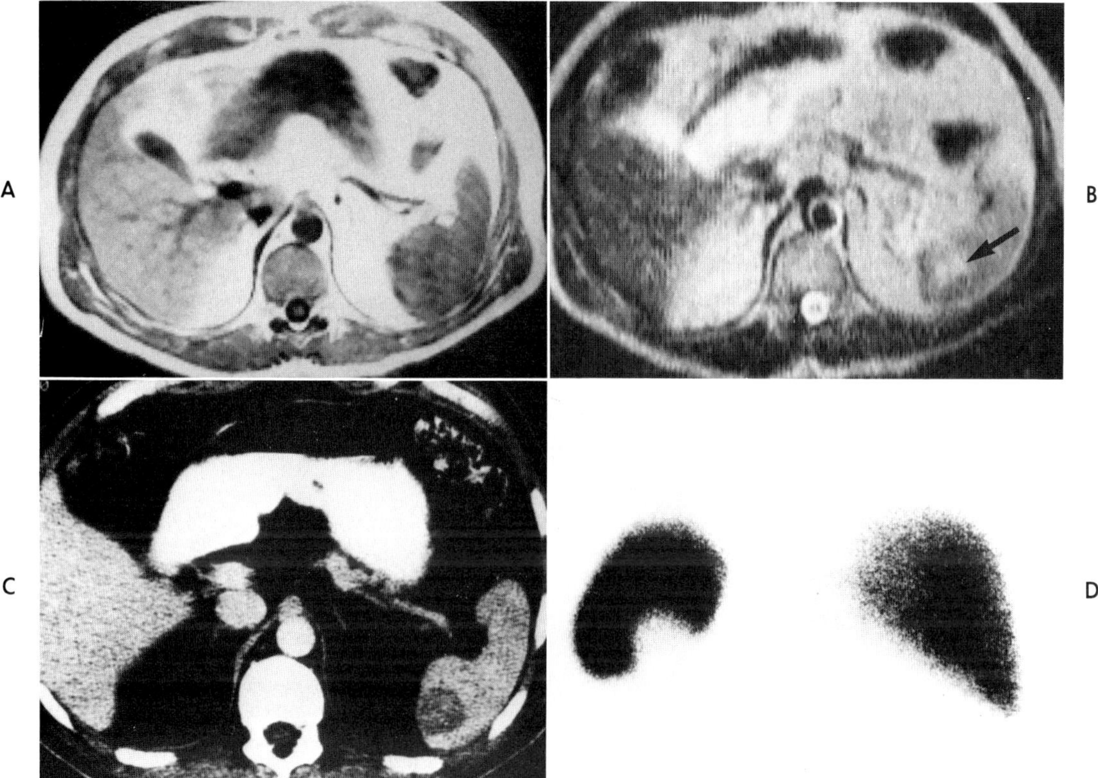

Fig. 23-4   Focal splenic lymphoma with central necrosis. **A,** Axial T1-weighted image (SE 300/14, 0.6 T) shows no abnormality. **B,** T2-weighted image (SE 2350/120) corresponding to **A** shows a small focal zone of increased signal intensity within the spleen *(arrow)*. **C,** Contrast CT scan shows a similar focal defect in the spleen. **D,** Posterior scintiscan shows a photopenic area larger than the lesion delineated by MR. MR underestimates the lesion size by demonstrating only the liquified, necrotic center. (From Hahn P.F., Weissleder, R., Stark, D.D., et al.: AJR 150:823-827, 1988.)

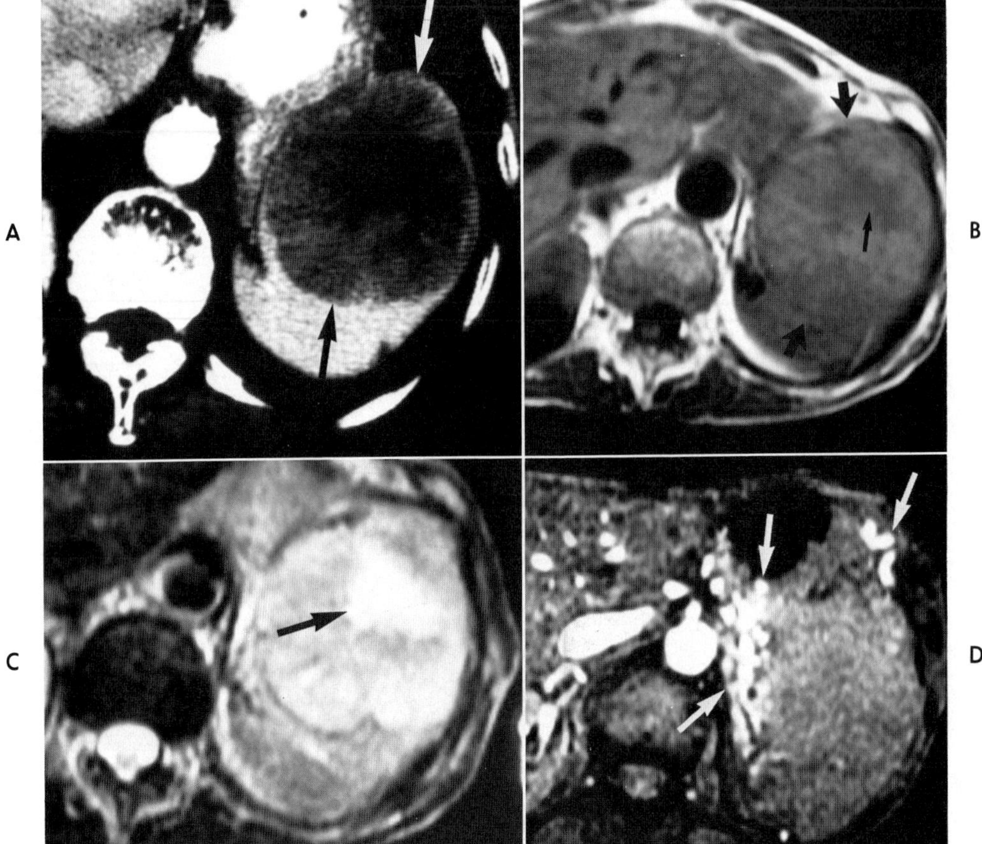

Fig. 23-5 Surgically proven splenic metastasis from carcinoma of the lung. *S* = spleen. **A,** Contrast enhanced CT scan reveals a low signal mass *(arrows)* at the anterior aspect of the spleen. **B,** SE 500/12 image reveals a large mass *(thick arrows)* in the hilum of the spleen, with central low signal *(thin arrow)*. **C,** SE 2500/100 image depicts the mass as high signal with central necrosis *(arrow)*. **D,** Gradient-echo image (TR/TE/flip angle = 25/13/20 degrees) reveals dilated gastroepiploic veins *(arrows)* suggestive of splenic vein obstruction. The splenic vein was not visualized.

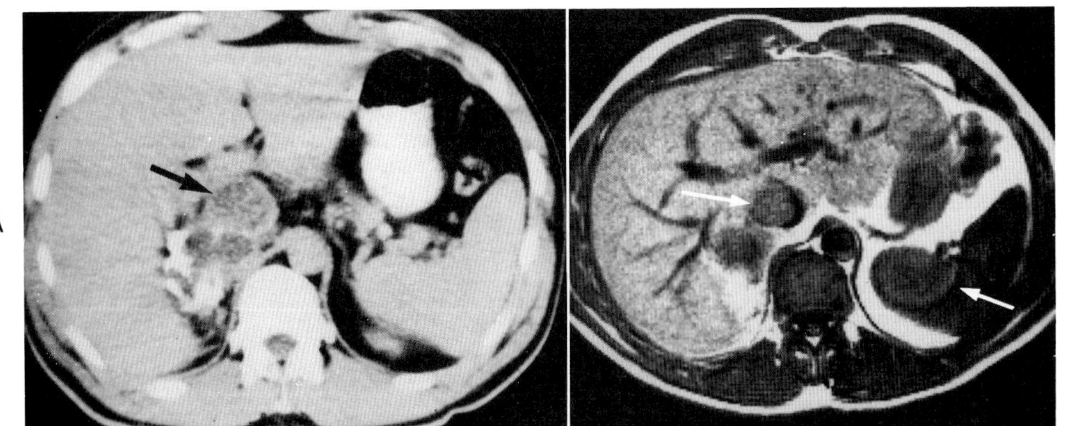

Fig. 23-6 Hemorrhagic renal cell carcinoma, metastatic to the spleen. **A,** CT shows extension of tumor into the inferior vena cava *(arrow)*. The spleen appears normal. **B,** SE 330/18 image shows the right renal carcinoma invading the inferior vena cava. A 5-cm splenic metastasis is present. (From Hahn, P.F., Weissleder, R., Stark, D.D., et al.: AJR 150:823-827, 1988.)

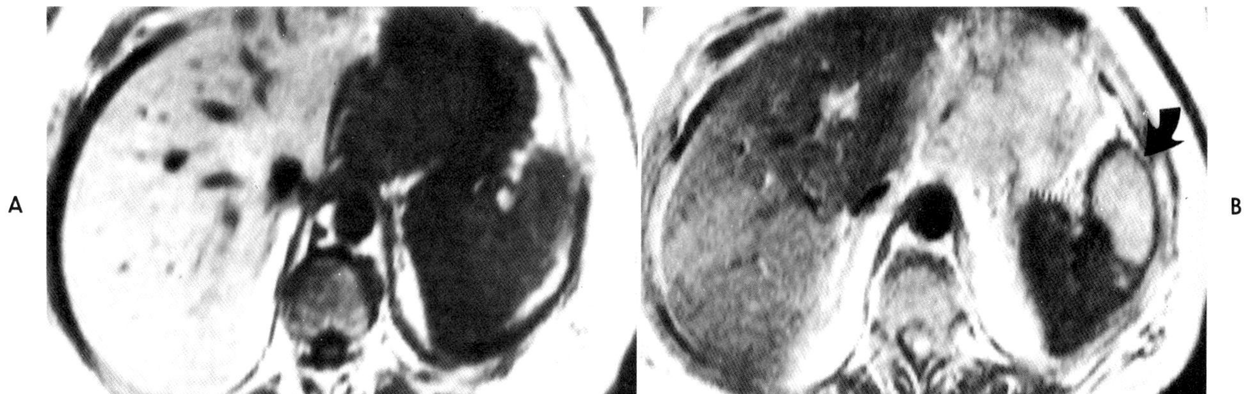

Fig. 23-7   Non-Hodgkin's lymphoma. The patient has severe anemia and recently received multiple blood transfusions. **A,** SE 300/14 image shows lymphoma invading the stomach. The spleen appears normal. **B,** 2300/60 image shows an unusually low signal intensity of the spleen relative to liver. This appearance is attributed to hemolysis and increased splenic iron content. Because of the abnormally low intensity of normal splenic tissue, focal splenic lymphoma is easily seen (arrow).

BENIGN LESIONS

Cysts are the most common benign tumors of the spleen. These may be congenital (true cysts, 20%) or traumatic (false cysts, 80%). Cysts may be multiple and should not be confused with abscesses, pseudocysts, and parasitic lesions. Cysts have smooth borders and homogeneous long T1 and very long T2 relaxation times (Fig. 23-8).

Splenic hemangiomas are less common than hepatic hemangiomas. MR features are similar, however, with long T1 and distinctively long T2 (Figs. 23-9 to 23-11). Therefore heavily T2-weighted images depict hemangiomas as smoothly marginated, well-defined, homogeneous, hyperintense lesions, similar to cysts. As in the liver, giant hemangiomas in the spleen can be heterogeneous, with hemorrhage, thrombosis, fibrosis, and hemosiderin deposition.[282,439]

The third most common benign splenic tumor is the lymphangioma. The spleen may be the primary site of involvement or may be involved as part of a diffuse abdominal lymphangiomatosis. In cystic lymphangiomatosis the lesions appear as clusters of cysts (Fig. 23-12). These may imitate simple cysts, with homogeneously long T1 and long T2. Occasionally, signal intensity may vary because of increased protein content or hemorrhage.[86]

Splenic infarcts are usually focal, since infarction of the entire spleen is very rare. Infarcts occur most often in blood dyscrasias, such as sickle cell disease or myeloproliferative disorders, or in systemic embolism from endocarditis or septal defects. Infarcts are depicted as peripheral, wedge-shaped lesions in only one third of cases; others present as multiple heterogeneous (42%) or massive (25%) lesions.[18]

Infarcts are visible on MR images most commonly in association with iron overload of the spleen, such as in patients with sickle cell disease or lymphoma. In this setting the infarct appears as a zone of high signal intensity within a low-signal spleen. Chronic infarcts, like focal lesions of lymphoma and sarcoid, have a lower signal intensity than surrounding uninvolved spleen on gradient-echo images, whereas the intensity of recent infarcts resembles the remainder of the spleen.[206]

Splenic granulomas are common but are often missed by MRI. In patients with granulomatous disease, the spleen may appear nodular rather than homogeneous (Fig. 23-13).

Siderotic nodules, also called Gamna-Gandy bodies, are brown, organized foci of hemorrhage present in the spleen of one eighth of patients with portal hypertension. The lesions appear as areas of low signal intensity on T2-weighted or gradient-echo images because of T2 shortening from hemosiderin. Because of its sensitivity to field inhomogeneity, MRI, especially at high field, is more sensitive than CT or ultrasound for detecting these nodules.[339,456]

LYMPHOMA AND LEUKEMIA

The spleen is a principal repository of lymphoma. Spleen size is an unreliable indicator of involvement; splenomegaly has a sensitivity of 36% and a specificity of 61% for splenic involvement in lymphoma patients.[165] Imaging studies have only marginally improved on the clinical staging of lymphoma in the spleen. Sonography, sulfur colloid scintigraphy, and CT have accuracy rates of 75%, 54% to 64%, and 58% to 65%, respectively.[62,312,486]

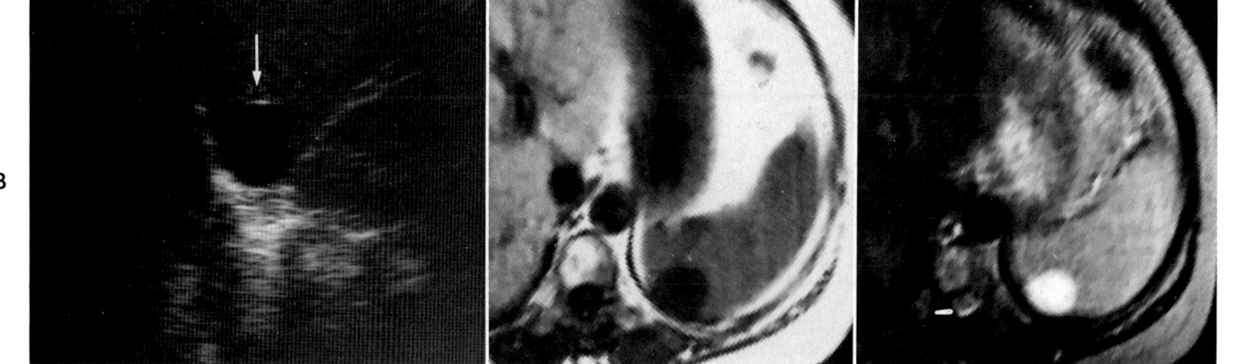

Fig. 23-8 Splenic cyst, surgically confirmed. **A,** Sonogram shows typical features of a simple splenic cyst: sharp margins, imperceptible wall, an echoic center, and good acoustic transmission. **B,** SE 300/14 image shows a sharply circumscribed low signal intensity lesion. **C,** SE 2400/120. Cyst signal intensity is greater than the intensity of cerebrospinal fluid. Note the incidental vertebral hemangioma, which has an increased signal intensity due to fatty stroma.

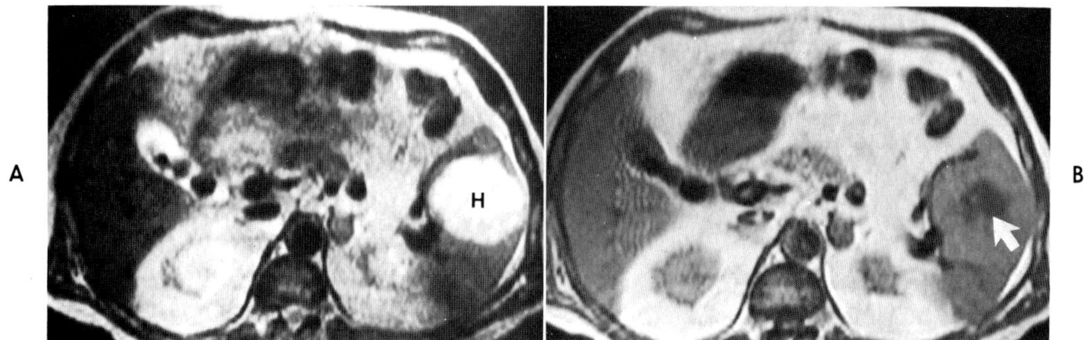

Fig. 23-9 Cavernous hemangioma of the spleen. **A,** T2-weighted image (SE 2091/100, 0.6 T) shows round hyperintense lesion *(H)* that is isointense to gallbladder bile. There are multiple low signal intensity gallstones. **B,** On intermediate image (SE 2091/20), the lesion is only slightly hyperintense. There is a central stellate low signal intensity scar *(arrow).*

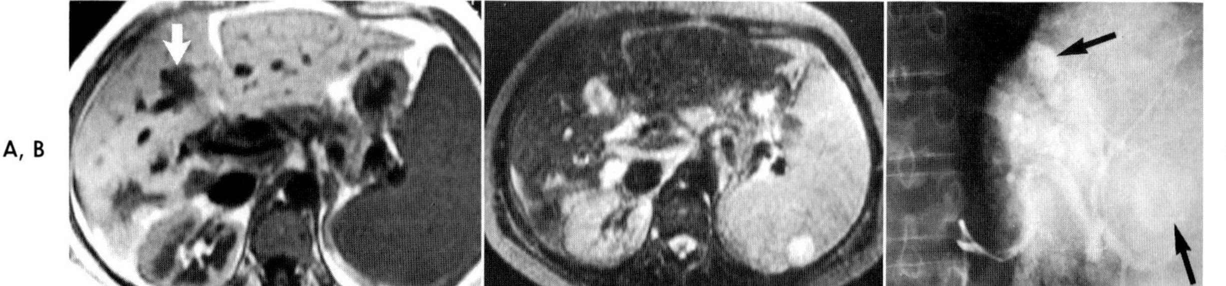

Fig. 23-10 Patient with hemangiomas of the liver and spleen. **A,** Axial T1-weighted MR image (SE 275/14, 0.6 T) shows focal hypointense lesion in the liver *(arrow).* **B,** T2-weighted (SE 2350/180) image at the same level as **A** shows intensely hyperintense lesion in the spleen in retrospect slightly hypointense on the T1-weighted image. Lesions in liver and in spleen are isointense. **C,** Selective splenic arteriogram shows multiple hypervascular splenic tumors *(arrows).*

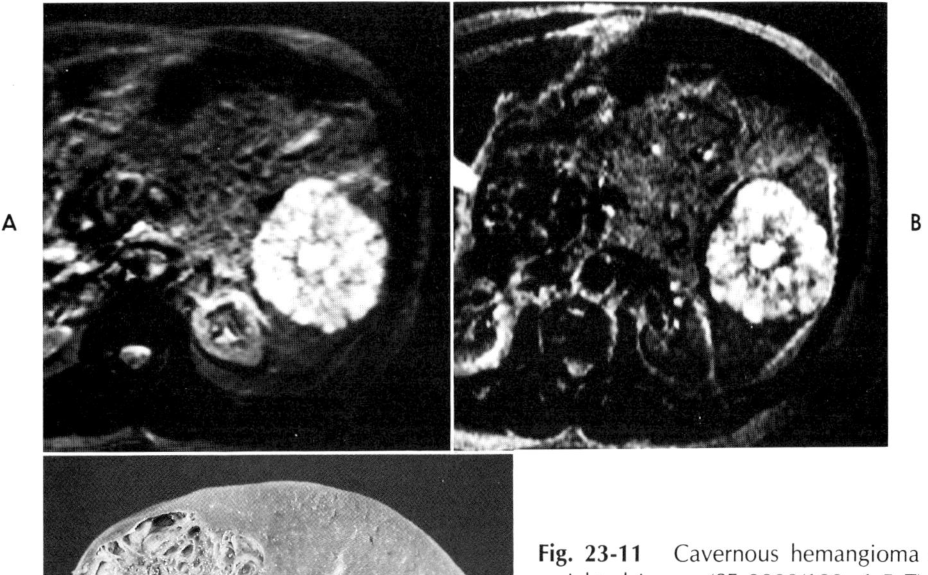

Fig. 23-11 Cavernous hemangioma of the spleen. **A,** T2-weighted image (SE 2000/100, 1.5 T) shows high signal intensity focal lesion in the spleen. **B,** Breath-holding gradient-echo image (33/10/90 degrees) more clearly demonstrates stellate internal septations. **C,** Splenectomy specimen. (Courtesy L. te Strake.)

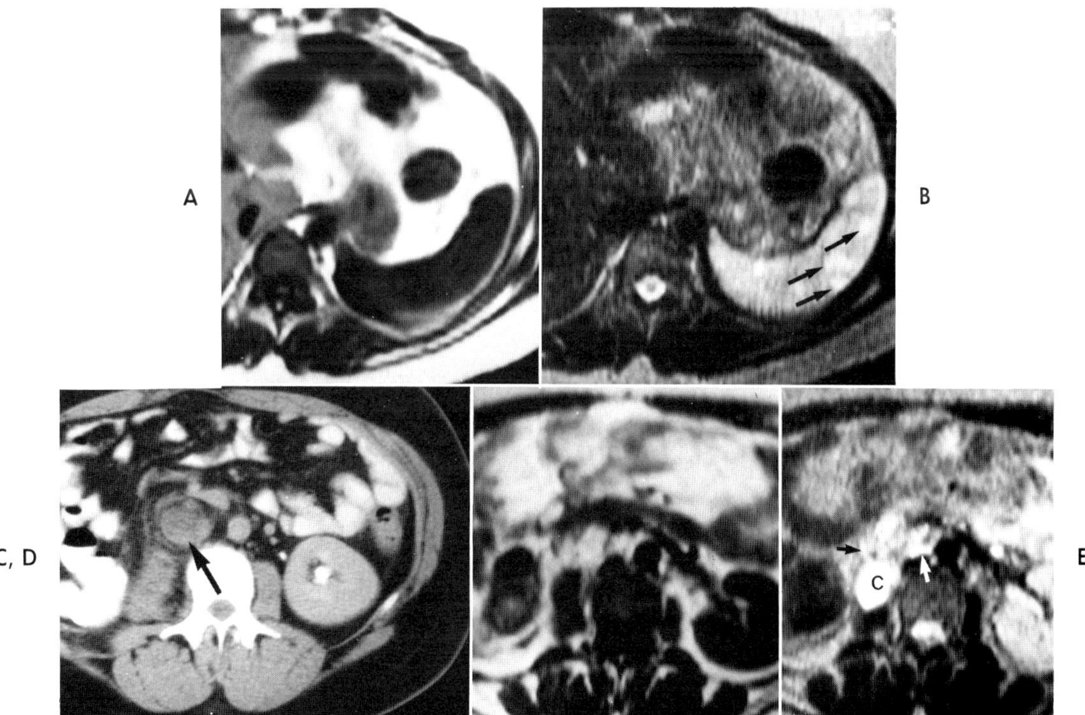

Fig. 23-12 Lymphangiomatosis with retroperitoneal and splenic involvement. **A,** Axial T1-weighted image (SE 270/14) shows no splenic abnormality. **B,** Corresponding heavily T2-weighted image (SE 2350/180) shows multiple foci of long T2 *(arrows),* indicating lymphangiomatous cysts within the spleen. **C,** Inferiorly, CT image shows retroperitoneal disease *(arrow)* around the inferior vena cava. A surgical debulking procedure had already been performed. **D** and **E,** T1- and T2-weighted images show that the retroperitoneal abnormality is composed of cysts *(C)* and channels *(small arrows).* There is evidence for T1 shortening, which could be the result of either a hemorrhage or a high protein content.

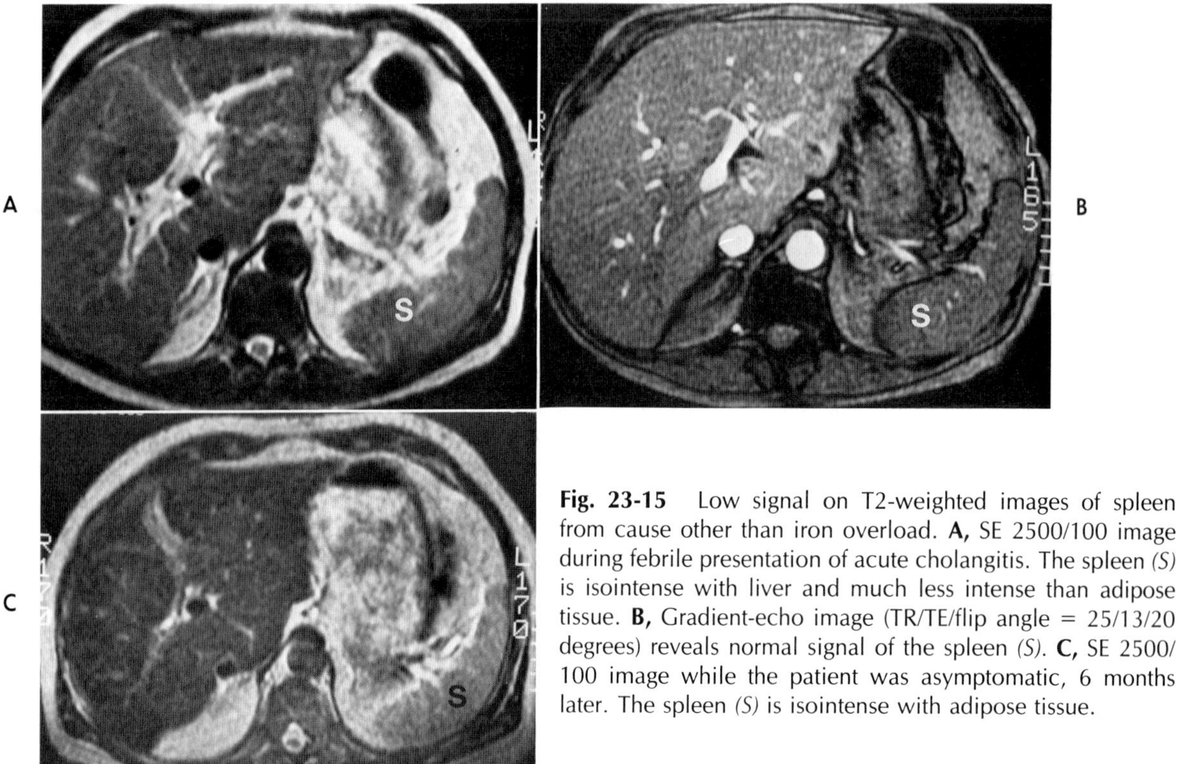

Fig. 23-15   Low signal on T2-weighted images of spleen from cause other than iron overload. **A,** SE 2500/100 image during febrile presentation of acute cholangitis. The spleen *(S)* is isointense with liver and much less intense than adipose tissue. **B,** Gradient-echo image (TR/TE/flip angle = 25/13/20 degrees) reveals normal signal of the spleen *(S)*. **C,** SE 2500/100 image while the patient was asymptomatic, 6 months later. The spleen *(S)* is isointense with adipose tissue.

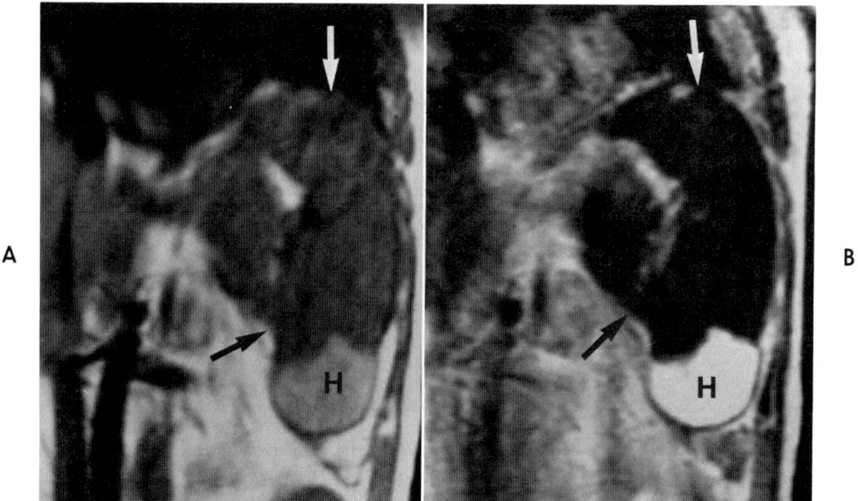

Fig. 23-16   Splenic hematoma in a patient with chronic myelogenous leukemia and transfusional siderosis. **A,** Coronal SE 500/20 image reveals a large spleen *(arrows)* with an expansile hematoma *(H)* inferiorly. **B,** Coronal SE 2400/100 image.

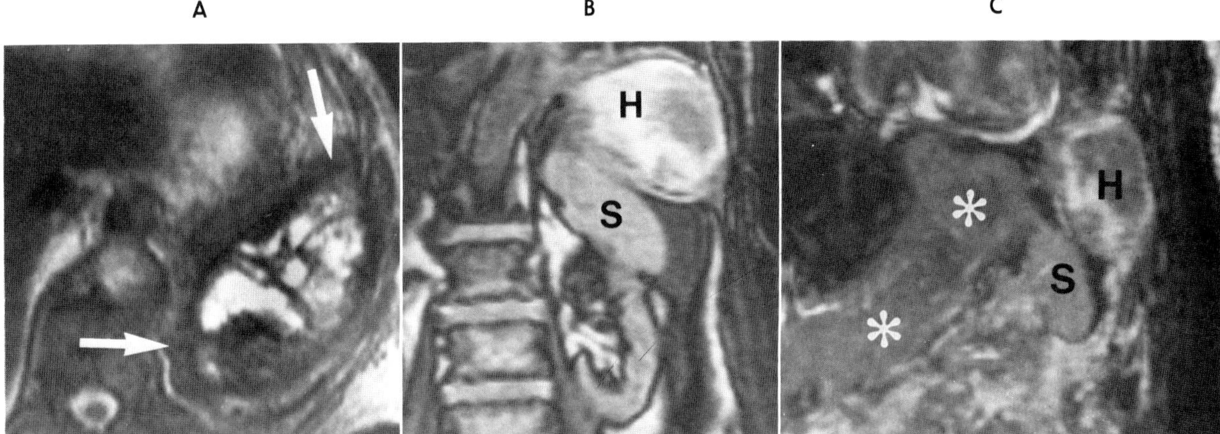

Fig. 23-17   Suprasplenic hematoma depicted as separate from spleen by coronal images. **A,** SE 2500/100 image reveals a heterogeneous collection in the left upper quadrant with a spleniform shape *(arrows)*. The margins have low signal, suggestive of hemosiderin. **B,** Coronal T1-weighted gradient echo image (T/TE/flip angle = 101/2.3/90 degrees). The hematoma *(H)* is clearly separate from the spleen *(S)*. **C,** Composite slab from technique as in **B,** demonstrating the relationship between hematoma *(H)*, spleen *(S)*, and stomach *(asterisks)*.

REFERENCES

1. Abbas, Y.A. and Kressel, H.Y.: MR of liver cirrhosis at 1.5 T, Society of Magnetic Resonance in Medicine 9th Annual Meeting, New York, NY, August 18-24, 1990, Book of Abstracts, p. 91.
2. Adler, D.D., Glazer, G.M., and Aisen, A.M.: MRI of the spleen: normal appearance and findings in sickle-cell anemia, AJR 147:843-845, 1986.
3. Adson, M.A.: Surgery symposium: mass lesions of the liver, Mayo Clin. Proc. 61:362-368, 1986.
4. Ahmann, D.L., Kiely, J.M., Harrison, E.G., et al.: Malignant lymphoma of the spleen. A review of 49 cases in which the diagnosis was made at splenectomy, Cancer 19:461-469, 1966.
5. Alderson, P.O., Adams, D.F., and McNeil, B.J.: Computed tomography, ultrasound, and scintigraphy of the liver in patients with colon or breast carcinoma: a prospective comparison, Radiology 149:225-230, 1983.
6. Alpern, M.B., Rubin, J.M., Williams, D.M, et al.: Porta hepatis: duplex Doppler US with angiographic correlation, Radiology 162:53-56, 1987.
7. Applegate, G.R., Wozney, P., Thaete, L., et al.: Blood flow in the portal vein: velocity quantitation with phase contrast evaluation, Society of Magnetic Resonance in Medicine 9th Annual Meeting, New York, NY, August 18-24, 1990, Book of Abstracts, p. 222.
8. Arai, K., Matsui, O., Takashima, T., et al.: Focal spared areas in fatty liver caused by regional decreased portal flow, AJR 151:300-302, 1988.
9. Arakawa, M., Kage, M., Sugihara, S., et al.: Emergence of malignant lesions within an adenomatous hyperplastic nodule in a cirrhotic liver, Gastroenterology 91:198-208, 1986.
10. Araki, T., Suda, K., Sekikawa, T., et al.: Portal venous tumor thrombosis associated with gastric adenocarcinoma, Radiology 174:811-814, 1990.
11. Arrive, L., Hricak, H, Goldberg, H.I., et al.: MR appearance of the liver after partial hepatectomy, AJR 152:1215-1220, 1989.
12. Atlas, S.W., Braffman, B.H., LoBrutto, R., et al.: Human malignant melanomas with varying degrees of melanin content in nude mice: MR imaging, histopathology, and electron paramagnetic resonance, J. Comput. Assist. Tomogr. 14:547-554, 1990.
13. Atri, M., de Stempel, J., Bret, P.M., et al.: Incidence of portal vein thrombosis complicating liver metastasis as detected by duplex ultrasound, J. Ultrasound Med. 9:285-289, 1990.
14. Bacon, B.R., Stark, D.D., Park, C.H., et al.: Ferrite particles, a new MRI contrast agent: lack of acute or chronic hepatotoxicity following intravenous administration, J. Lab. Clin. Med. 110:164-171, 1987.
15. Bagley, C.M. Jr., Young, R.C., Schein, P.S., et al.: Ovarian carcinoma metastatic to the diaphragm frequently undiagnosed at laparotomy, Am. J. Obstet. Gynecol. 116:397-400, 1973.
16. Bailes, D.R., Gilderdale, D.J., Bydder, G.M., et al.: Respiratory ordered phase encoding (ROPE): a method for reducing respiratory motion artifacts in MR imaging, J. Comput. Assist. Tomogr. 9:835-838, 1985.

17. Baker, M.E., Cohan, R.H., Nadel, S.N., et al.: Obliteration of the fat surrounding the celiac axis and superior mesenteric artery is not a specific CT finding of carcinoma of the pancreas, AJR 155:991-994, 1990.
18. Balcar, I., Seltzer, S.E., Davis, S., et al.: CT patterns of splenic infarction: a clinical and experimental study, Radiology 151:723-729, 1984.
19. Ballinger, R., Magin, R.L., Webb, A.G.: Sucrose polyester: a new oral contrast agent for MRI, Magn. Reson. Med. 19:199-202, 1991.
20. Balthazar, E.J., Robinson, D.L., Megibow, A.J., et al.: Acute pancreatitis: value of CT is establishing prognosis, Radiology 174:331-336, 1990.
21. Barakos, J., Goldberg, H., Brown, J.J., et al.: Comparison of computed tomography and magnetic resonance imaging in the evaluation of focal hepatic lesions, Gastrointest. Radiol. 15:93-101, 1990.
22. Barnes, P.A., Thomas, J.L., and Bernardino, M.E.: Pitfalls in the diagnosis of hepatic cysts by computed tomography, Radiology 141:129-133, 1981.
23. Baron, R.L., Kuyper, S.J., Lee, S.P., et al.: In vitro dissolution of gallstones with MTBE: correlation with characteristics at CT and MR imaging, Radiology 173:117-121, 1989.
24. Baron, R.L., Shuman, W.P., and Lee, S.P.: MR appearance of gallstones in vitro at 1.5 T: correlation with chemical composition, AJR 153:497-502, 1989.
25. Bassett, M.L., Halliday, J.W., Ferris, R.A., et al.: Diagnosis of hemochromatosis in young subjects: predictive accuracy of biochemical screening tests, Gastroenterology 87:628-633, 1984.
26. Bassett, M.L., Halliday, J.W., and Powell, L.W.: Value of hepatic iron measurements in early hemochromatosis and determination of the critical iron level associated with fibrosis, Hepatology 6:24-29, 1986.
27. Bell, J.D., Cox, I.J., Peden, C.J., et al.: In-vitro 1Hydrogen and 31Phosphorus (31P) magnetic resonance spectroscopy (MRS) studies on human liver extracts: normal and tumor biopsies, Society of Magnetic Resonance in Medicine 9th Annual Meeting, New York, NY, August 18-24, 1990, Book of Abstracts, p. 283.
28. Berland, L.L.: Focal areas of decreased echogenicity in the liver at the porta hepatis, J. Ultrasound Med. 5:157-159, 1986.
29. Bernadino, M.E., Chaloupka, J.C., Malko, J.A., et al.: Are hepatic and muscle T2 values different at 0.5 and 1.5 tesla? Magn. Reson. Imaging 7:363-367, 1989.
30. Bernardino, M.E., Erwin, B.C., Steinberg, H.V., et al.: Delayed hepatic CT scanning: increased confidence and improved detection of hepatic metastases, Radiology 159:71-74, 1986.
31. Bernardino, M.E., Steinberg, H.V., and Pearson, T.C.: Comparison of MRI and angiography in the determination of shunt patency for portal hypertension, Radiology 158:57-61, 1986.
32. Bernardino, M.E., Thomas, J.L., Barnes, P.A., et al.: Diagnostic approaches to liver and spleen metastases, Radiol. Clin. North. Am. 20:469-485, 1982.

33. Birnbaum, B.A., Weinreb, J.C., Megibow, A.J., et al.: Blinded retrospective comparison of MR imaging and Tc-99m-labeled red blood cell SPECT for definitive diagnosis of hepatic hemangiomas, Radiology 173(P): 270, 1989.

34. Bisceglie, A.M., Martin, P., Kasslanides, C., et al.: Recombinant interferon alfa therapy for chronic hepatitis C. A randomized, double-blind, placebo-controlled trial, N. Engl. J. Med. 321:1506-1510, 1989.

35. Bisset III, G.S., Strife, J.L., and Balistreri, W.F.: Evaluation of children for liver transplantation: value of MR imaging and sonography, AJR 155:351-356, 1990.

36. Boechat, M.I., Kangarloo, H., Ortega, J., et al.: Primary liver tumors in children: comparison of CT and MR imaging, Radiology 169:727-732, 1988.

37. Borg, S.A., Rubin, P., and DeWys, W.D.: Metastases and disseminated disease. In Clinical oncology: a multidisciplinary approach, ed. 6, New York, 1983, American Cancer Society, pp. 498-515.

38. Bottomley, P.A., Foster, T.H., Argersinger, R.E., and et al.: A review of normal tissue hydrogen NMR relaxation times and relaxation mechanisms from 1-100 MHz: dependence on tissue type, NMR frequency, temperature, species, excision, and age, Med. Phys. 11:425-448, 1984.

39. Bottomley, P.A., Hardy, C.J., Argersinger, R.E., et al.: A review of 1H nuclear magnetic resonance relaxation in pathology: are T1 and T2 diagnostic? Med. Phys. 14:1-37, 1987.

40. Brady, T.M., Gross, B.H., Glazer, G.M., et al.: Adrenal pseudomasses due to varices: angiographic-CT-MRI-pathologic correlations, AJR 145:301-304, 1985.

41. Brandt, D.J., Johnson, C.D., Stephens, D.H., et al.: Imaging of fibrolamellar hepatocellular carcinoma, AJR 151:295-299, 1988.

42. Bree, R.L., Schwab, R., Glazer, G.M., et al.: The varied appearances of hepatic cavernous hemangiomas with sonography, computed tomography, magnetic resonance imaging and scintigraphy, RadioGraphics 7:1153-1175, 1987.

43. Bressler, E.L., Alpern, M.B., Glazer, G.M., et al.: Hypervascular hepatic metastases: CT evaluation, Radiology 162:49-51, 1987.

44. Bret, P.M., Labadie, M., Bretangnolle, M., et al.: Hepatocellular carcinoma: diagnosis by percutaneous fine needle biopsy, Gastrointest. Radiol. 13:253-255, 1988.

45. Brick, S.H., Hill, M.C., and Lande, I.M.: The mistaken or indeterminate CT: diagnosis of hepatic metastases: the value of sonography, AJR 148:723-726, 1987.

46. Brittenham, G.M., Farrell, D.E., Harris, J.W., et al.: Magnetic-susceptibility measurement of human iron stores, N. Engl. J. Med. 307:1671-1675, 1982.

47. Brodsky, R.I., Friedman, A.C., Maurer, A.H., et al.: Hepatic cavernous hemangioma: diagnosis with ^{99m}Tc-labeled red cells and single-photon emission CT, AJR 148:125-129, 1987.

48. Brown, B.P., Abu-Yousef, M., Farner, R., et al.: Doppler sonography: a noninvasive method for evaluation of hepatic venocclusive disease, AJR 154:721-724, 1990.

49. Brown, J.J., Lee, J.M., Lee, J.K.T., et al.: Focal hepatic lesions: differentiation with MR imaging at 0.5 T, Radiology 179: 675-679, 1991.

50. Brown, R.K.J., Gomes, A., King, W., et al.: Hepatic hemangiomas: evaluation by magnetic resonance imaging and technetium-^{99m} red blood cell scintigraphy, J. Nucl. Med. 28:1683, 1987.

51. Bru, C., Maroto, A., Bruix, J., et al.: Diagnostic accuracy of fine-needle aspiration biopsy in patients with hepatocellular carcinoma, Dig. Dis. Sci. 34:1765-1769, 1989.

52. Buck, J.L. and Hayes, W.S.: Microcystic adenoma of the pancreas, RadioGraphics 10:313-322, 1990.

53. Butch, R.J., Stark, D.D., and Malt, R.A.: MR imaging of hepatic focal nodular hyperplasia, J. Comput. Assist. Tomogr. 10:874-877, 1986.

54. Buxton, R.B., Edelman, R.R., Rosen, B.R., et al.: Contrast in rapid MR imaging: T1- and T2-weighting, J. Comput. Assist. Tomogr. 11:7-16, 1987.

55. Bydder, G.M., Steiner, E., Blumgart, F.L.H., et al.: MR imaging of the liver using short T1 inversion recovery sequences, J. Comput. Assist. Tomogr. 9:1084-1089, 1985.

56. Bydder, G.M. and Young, I.R.: NMR imaging: clinical use of the inversion recovery sequence, J. Comput. Assist. Tomogr. 9:659-675, 1985.

57. Cameron, I.L., Ord, WV.A., and Fullerton, G.D.: Characterization of proton NMR relaxation times in normal and pathological tissues by correlation with other tissue parameters, Magn. Reson. Imag. 2:97-106, 1984.

58. Cancer facts and figures, New York, 1985, American Cancer Society.

59. Carr, D.H., Brown, J., Bydder, G.M., et al.: Gadolinium-DTPA as a contrast agent in MRI: initial clinical experience in 20 patients, AJR 143:215-224, 1984.

60. Carr, D.H., Hadjis, N.S., Banks, L.M., et al.: Computed tomography of hilar cholangiocarcinoma: a new sign, AJR 145:53-56, 1985.

61. Carvlin, M., Schultze-Haack, H., Le, C., et al.: Rethinking the design of oral contrast media, JMRI 1:188, 1991.

62. Castellino, R.A.: Imaging techniques for staging abdominal Hodgkin's disease, Cancer Treat. Rep. 66:697-700, 1982.

63. Caturelli, E., Costarelli, L., Giordano, M., et al: Hypoechoic lesions in fatty liver: quantitative study by histomorphology, Gastroenterol. 100:1678-1682, 1991.

64. Center for Disease Control: Deaths from chronic liver disease—United States, 1986, JAMA 263:355-360, 1990.

65. Chan, T.W., Listerud, J., and Kressel, H.Y.: Combined chemical-shift and phase-selective imaging for fat suppression: theory and initial clinical experience, Radiology 181:41-47, 1991.

66. Chang, Y.C., Nagasue, N., Kimura, N., et al.: Ultrasonographic features of hepatocellular pseudotumour in the cirrhotic liver, Clin. Radiol. 39:635-638, 1988.

67. Chapman, R.W.G., Marborgh, B.A., Rhodes, J.M., et al.: Primary sclerosing cholangitis: a review of its clinical features, cholangiography, and hepatic histology, Gut 21:870-877, 1980.

68. Chen, M.C., Tsang, Y., Stark, D.D., et al.: Hepatic metastases: rat models for imaging research, Magn. Reson. Imaging 7:1-8, 1989.

69. Chien, D., Atkinson, D.J., and Edelman, R.R.: Strategies to improve contrast in TurboFLASH imaging: reordered phase encoding and k-space segmentation, JMRI 1:63-70, 1991.

70. Chien, D. and Edelman, R.R.: Ultrafast imaging using gradient echoes, Magn. Reson. Quart. 7:31-56, 1991.

71. Chezmar, J.L. and Bernadino, M.E.: Mesoatrial shunt for the treatment of Budd-Chiari Syndrome: radiologic evaluation in eight patients, AJR 149:707-710, 1987.

72. Chezmar, J.L., Nelson, R.C., Malko, J.A., et al.: Hepatic iron overload: diagnosis and quantification by noninvasive imaging, Gastrointest. Radiol. 15:27-31, 1990.

73. Chezmar, J.L., Nelson, R.C., Small, W.C., et al.: Magnetic resonance imaging of the pancreas with gadolinium-DTPA, Gastrointest. Radiol. 16:139-142, 1991.

74. Chezmar, J.L., Rumancik, W.M., Megibow, A.J., et al.: Liver and abdominal screening in patients with cancer: CT versus MR imaging, Radiology 168:43-47, 1988.

75. Cho, K.H., Geisinger, K.R., Shields, J.J., et al.: Collateral channels and histopathology in hepatic vein occlusion, AJR 139:703-709, 1982.

76. Cho, J., Kim, E.E., Varma, D.G.K., et al.: MR imaging of hepatosplenic candidiasis superimposed on hemochromatosis, J. Comput. Assist. Tomogr. 14:774-776, 1990.

77. Choi, B.I., Han, M.C., Park, J.H., et al.: Giant cavernous hemangioma of the liver: CT and MR imaging in 10 cases, AJR 152:1221-1226, 1989.

78. Choi, B.I., Lee, G.K., Kim, S.T., et al: Mosaic pattern of encapsulated hepatocellular carcinoma: correlation of magnetic resonance imaging and pathology, Gastrointest. Radiol. 15:238-240, 1990.

79. Choji, K., Shinohara, T., Nojima, K., et al.: Significant reduction of the echogenicity of the compressed cavernous hemangioma, Acta Radiol. 29:317-320, 1988.

80. Claudon, M., Bessieres, M., Regent, D., et al.: Alveolar echinococcosis of the liver: MR findings, J. Comput. Assist. Tomogr. 14:608-614, 1990.

81. Clement, O., Frija, G., Chambon, C., et al.: Liver tumors in cirrhosis: experimental study with SPIO-enhanced MR imaging, Radiology 180:31-36, 1991.

82. Colina, F., Alberti, N., Solis, J.A., et al.: Diffuse nodular regenerative hyperplasia of the liver (DNRH). A clinicopathologic study of 24 cases, Liver 9:253-265, 1989.

83. Condon, B., Patterson, J., Jenkins, A., et al.: MR relaxation times of cerebrospinal fluid, J. Comput. Assist. Tomogr. 11:203-207, 1987.

84. Cuenod, C.A., Bellin, M.F., Bousquet, J.C., et al.: MRI of liver tumors using gadolinium-DOTA: prospective study comparing spin-echo long TR-TE sequence and CT, Magn. Reson. Imaging 9:235-245, 1991.

85. Curati, W.L., Halevy, A., Gibson, R.N., et al.: Ultrasound, CT, and MRI comparison in primary and secondary tumors of the liver, Gastrointest. Radiol. 13:123-128, 1988.

86. Cutillo, D.P., Swayne, L.C., Cucco, J., et al.: CT and MR imaging in cystic abdominal lymphangiomatosis, J. Comput. Assist. Tomogr. 13:534-536, 1989.

87. Cutillo, D.P., Swayne, L.C., Fasciano, M.G., et al.: Absence of fatty replacement in radiation damaged liver: CT demonstration, J. Comput. Assist. Tomogr. 13:259-261, 1989.

88. Dachman, A.H., Ros, P.R., Goodman, Z.D., et al.: Nodular regenerative hyperplasia of the liver: clinical and radiologic observations, AJR 148:717-722, 1987.

89. Dalen, K., Day, D.L., Ascher, N.L., et al.: Imaging of vascular complications after hepatic transplantation, AJR 150:1285-1290, 1988.

90. Davis, P.L., Kanal, E., Farnum, G.N., et al.: MR imaging of multiple hepatic cysts in a patient with polycystic liver disease, Magn. Reson. Imaging 5:407-411, 1987.

91. Davis, W.D., Ferrante, W.A., Tutton, R.H., et al.: Hepatic hemangioma with normal angiograms, JAMA 263:983-986, 1990.

92. de Lange, E.E., Mugler, J.P., Janus, C.L., et al.: Magnetization prepared rapid gradient echo (MP-RAGE) MR imaging of the liver, Society of Magnetic Resonance in Medicine 9th Annual Meeting, New York, NY, August 18-24, 1990, Book of Abstracts, p. 86.

93. DelMaschio, A., Vanzulli, A., Sironi, S., et al.: Pancreatic cancer versus chronic pancreatitis: diagnosis with CA 19-9 assessment, US, CT, and CT-guided fine-needle biopsy, Radiology 178:95-99, 1991.

94. Demas, B.E., Hricak, H., Goldberg, H.I., et al.: Magnetic resonance imaging diagnosis of hepatic metastases in the presence of negative CT studies, J. Clin. Gastroenterol. 7:553-560, 1985.

95. Demas, B.E., Hricak, H., Moseley, M., et al.: Gallbladder bile: an experimental study in dogs using MR imaging and proton MR spectroscopy, Radiology 157:453-455, 1985.

96. Demetris, A.J., Lasky, S., Van Thiel, D.H., et al.: Pathology of hepatic transplantation: a review of 62 adult allograft recipients immunosuppressed with a cyclosporine steroid regimen, Am. J. Pathol. 118:151-161, 1985.

97. Di Bisceglie, A.M., Martin, P., Kasslanides, C., et al.: Recombinant interferon alfa therapy for chronic hepatitis C, N. Engl. J. Med. 321:1506-1510, 1989.

98. Dietze, O., Vogel, W., Braunsperger, B., et al.: Liver transplantation in idiopathic hemochromatosis, Transplant. Proc. 22:1512-1513, 1990.

99. Dixon, W.T.: Simple proton spectroscopic imaging, Radiology 153:189-194, 1984.

100. Dodds, W.J., Erickson, S.J., Taylor, A.J., et al.: Caudate lobe of the liver: anatomy, embryology, and pathology, AJR 154:87-93, 1990.

101. Dooley, W.C., Cameron, J.L., Pitt, H.A., et al.: Is preoperative angiography useful in patients with periampullary tumors? Ann. Surg. 211:649-655, 1990.

102. Dooms, B.E., Fisher, M.R. Higgins, C.B., et al.: MR imaging of the dilated biliary tract, Radiology 158:337-341, 1986.

103. Dooms, G.C., Kerlan, R.K., Hricak, H.E., et al.: Cholangiocarcinoma: imaging by MR, Radiology 159:89-94, 1986.

104. Doppman, J.L., Cornbluth, M., Dwyer, A.J., et al.: Computed tomography of the liver and kidney in glycogen storage disease, J. Comput. Assist. Tomogr. 6:67-71, 1982.

105. Doppman, J.L., Dwyer, A., Vermess, M., et al.: Segmental hyperlucent defects in the liver, J. Comput. Assist. Tomogr. 8:50-57, 1984.

106. Dousset, M., Weissleder, R., Hendrick R.E., et al.: Short TI inversion-recovery imaging of the liver: pulse-sequence optimization and comparison with spin-echo imaging, Radiology 171:327-33, 1989.

107. DuBrow R.A., David C.L., Libshitz H.I., et al.: Detection of hepatic metastases in breast cancer: the role of nonenhanced and enhanced CT scanning, J. Comput. Assist. Tomogr. 14:366-369, 1990.

108. Dumoulin, C.L., Yucel, E.K., Vock, P., et al.: Two- and three-dimensional phase contrast MR angiography of the abdomen, J. Comput. Assist. Tomogr. 14:779-784, 1990.

109. Ebara, M., Ohto, M., Watanabe, Y., et al.: Diagnosis of small hepatocellular carcinoma: correlation of MR imaging and tumor histologic studies, Radiology 159:371-377, 1986.

110. Ebara, M., Watanabe, S., Kita, K., et al.: MR imaging of small hepatocellular carcinoma: effect of intratumoral copper content on signal intensity, Radiology 180:617-621, 1991.

111. Edelman, R.R., Atkinson, D.J., Silver, M.S., et al.: FRODO pulse sequences: a new means of eliminating motion, flow, and wraparound artifacts, Radiology 166:231, 1988.

112. Edelman, R.R., Hahn, P.F., Buxton, R., et al.: Rapid MR imaging with suspended respiration: clinical application in the liver, Radiology 161:125-131, 1986.

113. Edelman, R.R., Siegel, J.B.., Singer, A., et al.: Dynamic MR imaging of the liver with Gd-DTPA: initial clinical results, AJR 153:1213-1219, 1989.

114. Edelman, R.R., Wallner, B., Singer A., et al.: Segmented turbo-FLASH: method for breath-hold MR imaging of the liver with flexible contrast, Radiology 177:515-521, 1990.

115. Edelman, R.R., Zhao, B., Liu, C., et al.: MR angiography and dynamic flow evaluation of the portal venous system, AJR 153:755-760, 1989.

116. Edmondson, H.A.: Benign epithelial tumors and tumorlike lesions of the liver, In Okuda, J. and Peters, R.L. (eds.), Hepatocellular carcinoma, New York: 1976, Wiley, p. 309.

117. Egglin, T.K., Rummeny, E., Stark, D.D., et al.: Hepatic tumors: quantitative tissue characterization with MR imaging, Radiology 176:107-110, 1990.

118. Ehman, R.L. and Felmlee, J.P.: Adaptive techniques for high-definition MR imaging of moving structures, Radiology 173:255-263, 1989.

119. Ehman, R.L., McNamara, M.T., Brasch, R.C., et al.: Influence of physiologic motion on the appearance of tissue in MR images, Radiology 159:777-782, 1986.

120. Ehman, R.L., McNamara, M.T., Pallack, M., et al.: Magnetic resonance imaging with respiratory gating: techniques and advantages, AJR 143:1175-1182, 1984.

121. Elizondo, G., Fretz, C., Stark, D.D., et al.: Preclinical evaluation of MnDPDP: new paramagnetic hepatobiliary contrast agent for MR imaging, Radiology 178:73-78, 1991.

122. Elizondo, G., Weissleder, R., Stark, D.D., et al.: Amebic liver abscess: diagnosis and treatment evaluation with MR imaging, Radiology 165:795-800, 1987.

123. Elizondo, G., Weissleder, R., Stark, D.D., et al.: Hepatic cirrhosis and hepatitis: MR imaging enhanced with superparamagnetic iron oxide, Radiology 174:797-801, 1990.

124. Ellermann, J., Timm, G., Sauer, J., et al.: Effect of cytoprotective agents on rabbit liver bioenergetics monitored by 31-P magnetic resonance spectroscopy and ultrastructural studies, Society of Magnetic Resonance in Medicine 9th Annual Meeting, New York, NY, August 18-24, 1990, Book of Abstracts, p. 261.

125. Engelholm, E., de Toeuf, J., Zalcman, M., et al.: Computerized tomography and magnetic resonance in cancer of the pancreas. Comparison with cholangiopancreatography, Acta Gastroenterol. Belg. 50:195-210, 1987.

126. Fahlvik, A.K., Holtz, E., and Klaveness, J.: Relaxation efficacy of paramagnetic and superparamagnetic microspheres in liver and spleen, Magn. Reson. Imaging 8:363-369, 1990.

127. Farzaneh, F., Riederer, S.J., Lee, J.N., et al.: MR fluoroscopy: initial clinical studies, Radiology 171:545-549, 1989.

128. Feldman, G.B. and Knapp, R.C.: Lymphatic drainage of the peritoneal cavity and its significance in ovarian cancer, Am. J. Obstet. Gynecol. 119:991-994, 1974.

129. Felmlee, J.P. and Ehman, R.L.: Spatial presaturation: a method for suppressing flow artifacts and improving depiction of vascular anatomy in MR imaging, Radiology 164:559-564, 1987.

130. Felmlee, J.P., Ehman, R.L., Riederer, S.J., et al.: Adaptive motion compensation in MRI: accuracy of motion measurement, Magn. Reson. Med. 18:207-213, 1991.

131. Fernandez, M., Bernardino, M.E., Neylan, J., et al.: Diagnosis of pancreatic transplant dysfunction: value of gadopentatate dimeglumine-enhanced MR imaging, AJR 156:1171-1176, 1991.

132. Ferrucci, J.T. and Stark, D.D.: Iron oxide-enhanced MR imaging of the liver and spleen: review of the first 5 years, AJR 155:943-950, 1990.

133. Finlay, I.G., Meek, D.R., Gray, H.W., et al.: Incidence and detection of occult hepatic metastases in colorectal carcinoma, Br. Med. J. 284:803-805, 1982.

134. Finn, J.P., Edelman, R.R., Jenkins, R.L., et al.: Liver transplantation: MR angiography with surgical validation, Radiology 179:265-269, 1991.

135. Fischer, B., Szuch, P., Levine, M., et al.: The intestine as a scource of a portal blood factor responsible for liver regeneration, Surg. Gynecol. Obstet. 137:210-214, 1973.

136. Fisher, M.R., Wall, S.D., Hricak, H., et al.: Hepatic vascular anatomy on magnetic resonance imaging, AJR 144:739-746, 1985.

137. Fobbe, F., Hamm, B., and Schwarting, R.: Angiomyolipoma of the liver: CT, MR, and ultrasound imaging, J. Comput. Assist. Tomogr. 12:658-659, 1988.

138. Foley, W.D.: Dynamic hepatic CT, Radiology 170:617-622, 1989.

139. Foley, W.D., Berland, L.L., Lawson, T.L., et al.: Contrast enhancement technique for dynamic hepatic computed tomographic scanning, Radiology 147:797-803, 1983.

140. Foley, W.D., Kneeland, J.B., Cates, J.D., et al.: Contrast optimization for the detection of focal hepatic lesions by MR imaging at 1.5 T, AJR 149:1155-1160, 1987.

141. Frahm, J., Haase, A., Hanicke, W., et al.: Chemical shift MR imaging using a whole-body magnet, Radiology 156:441, 1985.

142. Franquet, T., Montes, M., de Azua, Y.R., et al.: Primary gallbladder carcinoma: imaging findings in 50 patients with pathologic correlation, Gastrointest. Radiol. 16:143-148, 1991.

143. Freeman, M.P., Vick, C.W., Taylor, K.J.W., et al.: Regenerating nodules in cirrhosis: sonographic appearance with anatomic correlation, AJR 146:533-536, 1986.

144. Freeny, P.C. and Marks, W.M.: Patterns of contrast enhancement of benign and malignant hepatic neoplasms during bolus dynamic and delayed CT, Radiology 160:613-618, 1986.

145. Freeny, P.C. and Marks, W.M.: Hepatic hemangioma: dynamic bolus CT, AJR 147:711-719, 1986.

146. Freeny, P.C., Marks, W.M., Ryan, J.A., et al.: Colorectal carcinoma evaluation with CT: preoperative staging and detection of postoperative recurrence, Radiology 158:347-353, 1986.

147. Fretz, C.J., Elizondo, G., Weissleder, R., et al.: Superparamagnetic iron oxide-enhanced MR imaging: pulse sequence optimization for detection of liver cancer, Radiology 172:393-397, 1989.

148. Fretz, C.J., Stark, D.D., Metz, C.E., et al.: Detection of hepatic metastases: comparison of contrast-enhanced CT, unenhanced MR imaging, and iron oxide-enhanced MR imaging, AJR 155:763-770, 1990.

149. Friedman, A.C., Lichtenstein, J.E., and Dachman, A.H.: Cystic neoplasms of the pancreas: radiological-pathological correlation, Radiology 149:45-50, 1983.

150. Friedman, A.C., Lichtenstein, J.E., Goodman, Z., et al.: Fibrolamellar hepatocellular carcinoma, Radiology 157:583-587, 1985.

151. Frucht, H., Doppman, J.L., Norton, J.A., et al.: Gastrinomas: comparison of MR imaging with CT, angiography, and US, Radiology 17:713-717, 1989.

152. Fugazzola, C., Procacci, C., Andreis, I.A.B., et al.: Cystic tumors of the pancreas: evaluation by ultrasonography and computed tomography, Gastrointest. Radiol. 16:53-61, 1991.

153. Fullerton, G.D., Cameron, K.L., and Ord, V.A.: Frequency dependence of magnetic resonance spin-lattice relaxation of protons in biological materials, Radiology 151:135-138, 1984.

154. Furui, S., Ohtomo, K., Itai, Y., et al.: Hepatocelluar carcinoma treated by transcatheter arterial embolization: progress evaluated by computed tomography, Radiology 150:773-778, 1984.

155. Furuya, K., Nakamura, M., Yamamoto, Y., et al.: Macroregenerative nodule of the liver: a clinicopathologic study of 345 autopsy cases of chronic liver disease, Cancer 61:99-105, 1988.

156. Gabata, T., Matsui, O., Kadoya, M., et al.: MR imaging of hepatic adenoma, AJR 155:1009-1011, 1990.

157. Garra, B.S, Shawker, T.H., Chang, R., et al.: The ultrasound appearance of radiation-induced hepatic injury, J. Ultrasound Med. 7:605-609, 1988.

158. Gehl, H., Bohndorf, K., Klose, K.C., et al.: Two-dimensional MR angiography in the evaluation of abdominal veins with gradient refocused sequences, J. Comput. Assist. Tomogr. 14:619-624, 1990.

159. Gehl, H., Vorwerk, D., Klose, K., et al.: Pancreatic enhancement after low-dose infusion of Mn-DPDP, Radiology 180:337-339, 1991.

160. Gerscovich, E.O., McGahan, J.P., Buonocore, M.H., et al.: The rediscovery of infant feeding formula with magnetic resonance imaging, Pediatric Radiol. 20:147-151, 1990.

161. Gibney, R.G., Hendin, A.P., and Cooperberg, P.L.: Sonographically detected hepatic hemangiomas: absence of change over time, AJR 149:953-957, 1987.

162. Giogio, A., Amoroso, P., Lettieri, G., et al.: Cirrhosis: value of caudate to right lobe ratio in diagnosis with US, Radiology 161:443, 1986.

163. Giorgio, A., Francica, F., de Stefano, G., et al.: Sonographic recongition of intraparenchymal regenerating nodules using high-frequency transducers in patients with cirrhosis, J. Ultrasound Med., 10:355-359, 1991.

164. Glatstein, E., Guernsey, J.M., Rosenberg, S.A., et al.: The value of laparotomy and splenectomy in the staging of Hodgkin's disease, Cancer 4:709-718, 1969.

165. Glazer, G.M., Aisen, A.M., Francis, I.R., et al.: Hepatic cavernous hemangioma: magnetic resonance imaging, Radiology 155:417-420, 1985.

166. Glazer, G.M., Aisen, A.M., Francis, I.R., et al.: Evaluation of focal hepatic masses: a comparative study of MRI and CT, Gastrointest. Radiol. 11:263-268, 1986.

167. Glover, G.H. and Schneider, E.: Three-point Dixon technique for true water/fat decomposition with B_0 inhomogeneity correction, Magn. Reson. Med. 18:371-383, 1991.

168. Glynn, M.J.: Isolated splenic vein thrombosis, Arch. Surg. 121:723-725, 1986.

169. Goldberg, H.I., Moss, A.A., Stark, D.D., et al.: Hepatic cirrhosis: magnetic resonance imaging, Radiology 153:737-739, 1984.

170. Gomori, J.M., Grossman, R.I., and Drott, H.R.: MR relaxation times and iron content of thalassemic spleens: an in vitro study, AJR 150:567-569, 1988.

171. Gomori, J.M., Horev, G., Tamary, H., et al.: Hepatic iron overload: quantitative MR imaging, Radiology 179:367-369, 1991.

172. Goodman, L.R. and Aprahamian, C.: Changes in splenic size after abdominal trauma, Radiology 176:629-632, 1990.

173. Goyal, A.K., Pokharna, D.S., and Sharma, S.K.: Ultrasonic diagnosis of cirrhosis: reference to quantitative measurements of hepatic dimensions, Gastrointest. Radiol. 15:32-34, 1990.

174. Grant, C.W.M., Karlik, S., and Florio, E.: A liposomal MRI contrast agent: phosphatidylethanolamine-DTPA, Magn. Reson. Med. 11:236-243, 1989.

175. Greif, W.L., Buxton, R.B., Lauffer, R.B., et al.: Pulse sequence optimization for MR imaging using a paramagnetic hepatobiliary contrast agent, Radiology 157:461-466, 1985.

176. Groszmann, R.J. and Atterbury, C.E.: The pathophysiology of portal hypertension: a basis for classification, Semin. Liver Dis. 2:177-186, 1982.

177. Gunther, R.W., Klose, K.J., Ruckert, K., et al.: Islet-cell tumors: detection of small lesions with computed tomography and ultrasound, Radiology 148:485-488, 1983.

178. Guyader, D., Gandon, Y., Deugnier, Y., et al.: Evaluation of computed tomography in the assessment of liver iron overload, Gastroenterology 97:737-743, 1989.

179. Haacke, E.M.: The effects of finite sampling in spin-echo or field-echo magnetic resonance imaging, Magn. Reson. Med. 4:407-421, 1987.

180. Haacke, E.M. and Lenz, G.W.: Improving MR image quality in the presence of motion by using rephasing gradients, AJR 148:1251-1258, 1987.

181. Haase, A., Matthaei, D., Bartkowski, R., et al.: Inversion recovery snapshot FLASH MR imaging, J. Comput. Assist. T 13:1036-1040, 1990.

182. Hackney, D.B., Lenkinski, R.E., Grossman, R.I., et al.: Initial experience with fast low-angle multiecho (FLAME) imaging of the central nervous system, J. Comput. Assist. Tomogr. 12:171-174, 1988.

183. Hadjis, N.S., Adam, A., Blenkharn, I., et al.: Primary sclerosing cholangitis associated with liver atrophy, Am. J. Surg. 158:43-47, 1989.

184. Hahn, P.F., Saini, S., Stark, D.D., et al.: Intraabdominal hematoma: the concentric ring sign in MR imaging, AJR 148:115-119, 1987.

185. Hahn, P.F., Stark, D.D., Lewis, J.M., et al.: First clinical trial of a new superparamagnetic iron oxide for use as an oral gastrointestinal contrast agent in MR imaging, Radiology 175:695-700, 1990.

186. Hahn, P.F., Stark, D.D., Saini, S., et al.: Ferrite particles for bowel contrast in MR imaging: design issues and feasibility studies, Radiology 164:37-41, 1987.

187. Hahn, P.F., Stark, D.D., Saini, S., et al.: The differential diagnosis of ringed hepatic lesions in MR imaging, AJR 154:287-290, 1990.

188. Hahn, P.F., Stark, D.D., Weissleder, R., et al.: Clinical application of superparamagnetic iron oxide to MR imaging of tissue perfusion in vascular liver tumors, Radiology 174:361-366, 1990.

189. Hahn, P.F., Weissleder, R., Stark, D.D., et al.: MR imaging of focal splenic tumors, AJR 150:823-827, 1988.

190. Halvorsen, R.A., Jr., Foster, W.L., Jr., Wilkinson, R.H., Jr., et al.: Hepatic abscess: sensitivity of imaging tests and clinical findings, Gastrointest. Radiol. 13:135-141, 1988.

191. Hamm, B., Fischer, E., and Taupitz, M.: Differentiation of hepatic hemangiomas from metastases by dynamic contrast-enhanced MR imaging, J. Comput. Assist. Tomogr. 14:205-216, 1990.

192. Hamm, B., Wolf, K.J., and Felix, R.: Conventional and rapid MR imaging of the liver with gadolinium-DTPA in clinical use, Radiology 164:313-320, 1987.

193. Hann, H.L., Kim, C.Y., London, W.T., et al.: Increased serum ferritin in chronic liver disease: a risk factor for primary hepatocellular carcinoma, Int. J. Cancer 43:376-379, 1989.

194. Hann, H.L., Stahlhut, M.W., Blumberg, B.S., et al.: Iron nutrition and tumor growth: decreased tumor growth in iron-deficient mice, Cancer Res. 48:4168-4170, 1988.

195. Hardy, P.A. and Henkelman, R.M.: Transverse relaxation rate enhancement caused by magnetic particulates, Magn. Reson. Imaging 7:265-275, 1989.

196. Harman, J.W. and Dacorso, P.: Spread of carcinoma to the spleen: its relation to generalized carcinomatous spread, Arch. Pathol. 45:179-186, 1948.

197. Hayashi, N., Yamamoto, K., Tamaki, N., et al.: Metastatic nodules of hepatocellular carcinoma: detection with angiography, CT, and US, Radiology 165:61-63, 1987.

198. Heiken, J.P., Lee, J.K.T., and Dixon, W.T.: Fatty infiltration of the liver: evaluation by proton spectroscopic imaging, Radiology 157:707-710, 1985.

199. Heiken, J.P., Lee, J.K.T.L., Glazer, H.S., et al.: Hepatic metastases studies with MR and CT, Radiology, 156:423-427, 1985.

200. Heiken, J.P., Weyman, P.J., Lee, J.K.T., et al.: Detection of focal hepatic masses: prospective evaluation with CT, delayed CT, CT during arterial portography, and MR imaging, Radiology 171:47-51, 1989.

201. Henderson, J.M., Campbell, J.D., Olson, R., et al.: Role of computed tomography in screening for hepatocellular carcinoma in patients with cirrhosis, Gastrointest. Radiol. 13:129-134, 1988.

202. Hendrick, R.E.: Sampling time effects on signal-to-noise and contrast-to-noise ratios in spin-echo MRI, Magn. Reson. Imaging 5:31-37, 1987.

203. Hendrick, R.E., Nelson, T.R., and Hendee, W.R.: Optimizing tissue contrast in magnetic resonance imaging, Magn. Reson. Imaging 2:193-204, 1984.

204. Hendrick, R.E., Stark, D.D., Weissleder, R., et al.: Maximizing liver lesion detection: a comparison of pulse sequence performance at different magnetic field strengths, Radiology 165(P):182, 1987.

205. Hennig, J., Nauerth, A., and Friedburg, H.: RARE imaging: a fast imaging method for clinical MR, Magn. Reson. Med. 3:823-33, 1986.

206. Henkelman, R.M., Hardy, P., Poon, P.Y., et al.: Optimal pulse sequence for imaging hepatic metastases, Radiology 161:727-734, 1986.

207. Hernandez, R.J., Sarnaik, S.A., Lande, I., et al.: MR evaluation of liver iron overload, J. Comput. Assist. Tomogr. 12:91, 1988.

208. Hess, C.F., Griebel, J., Schmiedl, U., et al.: Focal lesions of the spleen: preliminary results with fast MR imaging at 1.5T, J. Comput. Assist. Tomogr. 12:569-574, 1988.

209. Hess, C.F., Kurtz, B., Grodd, W., et al.: Hypoechoic lesions without halo in echogenic liver—a frequent sonographic dilemma, Acta Radiol. 29:541, 1988.

210. Higuchi, N., Oshio, K., Imai, Y., et al.: Clinical applications of multishot RARE in abdominal MR imaging, JMRI 1:150-151, 1991.

211. Hilpert, P.A., Friedman, A.C., Radecki, P.D., et al.: MRI of hemorrhagic renal cysts in polycystic kidney disease, AJR 146:1167-1172, 1986.

212. Hoener, B., Engelstad, B.L., Ramos, E.C., et al.: Comparison of Fe-HBED and Fe-EHPG as hepatobiliary MR contrast agents, JMRI 1:357-362, 1991.

213. Hoff, F.L., Aisen, A.M., Walden, M.E., et al.: MR imaging in hydatid disease of the liver, Gastrointest. Radiol. 12:39, 1987.

214. Holland, H.K. and Spivak, J.L.: Hemochromatosis, Med. Clin. N. Am. 73:831-845, 1989.

215. Holsinger, A.E., Riederer, S.J., Campeau, N.G., et al.: T1-weighted snapshot gradient-echo MR imaging of the abdomen, Radiology 181:25-32, 1991.

216. Holsinger, A.E., Wright, R.C., Riederer, S.J., et al.: Realtime interactive magnetic resonance imaging, Magn. Reson. Med. 14:547-553, 1990.

217. Hosoki, T.: Dynamic CT of pancreatic tumors, AJR 140:959-965, 1983.

218. Hosoki, T., Kuroda, C., Tokunaga, K., et al.: Hepatic venous outflow obstruction: evaluation with pulsed Duplex sonography, Radiology 170:733-737, 1989.

219. Housman, J.F., Chezmar, J.L., Nelson, R.C.: Magnetic resonance imaging in hemochromatosis: extrahepatic iron deposition, Gastrointest. Radiol. 14:59-60, 1989.

220. Hricak, H., Filly, R.A., Margulis, A.R., et al.: Work in progress: nuclear magnetic resonance imaging of the gallbladder, Radiology 147:481-484, 1983.

221. Imaeda, T., Inoue, A., Doi, H., et al.: Increased focal uptake of Tc-99m stannous phytate in an irregular fatty liver demonstrated by SPECT imaging, Clin. Nucl. Med. 15:504-506, 1990.

222. Intenzo, C., Kim, S., Madsen, M., et al.: Planar and SPECT Tc-99m red blood cell imaging in hepatic cavernous hemangiomas and other hepatic lesions, Clin. Nucl. Med. 13:237-240, 1988.

223. Ishikawa, I., Tateishi, K., Shinoda, A., et al.: Changes of the hepatic CT absorption value in hemodialysis patients, J. Comput. Assist. Tomogr. 8:701-703, 1984.

224. Israel, J., Unger, E., Buetow, K., et al.: Correlation between liver iron content and magnetic resonance imaging in rats, Magn. Reson. Imaging 7:629-634, 1989.

225. Itai, Y., Araki, T., Tasaka, A., et al.: Computed tomographic appearance of resectable pancreatic carcinoma, Radiology 143:719-726, 1982.

226. Itai, Y., Moss, A.A., and Goldberg, H.I.: Pancreatic cysts caused by carcinoma of the pancreas: a pitfall in the diagnosis of pancreatic carcinoma, J. Comput. Assist. Tomogr. 6:772-776, 1982.

227. Itai, Y., Ohnishi, S., Ohtomo, K., et al.: Regenerating nodules of liver cirrhosis: MR imaging, Radiology 165:419-423, 1987.

228. Itai, Y., Ohtomo, K., Araki, T., et al.: Computed tomography and sonography of cavernous hemangioma of the liver, AJR 141:315-320, 1983.

229. Itai, Y., Ohtomo, K., Furui, S., et al.: Lobar intensity differences of the liver on MR imaging, J. Comput. Assist. Tomogr. 10:236-241, 1986.

230. Itai, Y., Ohtomo, K., Furui, S., et al.: MR imaging of hepatocellular carcinoma, J. Comput. Assist. Tomogr. 10:963-968, 1986.

231. Itai, Y., Ohtomo, K., Furui, S., et al.: Noninvasive diagnosis of small cavernous hemangioma of the liver: advantage of MRI, AJR 145:1195-1199, 1985.

232. Itai, Y., Ohtomo, K., Kokubo, T., et al.: CT and MR imaging of fatty tumors of the liver, J. Comput. Assist. Tomogr. 11:253-257, 1987.

233. Itai, Y., Ohtomo, K., Kokubo, T., et al.: CT and MR imaging of postnecrotic liver scars, J. Comput. Assist. Tomogr. 12:971-975, 1988.

234. Itai, Y., Ohtomo, K., Kokubo, T., et al.: Segmental intensity differences in the liver on MR images: a sign of intrahepatic portal flow stoppage, Radiology 167:17-19, 1988.

235. Itoh, K., Nishimura, K., Togashi, K., et al.: Hepatocellular carcinoma: MR imaging, Radiology 164:21-25, 1987.

236. Itoh, K., Saini, S., Hahn, P.F., et al.: Differentiation between small hepatic hemangiomas and metastases on MR images: importance of size-specific quantitative criteria, AJR 155: 61-66, 1990.

237. Itoh, K., Weissleder, R., Hendrick, R.E., et al.: MR imaging contrast parameters: correlation with lesion detectability, Radiology 173(P): 228, 1989.

238. Jacobs, A. and Worwood, M.: Iron in biochemistry and medicine, II, New York, 1980, Academic Press.

239. Jafri, S.Z.H., Aisen, A.M., Glazer, G.M., et al.: Comparison of CT and angiography in assessing resectability of pancreatic carcinoma, AJR 142:525-529, 1984.

240. Jenkins, J.P.R., Braganza, J.M., Hickey, D.S., et al.: Quantitative tissue characterization in pancreatic disease using magnetic resonance imaging, Br. J. Radiol. 60:333-341, 1987.

241. Johnson, C.D., Stephens, D.H., Charboneau, J.W., et al.: Cystic pancreatic tumors: CT and sonographic assessment, AJR 151:1133-1138, 1988.

242. Johnson, G.A., Herfkens, R.J., and Brown, M.A.: Tissue relaxation time: in vivo field dependence, Radiology 156:805-810, 1985.

243. Johnston, D.L., Rice, L., Vick, G.W., et al.: Assessment of tissue iron overload by nuclear magnetic resonance imaging, Am. J. Med. 87:40-47, 1989.

244. Jones, E.C., Chezmar, J.L., Nelson, R.C., et al.: Variability of hepatic enhancement with regard to imaging time and location with gadolinium-enhanced MR imaging, Radiology 173(P): 271, 1989.

245. Josephson, L., Groman, E.V., Menz, E., et al.: A functionalized superparamagnetic iron oxide colloid as a receptor directed MR contrast agent, Magn. Reson. Imaging 8:637-646, 1990.

246. Josephson, L., Lewis, J., Jacobs, P., et al.: The effects of iron oxides on proton relaxivity, Magn. Reson. Imaging 6:647-653, 1988.

247. Kabalka, G.W., Buonocore, E., Hubner, K., et al.: Gadolinium-labeled liposomes: targeted MR contrast agents for the liver and spleen, Radiology 163:255-258, 1987.

248. Kaftori, J.K., Pery, M., Green, J., et al.: Thickness of the gallbladder wall in patients with hypoalbuminemia: a sonographic study of patients on peritoneal dialysis, AJR 148:1117-1118, 1987.

249. Kagen, L. Myoglobin, ed. 1. New York: 1973, Columbia University Press, p. 66.

250. Kaminsky, S., Laniado, M., Gogoll, M., et al.: Gadopentetate dimeglumine as a bowel contrast agent: safety and efficacy, Radiology 178:503-508, 1991.

251. Kaplan, S.B., Sumkin, J.H., Campbell, W.L., et al.: Periportal low-attenuation areas on CT: value as evidence of liver transplant rejection, AJR 152:285-287, 1989.

252. Kaurich, J.D., Coombs, R.J., and Zeiss, J.: Myelolipoma of the liver: CT features, J. Comput. Assist. Tomogr. 12:660-661, 1988.

253. Kawamura, Y., Endo, K., Watanabe, Y., et al.: Use of magnetite particles as a contrast agent for MR imaging of the liver, Radiology 174:357-360, 1990.

254. Keller, P.J., Hunter, W.W., and Schmalbrock, P.: Multisection fat-water imaging with chemical shift selective presaturation, Radiology 164:539, 1987.

255. Kenmochi, K., Sugihara, S., and Kojiro, M.: Relationship of histologic grade of hepatocellular carcinoma (HCC) to tumor size, and demonstration of tumor cells of multiple different grades in single small HCC, Liver 7:18-26, 1987.

256. Kerlin, P., Davis, G.L., McGill, D.B., et al.: Hepatic adenoma and focal nodular hyperplasia: clinical, pathologic, and radiologic features, Gastroenterology 84:994-1002, 1983.

257. Khuroo, M.S., Zargar, S.A., and Mahajan, R.: Echinococcus granulosus cysts in the liver: management with percutaneous drainage, Radiology 180:141-145, 1991.

258. Kitagawa, K., Matsui, O., Kadoya, M., et al.: Hepatocellular carcinomas with excessive copper accumulation: CT and MR findings, Radiology 180:623-628, 1991.

259. Korobkin, M., Stephens, D.H., Lee, J.K.T., et al.: Biliary cystadenoma and cystadenocarcinoma: CT and sonographic findings, AJR 153:507-511, 1989.

260. Kondo, Y., Niwa, Y., Akikusa, B., et al.: A histopathologic study of early hepatocellular carcinoma, Cancer 52:687-692, 1983.

261. Korin, H.W., Felmlee, J.P., Ehman, R.L., et al.: Adaptive technique for three-dimensional MR imaging of moving structures, Radiology 177:217-221, 1990.

262. Koslin, D.B., Stanley, R.J., Berland, L.L., et al.: Heptic perivascular lymphedema: CT appearance, AJR 150:111-113, 1988.

263. Koslow, S.A., Davis, P.L., DeMarino, G.B., et al.: MR, CT and US appearances of regenerating nodules in cirrhotic liver, Society of Magnetic Resonance in Medicine 7th Annual Meeting, San Francisco, Aug. 22-26, 1988, Program and Abstracts, p. 154.

264. Kronthal, A.J., Fishman, E.K., Kuhlman, J.E., et al.: Hepatic infarction in preeclampsia, Radiology 177:726-728, 1990.
265. Kudo, M., Ikekubo, K., Yamamoto, K., et al.: Distinction between hemangioma of the liver and hepatocellular carcinoma: value of labeled RBC-SPECT scanning, AJR 152:977-983, 1989.
266. Kuo, G., Choo, Q.L., Alter, H.J., et al.: An assay for circulating antibodies to a major etiolgic virus of human non-A, non-B hepatitis, Science 244:362-364, 1989.
267. Kurdziel, J.C., Dondelinger, R.F., Dicato, M.A., et al.: Magnetic resonance imaging (MRI) of the spleen and bone marrow in hematological disorders, JBR-BTR 71:211-229, 1988.
268. Laing, F.C., Jeffrey, R.B., Federle, M.P., et al.: Noninvasive imaging of unusual regenerating nodules in the cirrhotic liver, Gastrointest. Radiol. 7:245-249, 1982.
269. Lang, P., Steffen, R., Langer, M., et al.: Orthotopic liver transplantation: postoperative evaluation with MR imaging, Radiology 173(P):389, 1989.
270. Lapidot, A., Gopher, A., Korman, S.H., et al.: In vivo measurements of liver 6-phosphofructokinase activity in Down's Syndrome (Trisomy 21) by 13C NMR, Society of Magnetic Resonance in Medicine 9th Annual Meeting, New York, NY, August 18-24, 1990, Book of Abstracts, p. 282.
271. LaRusso, N.F., Wiesner, R.H., Ludwig, J., et al.: Medical intelligence. Primary sclerosing cholangitis, N. Engl. J. Med. 310:899-903, 1984.
272. Lauffer, R.B., Greif, W.L., Stark, D.D., et al.: Iron-EHPG as an hepatobiliary MR contrast agent: initial imaging and biodistribution studies, J. Comput. Assist. Tomogr. 9:431-438, 1985.
273. Lauffer, R.B., Vincent, A.C., Padmanabhan, S., et al.: Hepatobiliary MR contrast agents: 5-substituted iron-EHPG derivatives, Magn. Reson. Med. 4:582-590, 1987.
274. Le, C., Rajan, S.S., Francisco, J., et al.: Commonly administered products as oral contrast media for MR imaging: redux, JMRI 1:233, 1991.
275. Leander, P., Golman, K., Klaveness, J., et al.: MRI contrast media for the liver efficacy in conditions of acute biliary obstruction, Invest. Radiol. 25:1130-1134, 1990.
276. Lee, J.K.T., Heiken, J.P., and Dixon, W.T.: Detection of hepatic metastases by proton spectroscopic imaging: work in progress, Radiology 156:429-433, 1985.
277. Lee, M.J., Saini, S., Hamm, B., et al.: Focal nodular hyperplasia of the liver: MR findings in 35 proved cases, AJR 156:317-320, 1991.
278. Lehmann, B., Fanucci, E., Gigli, F., et al.: Signal suppression of normal liver tissue by phase corrected inversion recovery: a screening technique, J. Comput. Assist. Tomogr. 13:650-655, 1989.
279. LeSage, G.D., Baldus, W.P., Fairbanks, V.F., et al.: Hemochromatosis: genetic or alcohol-induced? Gastroenterology 84:1471-1477, 1983.
280. Levenson, H., Greensite, F., Hoefs, J., et al.: Fatty infiltration of the liver: quantification with phase-contrast MR imaging at 1.5 T vs biopsy, AJR 156:307-312, 1991.
281. Levine, E.: Carcinoma of the pancreas presenting as acute pancreatitis: CT diagnosis, Gastrointest. Radiol. 6:29-33, 1981.
282. Levine, E., Wetzel, L.H., and Neff, J.R.: MR imaging and CT of extrahepatic cavernous hemangiomas, AJR 147:1299-1304, 1986.
283. Levy, H.M. and Newhouse, J.H.: MR imaging of portal vein thrombosis, AJR 151:283-286, 1988.
284. Lewis, E., Bernardino, M.E., Barnes, P.A., et al.: The fatty liver: pitfalls in the CT and angiographic evaluation of metastatic disease, J. Comput. Assist. Tomogr. 7:235-241, 1983.
285. Li, K.C.P., Ang, P.G.P., Tart, R.P., et al.: Paramagnetic oil emulsions as oral magnetic resonance imaging contrast agents, Magn. Reson. Imaging 8:589-598, 1990.
286. Li, K.C.P., Tart, R.P., Fitzsimmons, J.R., et al.: Barium sulfate suspension as a negative oral MRI contrast agent: in vitro and human optimization studies, Magn. Reson. Imaging 9:141-150, 1991.
287. Lim, K.O., Stark, D.D., Leese, P.T., et al.: Hepatobiliary MR imaging: first human experience with MnDPDP, Radiology 178:79-82, 1991.
288. Lin, T., Ophir, J., and Potter, G.: Correlation of ultrasonic attenuation with pathologic fat and fibrosis in liver disease, Ultrasound Med. Biol. 14:729-734, 1988.
289. Listerud, J., Isaac, G., Chan, T., et al.: Aliphatic/olefinic fat cancellation: optimization and extension, Society of Magnetic Resonance in Medicine 9th Annual Meeting, New York, NY, August 18-24, 1990, Book of Abstracts, p. 590.
290. Listinsky, J.J. and Bryant, R.G.: Gastrointestinal contrast agents: a diamagnetic approach, Magn. Reson. Med. 8:285-292, 1988.
291. Liu, P., Uldall, P., Cronin, C., et al.: Magnetic resonance assessment of iron overload in renal failure: comparison with patients with thalassemia and normals, Society of Magnetic Resonance in Medicine 9th Annual Meeting, New York, NY, August 18-24, 1990, Book of Abstracts, p. 93.
292. Livraghi, T., Sangalli, G., and Vettori, C.: Adenomatous hyperplastic nodules in the cirrhotic liver: a therapeutic approach, Radiology 170:155-157, 1989.
293. Llauger, J., Perez, C., Coscojuela, P., et al.: Hepatic metastases: false-negative CT portography in cases of fatty infiltration, J. Comput. Assist. Tomogr. 15:320-322, 1991.
294. Loflin, T.G., Simeone, J.F., Mueller, P.R., et al.: Gallbladder bile in cholecystitis: in vitro MR evaluation, Radiology 157:457-459, 1985.
295. Lombardo, D.M., Baker, M.E., Spritzer, C.E., et al.: Hepatic hemangiomas vs metastases: MR differentiation at 1.5 T, AJR 155:55-59, 1990.
296. Lönnemark, M., Hemmingsson, A., Bach-Gansmo, T., et al.: Effect of superparamagnetic particles as oral contrast medium at magnetic resonance imaging, Acta Radiol. 30:193-196, 1989.
297. Lorigan, J.G., Charnsangavej, C., Carrasco, C.H., et al.: Atrophy with compensatory hypertrophy of the liver in hepatic neoplasms: radiographic findings, AJR 150:1291-1295, 1988.
298. Low, R.A., Kuni, C.C., and Letourneau, J.G.: Pancreas transplant imaging: an overview, AJR 155:13-21, 1990.
299. Lubbers, P.R., Ros, P.R., Goodman, Z.D., et al.: Accumulation of technetium-99m sulfur colloid by hepatocellular adenoma: scintigraphic-pathologic correlation, AJR 148:105-108.
300. MacDonald, R.A. and Mallory, G.K.: Hemochromatosis and hemosiderosis—a study of 211 autopsied cases, Arch. Intern. Med. 105:686-700, 1960.
301. Majumdar, S., Zoghbi, S., and Gore, J.D.: The influence of pulse sequence on the relaxation effects of superparamagnetic iron oxide contrast agents, Magn. Reson. Med. 10:289-301, 1989.
302. Majumdar, S., Zoghbi, S., Pope, C.F., et al.: A quantitative study of relaxation rate enhancement produced by iron oxide particles in polyacrylamide gels and tissue, Magn. Reson. Med. 9:185-202, 1989.
303. Majumdar, S., Zoghbi, S., Pope, C.F., et al.: Quantitation of MR relaxation effects of iron oxide particles in liver and spleen, Radiology 169:653-655, 1988.
304. Malt, R.A.: Current concepts—surgery for hepatic neoplasms, N. Engl. J. Med. 313:1591-1596, 1985.
305. Manas, K.J., Welsh, J.D., Rankin, R.A., et al.: Hepatic hemorrhage without rupture in preeclampsia, N. Engl. J. Med. 312:424-426, 1985.
306. Marincek, B., Barbier, P.A., Becker, C.D., et al.: CT appearance of impaired lymphatic drainage in liver transplants, AJR 147:519-523, 1986.
307. Mano, I., Yoshida, H., Nakabayaski, K., et al.: Fast spin echo imaging with suspended respiration: gadolinium enhanced MR imaging of liver tumors, J. Comput. Assist. Tomogr. 11:73-80, 1987.
308. Marchal, G., Demaerel, P., Decrop, E., et al.: Gadolinium-DOTA enhanced fast imaging of liver tumors at 1.5 T, J. Comput. Assist. Tomogr. 14:217-222, 1990.

309. Marchal, G., Tshibwabwa-Tuma, E., Verbeken, E., et al.: "Skip areas" in hepatic steatosis: a sonographic-angiographic study, Gastrointest. Radiol. 11:151-157, 1986.

310. Marchal, G., Van Hecke, P., Demaerel, P., et al.: Detection of liver metastases with superparamagnetic iron oxide in 15 patients: results of MR imaging at 1.5 T, AJR 152:771-775, 1989.

311. Marchal, G., Van Holsbeeck, M., Tshibwabwa-Ntumba, E., et al.: Dilatation of the cystic veins in portal hypertension: sonographic demonstration, Radiology 154:187-189, 1985.

312. Marglin, S.I. and Castellino, R.A.: Selection of imaging studies for the initial staging of patients with Hodgkin's disease, Semin. Ultrasound, CT, MR 7:2-8, 1985.

313. Marn, C.S., Glazer, G.M, Williams, D.M., et al.: CT-angiographic correlation of collateral venous pathways in isolated splenic vein occlusion: new observations, Radiology 175:375-380, 1990.

314. Marti-Bonmati, L., Menor, F., Vizcaino, I., et al.: Lipoma of the liver: US, CT, and MRI appearance, Gastrointest. Radiol. 14:5155-5157, 1989.

315. Marti-Bonmati, L., Vilar, J., Paniagua, J.C., et al.: High density barium sulphate as an MRI oral contrast, Magn. Reson. Imaging 9:259-261, 1991.

316. Martin, L.G., Henderson, J.M., Milikan, W.J., Jr., et al.: Angioplasty for long-term treatment of patients with Budd-Chiari syndrome, AJR 154:1007-1010, 1990.

317. Marymont J.H., Jr. and Gross, S.: Patterns of metastatic cancer in the spleen, Am. J. Clin. Pathol. 40:58-66, 1953.

318. Mathieu, D., Guinet, C., Cauquil, P., et al.: Intrahepatic calculi: imaging by MR, Radiat. Med. 6:108, 1988.

319. Mathieu, D., Rahmouni, A., Anglade, M-C., et al.: Focal nodular hyperplasia of the liver: assessment with contrast-enhanced Turbo-FLASH MR imaging, Radiology 180:25-30, 1991.

320. Mathieu, D., Vasile, N., Menu, Y., et al.: Budd-Chiari syndrome: dynamic CT, Radiology 165:409-413, 1987.

321. Matsui, O., Kadoya, M., Kameyama, T., et al.: Adenomatous hyperplastic nodules in the cirrhotic liver: differentiation from hepatocellular carcinoma with MR imaging, Radiology 173:123-126, 1989.

322. Matsui, O., Kadoya, M., Kameyama, T., et al.: Benign and malignant nodules in cirrhotic livers: distinction based on blood supply, Radiology 178:493-497, 1991.

323. Matsui, O., Kadoya, M., Takashima, T., et al.: Intrahepatic periportal abnormal intensity on MR images: an indication of various hepatobiliary diseases, Radiology 171:335-338, 1989.

324. Matsui, O., Takashima, T., Kadoya, M., et al.: Liver metastases from colorectal cancers: detection with CT during arterial portography, Radiology 165:65-69, 1987.

325. Mattison, G.R., Glazer, G.M., Quint, L.E., et al.: MR imaging of hepatic focal nodular hyperplasia: characterization and distinction from primary malignant hepatic tumors, AJR 148:711, 1987.

326. Mattrey, R.F., Hajek, P.C., Gylys-Morin, V.M., et al.: Perfluorochemicals as gastrointestinal contrast agents for MR imaging: preliminary studies in rats and humans, AJR 148:1259-1263, 1987.

327. Mattrey, R.F., Long, D.M., and Multer, F.: Perfluorooctylbromide: a reticuloendothelial-specific and tumor imaging agent for computed tomography, Radiology 145:755-758, 1982.

328. McCarthy, S., Hricak, H., Cohen, M., et al.: Cholecystitis: detection with MR imaging, Radiology 158:333-336, 1986.

329. McLaren, G.D., Muir, W.A., and Kellermeyer, R.W.: Iron overload disorders: natural history, pathogenesis, diagnosis, and therapy, CRC Crit. Rev. Clin. Lab. Sci. 19:205-266, 1984.

330. Megibow, A.J., Bosniak, M.A., Ambos, M.A., et al.: Thickening of the celiac axis and/or superior mesenteric artery: a sign of pancreatic carcinoma on computed tomography, Radiology 141:449-453, 1981.

331. Melki, P.S., Mulkern, R.V., Panych, L.P., et al.: Comparing the FAISE method with conventional dual-echo sequences, J. Magn. Reson. Imag. 1:319-326, 1991.

332. Menu, Y., Alison, D., Lorphelin, J.M., et al.: Budd-Chiari syndrome: US evaluation, Radiology 157:761-764, 1985.

333. Meyerhoff, D.J., Boska, M.D., Thomas, A.M., et al.: Alcoholic liver disease: quantitative image-guided P-31 MR spectroscopy, Radiology 173:393, 1989.

334. Meyerhoff, D.J., Karczmar, G.S., and Weiner, M.W.: Abnormalities of the liver evaluated by ^{31}P MRS, Invest. Radiol. 24:980-984, 1989.

335. Meyerhoff, D.J. and Weiner, M.W.: Magnetic resonance spectroscopy of the liver: a review, In Ferrucci, J.T. and Stark, D.D. (eds.), Liver imaging. Current trends and new techniques, Boston: 1990, Andover Medical Publishers, pp. 289-297.

336. Miller, D.L., Simmons, J.T., Chang, R., et al.: Hepatic metastasis detection: comparison of three CT contrast enhancement methods, Radiology 165:785, 1987.

337. Miller, D.L., Vermess, M., Doppman, J.L., et al.: CT of the liver and spleen with EOE-13: review of 225 examinations, AJR 143:235-243, 1984.

338. Minami, M., Itai, Y., Ohtomo, K., et al.: Cystic neoplasms of the pancreas: comparison of MR imaging with CT, Radiology 171:53-56, 1989.

339. Minami, M., Itai, Y., Ohtomo, K., et al.: Siderotic nodules in the spleen: MR imaging of portal hypertension, Radiology 172:681-684, 1989.

340. Mirowitz, S.A., Brown, J.J., Lee, J.K.T., et al.: Dynamic gadolinium-enhanced MR imaging of the spleen: normal enhancement patterns and evaluation of splenic lesions, Radiology 179:681-686, 1991.

341. Mirowitz, S.A., Heiken, J.P., and Lee, J.K.T.: Potential MR pitfall in relying on lesion/liver intensity ratio in presence of hepatic hemochromatosis, J. Comput. Assist. Tomogr. 12:323-324, 1988.

342. Mirowitz, S.A., Lee, J.K.T., Brown, J.J., et al.: Rapid acquisition spin-echo (RASE) MR imaging: a new technique for reduction of artifacts and acquisition time, Radiology 175:131-135, 1990.

343. Mirowitz, S.A., Lee, J.K.T., Gutierrez, E., et al.: Dynamic gadolinium-enhanced rapid acquisition spin-echo MR imaging of the liver, Radiology 179:371-376, 1991.

344. Mirvis, S.E., Whitley, N.O., and Miller, J.W.: CT diagnosis of acalculous cholecystitis, J. Comput. Assist. Tomogr. 11:83-87, 1987.

345. Mitchell, D.G., Blum, L., and Kurtz, A.B.: Ultrasound case of the day, RadioGraphics 10:366-368, 1990.

346. Mitchell, D.G., Burk, D.L., Vinitski, S., et al.: The biophysical basis of tissue contrast in extracranial MR imaging, AJR 149:831-837, 1987.

347. Mitchell, D.G., Hill, M.C., Cooper, R., et al.: The superior mesenteric artery fat plane: is obliteration pathognomic of pancreatic carcinoma? CT 11:247-253, 1987.

348. Mitchell, D.G., Kim, I., Chang, T.S., et al.: Fatty liver: chemical shift saturation and phase-difference MR imaging techniques in animals, phantoms and humans, Invest. Radiol. 26: 1041-1052, 1991.

349. Mitchell, D.G., Palazzo, J., Hann, H-W.Y.L., et al.: Hepatocellular tumors with high signal on T1 weighted MR images: chemical shift MRI and histologic correlation, J. Comput. Assist. Tomogr. 15:762-769, 1991.

350. Mitchell, D.G., Rubin, R., Siegelman, E., et al.: Hepatocellular carcinoma within siderotic regenerative nodules: The "nodule-within-nodule" sign on MR images, Radiology 178:101-103, 1991.

351. Mitchell, D.G., Siegelman, E.S., Rifkin, M.D., et al.: Hepatic cirrhosis: MR imaging diagnosis with histologic correlation, JMRI 1:210, 1991.

352. Mitchell, D.G. and Vinitski, S.: Principles of protocol optimization for MRI of the abdomen and pelvis, CRC Crit. Rev. Diag. Imag. 31:117-144, 1990.

353. Mitchell, D.G., Vinitski, S., Burk, D.L., et al.: Motion artifact reduction in MR imaging of the abdomen: gradient moment nulling versus respiratory-sorted phase encoding, Radiology 169:155-160, 1988.

288 References

446. Rossaro, L., Murase, N., Caldwell, C., et al.: ATP content and intracellular pH of rat liver during preservation monitored by 31P-NMR spectroscopy, Society of Magnetic Resonance in Medicine 9th Annual Meeting, New York, NY, August 18-24, 1990, Book of Abstracts, p. 285.

447. Rossman, M.D., Friedman, A.C., Radecki, P.D., et al.: MR imaging of gallbladder carcinoma, AJR 148:143-144, 1987.

448. Rubin, D.L., Herfkens, R.J., Pelc, N.J., et al.: MR measurement of portal blood flow in chronic liver disease: application to predicting clinical outcome, Society of Magnetic Resonance in Medicine 9th Annual Meeting, New York, NY, August 18-24, 1990, Book of Abstracts, p. 90.

449. Rubin, D.L., Muller, H.H., Nino-Murcia, M., et al.: Intraluminal contrast enhancement and MR visualization of the bowel wall: efficacy of PFOB, J. Magn. Reson. Imag. 1:371-380, 1991.

450. Rummeny, E., Saini, S., Stark, D.D., et al.: Detection of hepatic metastases with MR imaging: spin-echo vs phase-contrast pulse sequences at 0.6 T, AJR 153:1207-1211, 1989.

451. Rummeny, E., Saini, S., Wittenberg, J., et al.: MR imaging of liver neoplasms, AJR 152:493-499, 1989.

452. Rummeny, E., Weissleder, R., Sironi, S., et al.: Central scars in primary liver tumors: MR features, specificity, and pathologic correlation, Radiology 171:323-326, 1989.

453. Rummeny, E., Weissleder, R., Stark D.D., et al.: Primary liver tumors: diagnosis by MR imaging, AJR 152:63-72, 1989.

454. Rummeny, E., Wernecke, K., Bongartz, G., et al.: ROC analysis of high-field MR imaging versus CT for the detection of focal hepatic lesions, Magn. Reson. Imaging 8(S1):57, 1990.

455. Runge, V.M., Clanton, J.A., Herzer, W.A., et al.: Intravascular contrast agents suitable for magnetic resonance imaging, Radiology 153:171-176, 1984.

456. Sagoh, T., Itoh, K., Togashi, K., et al.: Gamna-Gandy bodies of the spleen: evaluation with MR imaging, Radiology 172:685-687, 1989.

457. Sagoh, T., Itoh, K., Togashi, K., et al.: Gallbladder carcinoma: evaluation with MR imaging, Radiology 174:131-136, 1990.

458. Saini, S., Modic, M.T., Hamm, B, et al.: Advances in contrast-enhanced MR imaging, AJR 156:235-254, 1991.

459. Saini, S., Stark, D.D., Brady, T.J., et al.: Dynamic spin-echo MRI of liver cancer using gadolinium-DTPA: animal investigation, AJR 147:357-362, 1986.

460. Saini, S., Stark, D.D., Hahn, P.PF., et al.: Are superparamagnetic ferrite particles cleared from the liver? Radiology 173(P): 175, 1989.

461. Saini, S., Stark, D.D., Hahn, P.F., et al.: Ferrite particles: a superparamagnetic MR contrast agent for the reticuloendothelial system, Radiology 162:211-216, 1987.

462. Saini, S., Stark, D.D., Hahn, P.F., et al.: Ferrite particles: a superparamagnetic MR contrast agent for enhanced detection of liver carcinoma, Radiology 162:217-222, 1987.

463. Saini, S., Stark, D.D., Rzedzian, R.R., et al.: Forty-millisecond MR imaging of the abdomen at 2.0 T, Radiology 173:111-116, 1989.

464. Saini, S., Wallner, B., Edelman, R.E., et al.: T1 and T2-weighted images provide similar contrast discrimination for hepatic MR imaging at 1.5 T, Society of Magnetic Resonance in Medicine 9th Annual Meeting, New York, NY, August 18-24, 1990, Book of Abstracts, p. 88.

465. Sauerbrei, E.E. and Lopez, M.: Pseudotumor of the quadrate lobe in hepatic sonography: a sign of generalized fatty infiltration, AJR 147:923-927, 1986.

466. Savoca, P.E., Longo, W.E., Zucker, K.A., et al.: The increasing prevalence of acalculous cholecystitis in outpatients: results of a 7-year study, Ann. Surg. 211:433-437, 1990.

467. Schafer, A.I., Cheron, R.G., Dluhy, R., et al.: Clinical consequences of acquired transfusional iron overload in adults, N. Engl. J. Med. 304:319-324, 1981.

468. Schertz, L.D., Lee, J.K.T., Heiken, J.P., et al.: Proton spectroscopic imaging (Dixon method) of the liver: clinical utility, Radiology 173:401-405, 1989.

469. Schiebler, M.L., Kressel, H.Y., Saul, S.H., et al.: MR imaging of focal nodular hyperplasia of the liver, J. Comput. Assist. Tomogr. 11:651-654, 1987.

470. Schlumpf, R., Marincek, B., Von-Schulthess, G., et al.: Magnetic resonance imaging and computed tomography in long-term-functioning duct-occluded pancreas allotransplants, Diabetes 39(S1):24-26, 1989.

471. Schmiedl, U., Kolbel, G., Hess, C.F., et al.: Dynamic sequential MR imaging of focal liver lesions: initial experience in 22 patients at 1.5 T, J. Comput. Assist. Tomogr. 14:600-607, 1990.

472. Schmiedl, U., Moseley, M.E., Ogan, M.D., et al.: Comparison of initial biodistribution patterns of Gd-DTPA and albumin-(Gd-DTPA) using rapid spin echo MR imaging, J. Comput. Assist. Tomogr. 11:306-313, 1987.

473. Schmiedl, U., Paajanen, H., Arakawa, M., et al.: MR imaging of liver abscesses; application of Gd-DTPA, Magn. Reson. Imaging 6:9-16, 1988.

474. Schneider, S., Wrazidlo, W., Brambs, H.J., et al.: Correlation of bioptic findings and MR imaging in the follow-up of liver transplants, Radiology 173(P): 389, 1989.

475. Schulte, S.J., Baron, R.L., Teefey, S.A., et al.: CT of the extrahepatic bile ducts: wall thickness and contrast enhancement in normal and abnormal ducts, AJR 154:79-85, 1990.

476. Schwartz, S.I.: Primary sclerosing cholangitis: a disease revisited, Surg. Clin. N. Am. 53:1161-1167, 1973.

477. Seltzer, S.E. and Holman, B.L.: Imaging hepatic metastases from colorectal carcinoma: identification of candidates for partial hepatectomy, AJR 152:917-923, 1989.

478. Semelka, R.C., Chew, W.M., Hricak, H., et al.: Fat-saturation MR imaging of the upper abdomen, AJR 155: 1111-1116, 1990.

479. Sharp, J.T., Goldberg, N.B., Druz, W.S., et al.: Relative contributions of rib cage and abdomen to breathing in normal subjects, J. Appl. Physiol. 39:608-618, 1975.

480. Shea Jr, W.J., Demas, B.E., Goldberg, H.I., et al.: Sclerosing cholangitis associated with hepatic arterial FUDR chemotherapy: radiographic-histologic correlation, AJR 146:717-721, 1986.

481. Shiina, S., Tagawa, K., Unuma, T., et al.: Percutaneous ethanol injection therapy of hepatocellular carcinoma: analysis of 77 patients, AJR 155:1221-1226, 1990.

482. Shtern, F., Garrido, L., Compton, C., et al.: MR imaging of blood-borne liver metastases in mice: contrast enhancement with Fe-EHPG, Radiology 178:83-89, 1991.

483. Siegelman, E.S., Mitchell, D.G., Rubin, R., et al.: Parenchymal versus reticuloendothelial iron overload in the liver: distinction with MR imaging, Radiology 179:361-366, 1991.

484. Silverman, P.M., Feuerstein, I.M., Garra, B.S., et al.: Evaluation of STIR imaging as a complement to spin-echo MR and CT of the porta hepatis/hepatoduodenal ligament, Magn. Reson. Imaging 9:73-777, 1991.

485. Silverman, P.M., Patt, R.H., Garra, B.S., et al.: MR imaging of the portal venous system: value of gradient-echo imaging as an adjunct to spin-echo imaging, ARJ 157:297-302, 1991.

486. Silverman, S., DeNardo, G.L., Glatstein, E., et al.: Evaluation of the liver and spleen in Hodgkin's disease. II. The value of splenic scintigraphy, Am. J. Med. 52:362-366, 1972.

487. Sironi, S., Livraghi, T., and DelMaschio, A.: Small hepatocellular carcinoma treated with percutaneous ethanol injection: MR imaging findings, Radiology 180:333-336, 1991.

488. Solbiati, L., Bossi, M.C., Bellotti, E., et al.: Focal lesions in the spleen: sonographic patterns and guided biopsy, AJR 140:59-65, 1983.

489. Sonoda, T., Shirabe, K., Takenaka, K., et al.: Angiographically undetected hepatocellular carcinoma: clinicopathologic characteristics, follow-up and treatment, Hepatology 10:1003-1007, 1989.

490. Spritzer, C., Kressel, H.Y., Mitchell, D., et al.: MR imaging of normal extrahepatic bile ducts, J. Comput. Assist. Tomogr. 11:248-252, 1987.

491. Stanley, P.: Budd-Chiari syndrome, Radiology 170:625-627, 1989.

492. Stark, D.D., Bass, N.M., Moss, A.A., et al.: Nuclear magnetic resonance imaging of experimentally induced liver disease, Radiology 148:743-751, 1983.

493. Stark, D.D., Felder, R.C., Wittenberg, J., et al.: Magnetic resonance imaging of cavernous hemangioma of the liver: tissue specific characterization, AJR 145:213-220, 1985.

494. Stark, D.D., Goldberg, H.I., Moss, A.A., et al.: Chronic liver disease: evaluation by magnetic resonance, Radiology 150:149-151, 1984.

495. Stark, D.D., Hahn, P.F., Trey, C., et al.: MRI of the Budd-Chiari syndrome, AJR 146:1141-1148, 1986.

496. Stark, D.D., Hendrick, R.E., Hahn, P.F., et al.: Motion artifact suppression by fast spin echo imaging, Radiology 164:183-191, 1987.

497. Stark, D.D., Moseley, M.E., Bacon, B.R., et al.: Magnetic resonance imaging and spectroscopy of hepatic iron overload, Radiology 154:137-142, 1985.

498. Stark, D.D., Moss, A.A., Goldberg, H.I., et al.: Magnetic resonance imaging and CT of the normal and diseased pancreas: a comparative study, Radiology 150:153-162, 1984.

499. Stark, D.D., Weissleder, R., Elizondo, G., et al.: Superparamagnetic iron oxide: clinical application as a contrast agent for MR imaging of the liver, Radiology 168:297-301, 1988.

500. Stark, D.D., Wittenberg, J., Butch, R.J., et al.: Hepatic metastases: randomized, controlled comparison of detection with MR imaging and CT, Radiology 165:399-406, 1987.

501. Stark, D.D., Wittenberg, J., Edelman, R.R., et al.: Detection of hepatic metastases: analysis of pulse sequence performance in MR imaging, Radiology 159:365-370, 1986.

502. Stark, D.D., Wittenberg, J., Middleton, M.S., et al.: Liver metastases: detection by phase-contrast MR imaging, Radiology 158:327-332, 1986.

503. Starzl, T.E., Halgrimson, C.G., Francavilla, F.R., et al.: The origin, hormonal nature and action of hepatotrophic substances in portal venous blood, Surg. Gynecol. Obstet. 137:179-199, 1973.

504. Starzl, T.E., Francavilla, A., Porter, K.A., et al.: The effect of splanchnic viscera removal upon canine liver regeneration, Surg. Gynecol. Obstet. 147:193-207, 1978.

505. Stehling, M.K., Coxon, R., Blamire, A.M., et al.: High-resolution, contrast-optimized echo-planar MR imaging of the liver, Radiology 173(P): 337, 1989.

506. Steinberg, H.V., Alarcon, J.J., and Bernardino, M.E.: Focal hepatic lesions: comparative MR imaging at 0.5 and 1.5 T, Radiology 174:153-156, 1990.

507. Steiner, E., Stark, D.D., Hahn, P.F., et al.: Imaging of pancreatic neoplasms: comparison of MR and CT, AJR 152:487-491, 1989.

508. Stone, M.D., Cady, B., Jenkins, R.L., et al.: Surgical therapy for recurrent liver metastases from colorectal cancer, Arch. Surg. 125:718-722, 1990.

509. Stromeyer, F.W. and Ishak, K.G.: Nodular transformation (nodular "regenerative" hyperplasia) of the liver, Human Path. 12:60-71, 1981.

510. Stuck, K.J. and Kuhns, L.R.: Improved visualization of the pancreatic tail after maximum distension of the stomach, J. Comput. Assist. Tomogr. 5:509-512, 1981.

511. Subramanyam, B.R., Balthazar, E.J., Madamba, M.R., et al.: Sonography of portosystemic venous collaterals in portal hypertension, Radiology 146:161-166, 1983.

512. Sugarbaker, P.H.: Surgical decision making for large bowel cancer metastatic to the liver, Radiology 174:621-626, 1990.

513. Sugarbaker, P.H., Vermess, M., Doppman, J.L., et al.: Improved detection of focal lesions with computerized tomographic examination of the liver using ethiodized oil emulsion (EOE-13) liver contrast, Cancer 54:1489-1495, 1976.

514. Sumida, M., Ohto, M., Ebara, M., et al.: Accuracy of angiography in the diagnosis of small hepatocellular carcinoma, AJR 147:531-536, 1986.

515. Suramo, I., Paivansalo, M., and Myilyla, V.: Cranio-caudad movements of the liver, pancreas, and kidneys in respiration, Acta Radiol. [Daign] (Stockh) 25:129-131, 1984.

516. Suzuki, T., Shibuya, H., Yoshimatsu, S., et al: Ultrasonically guided staging splenic tissue core biopsy in patients with non-Hodgkin's lymphoma, Cancer 60:879-882, 1987.

517. Szumowski, J., Eisen, J.K., Vinitski, S., et al.: Hybrid methods of chemical-shift imaging, Magn. Reson. Med. 9:379, 1989.

518. Szumowski, J. and Plewes, D.B.: Separation of lipid and water MR imaging signals by Chopper averaging in the time domain, Radiology 165:247-250, 1987.

519. Takayasu, K., Makuuchi, M., and Takayama, T.: Computed tomography of a rapidly growing hepatic hemangioma, J. Comput. Assist. Tomogr. 14:143-145, 1990.

520. Takayasu, K., Moriyama, N., Muramatsu, Y., et al.: Intrahepatic venous collaterals forming via the inferior right hepatic vein in 3 patients with obstruction of the inferior vena cava, Radiology 154:323-328, 1985.

521. Takayasu, K., Moriyama, N., Muramatsu, Y., et al.: The diagnosis of small hepatocellular carcinomas: efficacy of various imaging procedures in 100 patients, AJR 155:49-54, 1990.

522. Takayasu, K., Moriyama, N., Shima, Y., et al.: Atypical radiographic findings in hepatic cavernous hemangioma: correlation with histologic features, AJR 146: 1149-1153, 1986.

523. Takayasu, K., Muramatsu, Y., Shima, Y., et al.: Hepatic lobar atrophy following obstruction of the ipsilateral portal vein from hilar cholangiocarcinoma, Radiology 160:389-393, 1986.

524. Takayasu, K., Shima, Y., Muramatsu, Y., et al.: Angiography of small hepatocellular carcinomas: analysis of 105 resected tumors, AJR 147:525-529, 1986.

525. Takayasu, K., Shima, Y., Muramatsu, Y., et al.: Hepatocellular carcinoma: treatment with intraarterial iodized oil with and without chemotherapeutic agents, Radiology 162:345-351, 1987.

526. Takayasu, K., Shima, Y., Muramatsu, Y., et al.: Imaging characteristics of large lipoma and angiomyolipoma of the liver, Cancer 59:916-921, 1987.

527. Tamada, T., Moriyasu, F., Ono, S., et al.: Portal blood flow: measurement with MR imaging, Radiology 173:639-644, 1989.

528. Tanimoto, A., Baba, Y., Kreft, B.P., et al.: Receptor targeted iron oxide fails to detect diffuse liver disease, Society of Magnetic Resonance in Medicine, 10th Annual Meeting, San Francisco, August 10-16, 1991, Book of Abstracts, p. 56.

529. Teefey, S.A., Baron, R.L., Rohrmann, C.A., et al.: Sclerosing cholangitis: CT findings, Radiology 169:635-639, 1988.

530. Teitelbaum, G.P., Ortega, H.V., Vinitski, S., et al.: Optimization of gradient-echo imaging parameters for intracaval filters and trapped thromboemboli, Radiology 174:1013-1019, 1990.

531. Terada, T., Kadoya, M., Nakanuma, Y., et al.: Iron-accumulating adenomatous hyperplastic nodule with malignant foci in the cirrhotic liver, Cancer 65:1994-2000, 1990.

532. Terada, T. and Nakanuma, Y.: Iron-negative foci in siderotic macroregenerative nodules in human cirrhotic liver, Arch. Pathol. Lab. Med. 113:916-920, 1989.

533. Terada, T. and Nakanuma, Y.: Survey of iron-accumulative macroregenerative nodules in cirrhotic livers, Hepatology 10:851-854, 1989.

534. Terada, T., Nakanuma, Y., Hoso, M., et al.: Fatty macroregenerative nodule in non-steatotic liver cirrhosis. A morphologic study, Virchows Archiv. A. Pathol. Anat. 415:131-136, 1989.

535. Terpstra, O.T., Metselaar, H.J., Hesselink, E.J., et al.: Auxiliary partial liver transplantation for acute and chronic liver disease, Transplant. Proc. 22:1564, 1990.

536. Terrier, F., Vock, P., Cotting, J., et al.: Effect of intravenous fructose on the P-31 MR spectrum of the liver: dose response in healthy volunteers, Radiology 171:557-563, 1989.

537. The Clinical NMR Group, Aberdeen: Magnetic resonance imaging of parenchymal liver disease: a comparison with ultrasound, radionuclide scintigraphy and x-ray computed tomography, Clin. Radiol. 38:495, 1987.

538. Thickman, D., Hendrick, R.E., Jerjian, K.A., et al.: Liver-lesion tissue contrast on MR images: effect of iron oxide concentration and magnetic field strength, Radiology 176:557-562, 1990.

539. Thoeni, R.F., Werthmuller, W.C., Warren, R.S., et al.: Lesion detection and vascular assessment with modified CTAP and MR imaging of liver: no need for angiographic portogram? Radiology 177(P):92, 1990.

540. Thomas, J.L., Bernardino, M.E., Vermess, M., et al.: EOE-13 in the detection of hepatosplenic lymphoma, Radiology 145:629-634, 1982.

541. Thomsen, C., Christoffersen, P., Henriksen, O., et al.: Prolonged *T1* in patients with liver cirrhosis: an in vivo MRI study, Magn. Reson. Imaging 8:599-604, 1990.

542. Thomsen, C., Josephsen, P., Karle, H., et al: Determination of T1- and T2-relaxation times in the spleen of patients with splenomegaly, Magn. Reson. Imaging 8:39-42, 1990.

543. Tilcock, C., Unger, E.C., Ahkong, Q.F., et al.: Polymeric oral contrast agents for MR imaging of the gastrointestinal tract, J. Magn. Reson. Imaging 1:463-468, 1991.

544. Tilcock, C., Unger, E., Cullis, P., et al.: Liposomal Gd-DTPA: preparation and characterization of relaxivity, Radiology 171:77-80, 1989.

545. Titelbaum, D.S., Hatabu, H., Schiebler, M.L., et al.: Fibrolamellar hepatocellular carcinoma: MR appearance, J. Comput. Assist. Tomogr. 12:588-591, 1988.

546. Tjon A Tham, R.T.O., Falke, T.H.M., Jansen, J.B.M.J., et al.: CT and MR imaging of advanced Zollinger-Ellison syndrome, J. Comput. Assist. Tomogr. 13:821-828, 1989.

547. Tkach, J.A. and Haacke, E.M.: A comparison of fast spin echo and gradient field echo sequences, Magn. Reson. Imaging 6:373-389, 1988.

548. Torres, W.E., Gaylord, G.M., Whitmire, L.F., et al.: Correlation between MR and angiography in portal hypertension, AJR 148:1109, 1988.

549. Tsang, Y., Stark, D.D., Chen, M.C., et al.: Hepatic micrometastases in the rat: ferrite-enhanced MR imaging, Radiology 167:21-24, 1988.

550. Tscholakoff, D., Hricak, H., Thoeni, R., et al.: MR imaging in the diagnosis of pancreatic disease, AJR 148:703-709, 1987.

551. Tsujimoto, F., Miyamoto, Y., and Tada, S.: Differentiation of benign from malignant ascites by sonographic evaluation of gallbladder wall, Radiology 157:503-504, 1985.

552. Tumeh, S.S., Benson, C., Nagel, J.S., et al.: Cavernous hemangioma of the liver: detection with single-photon emission computed tomography, Radiology 164:353-356, 1987.

553. Tyrrel, R.T., Kaufman, S.L., and Bernardino, M.E.: Straight line sign: appearance and significance during CT portography, Radiology 173:635-637, 1989.

554. Unger, E.C., Lee, J.K.T., and Weyman, P.J.: CT and MR imaging of radiation hepatitis, J. Comput. Assist. Tomogr. 11:264-268, 1987.

555. Unger, E.C., MacDougall, P., Cullis, P., et al.: Liposomal Gd-DTPA: effect of encapsulation on enhancement of hepatoma model by MRI, Magn. Reson. Imaging 7:417-423, 1989.

556. Unger, E.C., Needleman, P., Cullis, P., et al.: Gadolinium-DTPA liposomes as a potential MRI contrast agent: work in progress, Invest. Radiol. 23:928-932, 1988.

557. Unger, E.C., Winokur, T., MacDougall, P., et al.: Hepatic metastases: liposomal Gd-DTPA-enhanced MR imaging, Radiology 171:81-85, 1989.

558. Unger, E.C., Zerella, A., and Tilcock, C.: Biodistribution, clearance, and MR imaging of Gd-DTPA liposomes, Radiology 173(P): 274, 1989.

559. Vahey, T.N., Glazer, G.M., Francis, I.R., et al.: MR diagnosis of pancreatic transplant rejection, AJR 150:557-560, 1988.

560. Van Beers, B., Demeure, R., Pringot, J., et al.: Dynamic spin-echo imaging with Gd-DTPA: value in the differentiation of hepatic tumors, AJR 154:515-519, 1990.

561. Van Beers, B., Pringot, J., Trigaux, J.P., et al.: Hepatic heterogeneity on CT in Budd-Chiari syndrome: correlation with regional disturbances in portal flow, Gastoinest. Radiol. 13:61-66, 1988.

562. Van Hecke, P., Marchal, G., Decrop, E., et al.: Experimental study of the pharmacokinetics and dose response of ferrite particles used as a contrast agent in MRI of the normal liver of the rabbit, Invest. Radiol. 24:397-399, 1989.

563. Van Lom, K.J., Brown, J.J., Perman, W.H., et al.: Liver imaging at 1.5 tesla: pulse sequence optimization based on improved measurement of tissue relaxation times, Magn. Reson. Imaging 9:165-171, 1991.

564. Vassiliades, V.G., Foley, W.D., Alarcon, J., et al.: Hepatic metastases: CT versus MR imaging at 1.5 T, Gastrointest. Radiol. 16: 159-163, 1991.

565. Vermess, M., Leung, A.W., Bydder, G.M., et al.: MR imaging of the liver in primary hepatocellular carcinoma, J. Comput. Assist. Tomogr. 9:749-754, 1985.

566. Vinitski, S., Albert, S., Mitchell, D.G., et al.: Partial angle inversion recovery (PAIR) imaging, Magn. Reson. Imaging 10: 207-215, 1992.

567. Vinitski, S., Griffey, R., Fuka, M., et al.: Effect of the sampling rate on magnetic resonance imaging, AJR 5:278-285, 1987.

568. Vlachos, L., Trakadas, S., Gouliamos, A., et al.: Comparative study between ultrasound, computed tomography, intra-arterial digital subtraction angiography, and magnetic resonance imaging in the differentiation of tumors of the liver, Gastrointest. Radiol. 15:102-106, 1990.

569. Wada, K., Kondo, F., and Kondo, Y.: Large regenerative nodules and dysplastic nodules in cirrhotic livers: a histopathologic study, Hepatology 8:1684-1688, 1988.

570. Wallner, B., Edelman, R.R., Finn, J.P., et al.: Bright pleural effusion and ascites on gradient-echo MR images: a potential source of confusion in vascular MR studies, AJR 155:1237-1240, 1990.

571. Wang, Z., Zhu, Y., Wang, S., et al.: Recognition and management of Budd-Chiari syndrome: report of one hundred cases, J. Vasc. Surg. 10:149-156, 1989.

572. Wanless, I.R., Peterson, P., Das, A., et al.: Hepatic vascular disease and portal hypertension in polycythemia vera and agnogenic myeloid metaplasia: a clinicopathological study of 145 patients examined at autopsy, Hepatology 12:1166-1174, 1990.

573. Wanless, I.R. and Lentz, J.S.: Fatty liver hepatitis (Steatohepatitis) and obesity: an autopsy study with analysis of risk factors, Hepatology 12:1106-1110, 1990.

574. Ward, B.A., Miller, D.L., Frank, J.A., et al.: Prospective evaluation of hepatic imaging studies in the detection of colorectal metastases: correlation with surgical findings, Surgery 105:180, 1989.

575. Warren, S. and Davis, A.H.: Studies on tumor metastasis. V. The metastases of carcinoma to the spleen, Am. J. Cancer 21:517-533, 1934.

576. Warshaw, A.L., Compton, C.C., Lewandrowski, K., et al.: Cystic tumors of the pancreas: new clinical, radiologic, and pathologic observations in 67 patients, Ann. Surg. 212:432-445, 1990.

577. Watanabe, T. and Tanaka, K.: Effect of carcinostatic agents on carcinomatous metastasis in the spleen, Gann. 60:611-616, 1969.

578. Wechsler, R.J., Munoz, S.J., Needleman, L., et al.: The periportal collar: a CT sign of liver transplant rejection, Radiology 165:57-60, 1987.

579. Wehrli, F.W.: Fast-scan magnetic resonance: principles and applications, Magn. Reson. Quarterly 6:165-236, 1990.

580. Wehrli, F.W., MacFall, J.R., Glover, G.H., et al.: The dependence of nuclear magnetic resonance (NMR) image contrast on intrinsic and pulse sequence timing parameters, Magn. Reson. Imaging 2:3-16, 1984.

581. Wehrli, F.W., Perkins, T.G., Shimakawa, A., et al.: Chemical shift-induced amplitude modulations in images obtained with gradient refocusing, Magn. Reson. Imaging 5:157-158, 1987.

582. Wehrli, F.W., Shaw, D., and Kneeland, J.B.: Biomedical magnetic resonance imaging: principles, methodology, and applications, VCH Publishers, New York, 1988.

583. Weinmann, H.J., Brasch, R.C., Press, W.R., et al.: Characteristics of gadolinium-DTPA complex: a potential NMR contrast agent, AJR 142:619-624, 1984.

584. Weinreb, J.C., Brateman, L., and Maravilla, K.R.: Magnetic resonance imaging of hepatic lymphoma, AJR 143:1211-1214, 1984.

585. Weinreb, J.C., Hodges, S., and Garcia, R.: Magnetic resonance imaging of patent umbilical veins, AJR 144:747-748, 1985.

586. Weissleder, R., Elizondo, G., Stark, D.D., et al.: The diagnosis of splenic lymphoma by MR imaging: value of superparamagnetic iron oxide, AJR 152:175-180, 1989.

587. Weissleder, R., Hahn, P.F., and Stark, D.D.: Spleen. Magnetic resonance imaging. In Margulis, A.R. and Burhenne, H.J. (eds.), Alimentary tract radiology, St. Louis, 1989, Mosby–Year Book, pp. 1435-1448.

588. Weissleder, R., Hahn, P.F., Stark, D.D., et al.: Superparamagnetic iron oxide: enhanced detection of focal splenic tumors with MR imaging, Radiology 169:399-403, 1988.

589. Weissleder, R., Reimer, P., Lee, A.S., et al.: MR receptor imaging: ultrasmall iron oxide particles targeted to asialoglycoprotein receptors, AJR 155:1161-1167, 1990.

590. Weissleder, R., Saini, S., Stark, D.D., et al.: Dual-contrast MR imaging of liver cancer in rats, AJR 150:561-566, 1988.

591. Weissleder, R., Saini, S., Stark, D.D., et al.: Pyogenic liver abscess: contrast-enhanced MR imaging in rats, AJR 150:115-120, 1988.

592. Weissleder, R., Stark, D.D., Compton, C.C., et al.: Ferrite-enhanced MR imaging of hepatic lymphoma: an experimental study in rats, AJR 149:1161-1165, 1987.

593. Weissleder, R., Stark, D.D., Compton, C., et al.: Cholecystitis: diagnosis by MR imaging, Magn. Reson. Imaging 6:345-348, 1988.

594. Weissleder, R., Stark, D.D., Elizondo, G., et al.: MRI of hepatic lymphoma, Magn. Reson. Imaging 6:675-681, 1988.

595. Weltin, G., Taylor, K.J.W., Carter, A.R., et al.: Duplex Doppler: identification of cavernous transformation of the portal vein, AJR 144:999-1001, 1985.

596. Wenker, J.C., Baker, M.K., Ellis, J.H., et al.: Focal fatty infiltration of the liver: demonstration by magnetic resonance imaging, AJR 143:573-574, 1984.

597. Wesbey, G.E., Brasch, R.C., Engelstad, B.L., et al.: Nuclear magnetic resonance contrast enhancement study of the gastrointestinal tract of rats and a human volunteer using nontoxic oral iron solutions, Radiology 149:175-180, 1983.

598. West, M.S., Garra, B.S., Horii, S.C., et al.: Gallbladder varices: imaging findings in patients with portal hypertension, Radiology 179:179-182, 1991.

599. White, E.M., Simeone, J.F., Mueller, P.R., et al.: Focal periportal sparing in hepatic fatty infiltration: a cause of hepatic pseudomass on US, Radiology 162:57-59, 1987.

600. Widrich, W.C., Srinivasan, M., Semine, M.C., et al.: Collateral pathways of the left gastric vein in portal hypertension, AJR 142:375-382, 1984.

601. Wiesner, R.H. and LaRusso, N.F.: Clinicopathologic features of the syndrome of primary sclerosing cholangitis, American Gastroenterological Association 200-206, 1980.

602. Wilbur, A.C. and Gyi, B.: Hepatocellular carcinoma: MR appearance mimicking focal nodular hyperplasia, AJR 149:721-722, 1987.

603. Wilbur, A.C., Gyi, G., and Renigers, S.A.: High-field MRI of primary gallbladder carcinoma, Gastrointest. Radiol. 13:142-144, 1988.

604. Williams, D.M., Cho, K.J., Aisen, A.M., et al.: Portal hypertension evaluated by MR imaging, Radiology 157:703-706, 1985.

605. Williams, R., Williams, H.S., Scheuer, P.J., et al.: Iron absorption and siderosis in chronic liver disease, Quarterly J. Med. 36(141):151-165, 1967.

606. Wintrobe, M.M. (ed.): Clinical hemotology, ed 8. Philadelphia: 1981, Lea and Febiger, pp. 171-191.

607. Wittenberg, J., Stark, D.D., Forman, B.H., et al.: Differentiation of hepatic metastases from hepatic hemangiomas and cysts by using MR imaging, AJR 151:79-84, 1988.

608. Wittenberg, J., Tosteson, A.A., Karstaedt, N., et al.: MR imaging versus CT: a multi-institutional comparison of hepatic metastatic tumor detection accuracy, Radiology 169(P):63, 1988.

609. Wojtasek, D.A. and Teixidor, H.S.: Echinococcal hepatic disease: magnetic resonance appearance, Gastrointest. Radiol. 14:158, 1989.

610. Wolf, G.L.: Opinion. Safer, more expensive iodinated contrast agents: how should we decide? Radiology 159:557-558, 1986.

611. Wolf, G.L., Burnett, K.R., Goldstein, E.J., et al.: Contrast agents for magnetic resonance imaging, In Kressel, H., (ed.), Magnetic resonance annual, New York, Raven Press, 1985, pp. 231-266.

612. Wolf, G.L., and Fobben, E.S.: Tissue proton T1 and T2 response to gadolinium-DTPA injection in rabbits: a potential contrast agent for MR imaging, Invest. Radiol. 19:324-328, 1984.

613. Wolf, G.L., Joseph, P.M., and Goldstein, E.J.: Optimal pulsing sequences for MR contrast agents, AJR 147:367-371, 1986.

614. Wood, M.L., Runge, V.M., and Henkelman, R.M.: Why are respiratory motion artifacts more conspicuous in high field MRI? Magn. Reson. Imaging 5(S1):73, 1987.

615. Wozney, P., Zajko, A.B., Bron, K.M., et al.: Vascular complications after liver transplantation: a 5-year experience, AJR 147:657-663, 1986.

616. Yankelevitz, D., Henschke, C.I., Chu, F., et al.: Serial MR imaging evaluation of effects of radiation therapy on bone marrow and liver, Radiology 173(P): 274, 1989.

617. Yates, C.H. and Streight, R.A.: Focal fatty infiltration of the liver simulating metastatic disease, Radiology 159:83-84, 1986.

618. Yoshida, H., Itai, Y., Ohtomo, K., et al.: Small hepatocellular carcinoma and cavernous hemangioma: differentiation with dynamic FLASH MR imaging with Gd-DTPA, Radiology 171:339-342, 1989.

619. Yoshikawa, J., Matsui, O., Takashima, T., et al.: Fatty metamorphosis in hepatocellular carcinoma: radiologic features in 10 cases, AJR 151:717-720, 1988.

620. Yoshikawa, J., Matsui, O., Takashima, T., et al.: Focal fatty change of the liver adjacent to the falciform ligament: CT and sonographic findings in five surgically confirmed cases, AJR 149:491-494, 1987.

621. Yoshimatsu, S., Inouse, Y., Ibukuro, K., et al.: Hypovascular hepatocellular carcinoma undetected at angiography and CT with iodized oil, Radiology 171:343-347, 1989.

622. Yuh, W.T.C., Hunsicker, L.G., Nghiem, D.D., et al.: Pancreatic transplants: evaluation with MR imaging, Radiology 170:171-177, 1989.

623. Yuh, W.T.C., Wiese, J.A., Abu-Yousef, M.M., et al.: Pancreatic transplant imaging, Radiology 167:679-683, 1988.

624. Yumoto, Y., Jinno, K., Tokuyama, K., et al.: Hepatocellular carcinoma detected by iodized oil, Radiology 154:19-24, 1985.

625. Zajko, A.B., Bennett, M.J., Campbell, W.L., et al.: Mucocele of the cystic duct remnant in eight liver transplant recipients: findings at cholangiography, CT and US, Radiology 177:691-693, 1990.

626. Zeman, R.K., Dritschilo, A., Silverman, P.M., et al.: Dynamic CT vs 0.5 T MR imaging in the detection of surgically proven hepatic metastases, J. Comput. Assist. Tomogr. 13:637-644, 1989.

627. Zirinsky, K., Markisz, J.A., Rubenstein, W.A., et al.: MR imaging of portal venous thrombosis: correlation with CT and sonography, AJR 150:283-288, 1988.

628. Zonderland, H.M., Lameris, J.S., Terpstra, O.T., et al.: Auxilliary partial liver transplantation: imaging evaluation in 10 patients, AJR 153:981-985, 1989.

629. Zornoza, J. and Ginaldi, S.: Computed tomography in hepatic lymphoma, Radiology 138:405-410, 1981.

Index